# Practice Management
# for Dental Hygienists

# Practice Management for Dental Hygienists

ESTHER K. ANDREWS, CDA, RDA, RDH, MA

⊞. Lippincott Williams & Wilkins
a Wolters Kluwer business
Philadelphia · Baltimore · New York · London
Buenos Aires · Hong Kong · Sydney · Tokyo

*Senior Acquisitions Editor:* John Goucher
*Managing Editor:* Kevin C. Dietz
*Marketing Manager:* Hilary Henderson
*Production Editor:* Eve Malakoff-Klein
*Designer:* Risa Clow
*Compositor:* Circle Graphics, Inc.
*Printer:* Courier Corporation—Kendallville

Cover images courtesy of Hu-Friedy

**Library of Congress Cataloging-in-Publication Data**

Andrews, Esther K.
    Practice management for dental hygienists / Esther K. Andrews.
        p. ; cm.
    Includes bibliographical references.
    ISBN-13: 978-0-7817-5359-3
    ISBN-10: 0-7817-5359-7
    1. Dentistry—Practice. 2. Dental offices—Management. 3. Dental
hygienists. I. Title.
    [DNLM: 1. Practice Management, Dental—organization & admin-
istration. 2. Dental Hygienists. WU 77 A565p 2007]
RK58.A63 2007
617.6068—dc22

                                2005037381

# About the Author

Esther K. Andrews earned an MA from Michigan State University (East Lansing), an AAAS from Grand Rapids (Michigan) Community College, and a BS and an AAS from Ferris State University (Big Rapids, Michigan). With more than 25 years of teaching and scholarship experience, she was previously a member of the faculty at the University of Illinois—Chicago/Kennedy King College, Minnesota State University (Mankato), Old Dominion University, University of Kentucky (Lexington), and Lane Community College (Eugene, Oregon).

Ms. Andrews has comprehensive clinical experience in dental assisting and dental hygiene. She started her education at the Oakland (Michigan) Technical Center—Southwest Campus in the dental office assisting program. She worked in private dental practice as a certified dental assistant and, later, as a registered dental assistant in Michigan, where she was actively involved in the American Dental Assistants Association (ADAA). After 15 years of clinical practice and teaching dental assistants, she completed a dental hygiene program, taught, and maintained membership in the American Dental Hygienists' Association (ADHA). This blend of experiences enabled her to complete this book while working in private practice as a dental hygienist.

Ms. Andrews' honors and awards include the 2004 ADAA Journal Award, 2000 ADAA life membership, the 1990 Grand Rapids (Michigan) Community College's Daniel A. Kemp DDS Memorial Award for Excellence in Dental Assisting and Dental Hygiene, and the 1988 Michigan Dental Assistants' Association Impact Award.

Publications include "Dental Specialization," *The Dental Assistant Journal* (September/October 2003); "Impressions, Study Casts, and Oral Stents" in *Dental Hygiene Theory and Practice* (2nd Ed.); Continuing Education: "Insurance Cross Coding: Submitting Medical Insurance," *Journal of Contemporary Dental Practice* [online journal: www.thejcdp.com/issue012/index.shtml] (fall 2002); Continuing Education: "Submitting Dental Insurance Claims" (with L. G. Semple), *Journal of Contemporary Dental Practice* [online journal: www.thejcdp.com/issue011/index.shtml] (summer 2002); and *Case Based Learning in Dental Hygiene* (2002) (with E. Thomson, D. Bauman, and D. Shuman).

# Dedication and Acknowledgments

## DEDICATION

To my family, we're having fun when we're not having fun.

## ACKNOWLEDGMENTS

A considerable number of people have supplied encouragement, enlightenment, and support to my life and the process of my scholarly pursuits. As a second-generation American, I am the first female in the Andrews family to complete a college degree. The educational system in Michigan, from West Bloomfield High School to Oakland Technical Center—Southwest Campus, Ferris State University, Grand Rapids Community College, and Michigan State University provided me with an outstanding education that allowed me to develop this book. Thank you to the many inspiring teachers from these institutions, who delivered exceptional, quality instruction.

*Practice Management for Dental Hygienists* would not have been possible without the help of many friends, colleagues, and business associates. The following individuals contributed their expert knowledge, opinions, and assistance: Bunny Bookwalter, CDA, RDA, RDH, MS, of Grand Rapids Community College (Michigan) for long-term friendship and encouragement and for having a profound influence on the course of my life; Louise Dube (Bloomfield Hills, Michigan) for teaching me employability skills at the Oakland Technical Center—Northwest Campus (Clarkston, Michigan); Vicki Sanco (Turner) of Jameson and Associates for insight into insurance and practice management issues; Carol Tekavec, CDA, RDH, of Stepping Stones to Success for allowing us to reprint the copyrighted dental hygiene forms found in Chapter 22; Lynnette Engeswick, RDH, MS, department chair of the dental hygiene program at Minnesota State University, for her expertise on geriatric clients used in the case study in Chapter 6; the reference librarians of the Berwyn Public Library (Illinois) and the Chicago Library system; Dr. Jim Hull and Nancy Richter of Procter and Gamble (Cincinnati, Ohio) for helping me become a better writer; Sharon Stull, CDA, BSDH, MS, of Old Dominion University for referring me to Lippincott Williams & Wilkins; the National Library of Medicine staff (Bethesda, Maryland) for assistance with art identification; Patrick Ryan of Safeguard Printing and Promotional Products for providing business forms and allowing us to reprint them here; Paige Marshall of Werner Consulting for the referral to Dr. Patrick Healy (Lockport, Illinois), who shared photographs of his office design; Dr. Lee Baker (Augusta, Georgia) for the photograph of the reception area in his dental office (photographed by Jeff Barnes); the Ottawa Dental Lab (Illinois); and Wayne Coyne of CollaGenex Pharmaceuticals for allowing us to use their promotional oral risk assessment form.

Many thanks and appreciation go to my eclectic family and friends whose contributions of love and support are greatly appreciated. Sarah Dudak helped with encouragement and clerical duties. A heartfelt word of thanks goes to Laurie Semple, CDA, RDA, CDPMA, BS, for encouraging me to become a teacher and to keep working at it. She also contributed the section on the use of computers in dental practice (Chapter 8). Recognition goes to my past students, who are now pursuing their life's work in the field of dentistry and helping others.

A special thank you to Lippincott Williams & Wilkins for the acceptance of this proposal; John Goucher, acquisitions editor, for his assistance and guidance during the proposal stages; Kevin C. Dietz, managing editor, for his assistance during the development process; the reviewers of the text for their constructive suggestions; Eve Malakoff-Klein, production editor, for her assistance in polishing this book; and the art team and copy editor for their efforts during the final stages of production.

## REVIEWERS

The publisher and author gratefully acknowledge the many professionals who shared their expertise and assisted in developing this textbook, appropriately targeting our marketing efforts, creating useful ancillary products, and setting the stage for subsequent editions. Three of these individuals are

**Barbara Bennett**
Program Chair, Dental Hygiene
Texas State Technical College
Harlingen, Texas

**Sharon Compton**
Associate Professor/Director
University of Alberta
Edmonton, Alberta, Canada

**Brenda Frisher**
Asheville-Buncombe Technical Community College
Asheville, North Carolina

# Preface

This book is written primarily for dental hygiene students; however, it contains information that can be used by dental assisting students and practicing clinicians. The sections of this text address the four areas of dental hygiene practice that most closely relate to dental hygiene practice management:

- Basics of dentistry and dental law
- Office management
- Applied communications
- Employability skills

Each section is focused on core dental practice management principles and techniques to help you, the student, use critical thinking skills when learning the content of a variety of courses, such as introduction to health occupations, ethics and jurisprudence, dental hygiene theory and practice, teaching strategies, practice management, dental hygiene seminar, communication, and dental specialties. The applicable competencies from the American Dental Education Association's "Competencies for Entry into the Profession of Dental Hygiene" online document are listed in each section summary. Although these competencies are not used verbatim in all dental hygiene programs, they serve as principles for competent practice to help students and faculty. References for each section are also provided in the section summary.

The critical thinking "Learning Outcomes" and "Key Terms," listed at the beginning of each chapter, guide you through the text. At the end of each chapter, the "Concept Summary" section reviews the content covered. Each chapter also includes a variety of learning activities designed for individuals and/or groups and can be used during or after class. The study questions and answers provide a review of the chapter's content to reinforce the main ideas. Critical thinking activities allow you to apply your knowledge of the subject matter within large or small groups. Assignments provide you with real-world practice of the business tasks performed in professional offices. The assignments found in Chapter 19 are typical projects that dental hygiene students prepare during a course of study. For each type of assignment, you will use writing skills to develop higher level cognitive critical thinking skills and to actively participate in the learning process. The oral presentation of these assignments provides public speaking practice and experience.

Selected case studies allow you to apply the concepts found in the chapter. Other assignments direct you to locate information related to subject areas on the Internet. Role-playing activities prepare you to better interact with patients by helping you synthesize and apply critical thinking skills. Calculation of practice management formulas and business math applications further reinforce the use of critical thinking skills. The final piece in the application of critical thinking skills is the listing of Internet resources on selected concepts in the section summaries; these can be used as a guide to further study.

As a dental assisting and dental hygiene instructor, I hope this book provides you with the skills necessary to complete your education before entering the industry. The role of the dental hygienist exceeds that of a technical clinician; it includes the application of business concepts, communication, and employability skills for success and happiness on the job.

# Contents

## SECTION IV: EMPLOYABILITY SKILLS

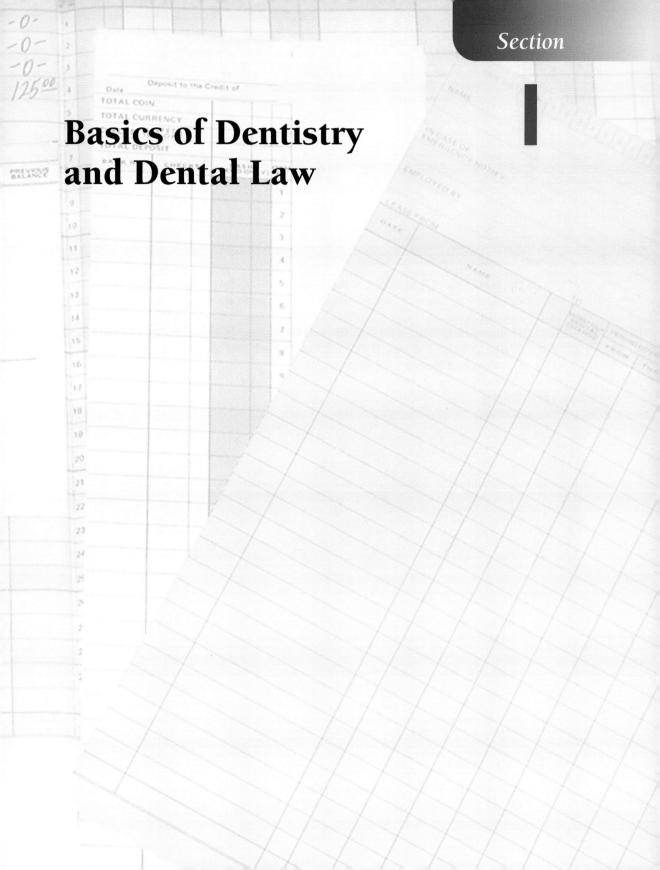

# Basics of Dentistry
# and Dental Law

# History of Dentistry

## LEARNING OUTCOMES

Upon mastery of the content of this chapter, the student should be able to:
- Identify ancient and modern beliefs in oral healthcare practices and beautification procedures.
- Acknowledge individual contributions to the field of dentistry.
- Recognize that all people on earth have contributed to human history.
- Value the differences between people.

## KEY TERMS

al-Qasim, Abu
Apollonia
Black, Greene Vardiman (GV)
caduceus
Fauchard, Pierre
Galen
Hippocrates
Newman, Irene

Pasteur, Louis
Revere, Paul
Roentgen, Wilhelm
Southard, Juliette A.
tooth worm
van Leeuwenhoek, Anton
Wells, Horace

## HISTORY OF DENTISTRY

Throughout history, people have practice many unusual oral healthcare and beautification practices and procedures. Among early cultures, disease was often regarded as the supernatural work of a demon or angry deity. Attempts to rid the body of disease included making sacrifices to the gods, asking penance for one's sins, seeking intervention from friendly spirits, or making the body unpleasant for evil spirits by inducing vomiting, using smoke fumigation (*Fig. 1.1*), or starving, beating, bleeding, or torturing the disease sufferer. These rudimentary "cures" often caused more harm than the disease.

## ANCIENT HISTORY

One of the most widespread ancient theories regarding the cause of tooth pain was the **tooth worm**. Documentation from nearly 7,000 years ago found on a Sumerian clay tablet

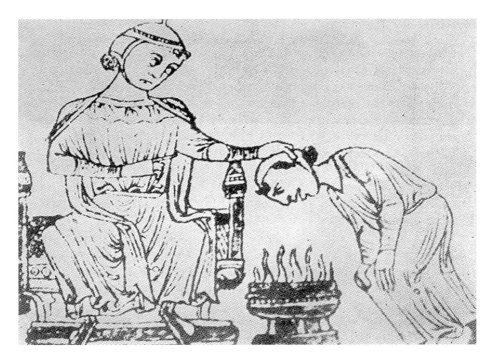

**Figure 1.1** An early image of the fumigation procedure. Courtesy ADA Dental Cosmos.

excavated along the Euphrates River states that small gnawing worms located within the tooth cause toothache. This theory developed because the tooth nerve is similar in appearance to that of a small worm. When ancient oral healthcare practitioners opened the pulpal chamber, they believed that the tooth "worm" was revealed. Early oral health-care practice involved removing or destroying the tooth worm, providing relief to the individual with a toothache. The Babylonian culture, in what is now modern-day Iraq, used incantations, rituals/regimens, and herbal and mineral remedies, and established fees for dental services rendered and penalties for practitioner error (e.g., a tooth for a tooth).

Oral healthcare practices and procedures used by Bronze Age cultures in what is now India included therapeutics and surgery. Herbal, botanical, and mineral (Ayurvedic) reme-dies were used to treat gingival inflammation, along with laxatives, emetics, scarification, medicinal pastes, gargles, and herbal infusions. Surgical instruments from this era designed for extractions, calculus removal, and cauterization of tumors have also been documented. These cultures treated tooth worm infection with a heated probe to burn and destroy the tooth worm. Instructions for oral hygiene called for the use of a frayed twig to brush the teeth along with a dentifrice mixture of honey, oil, pepper, cinnamon, ginger, and salt.

The hieroglyphics recorded on ancient Egyptian papyri document oral healthcare pro-cedures used by that culture. The Ebers papyrus contains directions for an oral remedy, while other papyri record regimens for morning mouth cleansing, strengthening teeth, and treatment of caries and alveolar abscesses using chemicals, herbs, plasters, and mouthwashes. Radiographic examination of Egyptian mummies shows evidence of severe occlusal tooth abrasion due to the consumption of foods made from coarsely milled flour. Dental treatment in this culture involved drilling the bone for draining abscesses, extracting teeth, and placing gold wiring to hold teeth together.

The hygienic code of the ancient Hebrew culture outlined acceptable foods to be eaten, rules for personal cleanliness, community sanitation, disinfection following illness, isolation of lepers, prayers for healing, toothache remedies, and beautification rituals to replace missing anterior teeth with carved ivory or gold.

Ancient Greek priests treated patients in the temples of Asclepius, the Greek god of healing. Statues of Asclepius depict the deity holding a staff with a serpent coiled around it (*Fig. 1.2[left]*), from which the familiar symbol for the healthcare professions, the caduceus (a winged staff with a snake coiled around it), evolved (*Fig. 1.2[right]*). Asclepius' priests, who carried a staff and snakes, conducted healthcare rituals in more than 200 temples. They practiced massage, bathing, and exercise, and administered sleeping potions to semihypnotize their patients while advising them on their course of treatment. Today, the caduceus icon is used as a symbol of the healthcare professions as well as the medical branches of the U.S. military, on jewelry (especially medical-alert jewelry), and on publications.

The famous Greek physician **Hippocrates** (460–377 B.C.) treated diseases by observation. He believe that a proper diet and regimen assisted healing and that nature should be allowed to do the rest. His greatest contribution may have been to set illness apart from superstition and supernatural forces, basing treatment instead on the facts presented by the patient. He also authored a code of moral standards known as the Hippocratic Oath, designed to guide ethical conduct of physicians. In modern times, practitioners in each

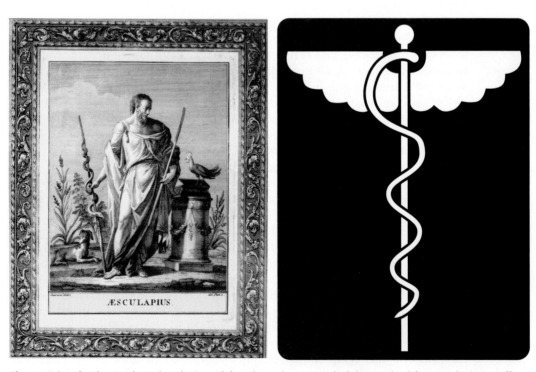

**Figure 1.2 Left.** The Greek God Asclepius. **Right.** The caduceus symbol that evolved from Asclepius' staff.

branch of medicine and allied health field set and revise the ethical standards that relate to new and veteran professionals who practice in the healthcare arena.

Pre-Roman civilization developed the alphabet, invented glass, and perfected metal-working for the repair and replacement of teeth. The Roman Empire's body of laws, known as the Laws of Twelve Tables (450 B.C.) contained rules relating to the practice of dentistry. In ancient Rome, dentistry was not separated from medicine but was included in medical practice. Native Romans for the most part did not practice medicine but relied on Greeks, slaves, and freedmen from other areas of their empire. For example, the Greek physician Galenos of Pergamon (**Galen**) served Roman Emperor Marcus Aurelius. Galenos was an avid student of the knowledge set forth by Hippocrates and combined all the ancient texts into one work, written in Latin, that included drugs, dietary recommendations, description of diseases, and the study of human anatomy, particularly the skeleton.

Early Christians suffered persecution during and after the reign of Roman Emperor Nero. In 249 A.D., **Apollonia**, the daughter of an Egyptian magistrate in Alexandria, was arrested and offered the choice to either renounce Christianity and accept pagan beliefs or be burned at the stake. When she refused to recant her religion, a mob seized her, broke her teeth, and lit a fire to burn her alive (*Fig. 1.3*). She knelt and prayed, then jumped into the fire of her own free will, a martyr to her faith. She was eventually canonized and

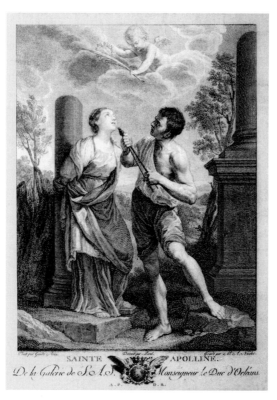

**Figure 1.3** St. Apollonia's martyrdom. Courtesy National Library of Medicine.

became the patron saint of dentistry; in medieval times, people prayed to her for relief of dental pain.

Medieval medical science advanced further in Asia than Europe after the fall of the Roman Empire. Arabian populations, for whom the pursuit of scientific knowledge was important, dominated northern Africa and southern Europe from the 8th through the 12th centuries. Arabian physicians preserved Hippocrates' early teachings; and by the end of the 9th century, Arabian medicine described diseases and remedies. **Abu al-Qasim**, also known as Abulcasis, wrote an encyclopedia of medicine and surgery (al-Tasrif) that is now kept at Oxford University. His unique contribution to dentistry reported the relationship between calculus and periodontal disease. He promoted prevention by recommending scaling calculus above and below the gums until all accretions were removed even if it takes multiple visits. *Figure 1.4* illustrates early dental scaler instruments.

Healthcare practices among African peoples are well-documented in the scientific literature. Two principal precepts are relevant to oral healthcare. The first is related to the tradition that one uses the right hand for food preparation because it is clean, and uses the left hand for handling anything dirty or unclean. This is still practiced by many modern populations in Africa and the Mideast. Oral healthcare practices are performed using the left hand because it is designated for cleansing. The second is the miswak or siwak, also known as the African Chewing Stick, which is used for cleaning the teeth. A twig cut from the araac tree (Salvadora persea) or mastic tree (Pistacia lentiscus) is washed, then chewed on one end until it frays slightly. Once softened, the frayed twig is used to scrub the teeth, gingival, and tongue. Miswaks contain plant oils and minerals that deodorize the mouth and whiten teeth; they also have antibacterial properties. Substances such as bicarbonate of soda, charcoal, and salt were used with the miswak to enhance these properties.

Ancient Chinese culture used plants and minerals in oral healthcare practices, placing arsenic into decayed teeth to destroy tooth worms, filling teeth with silver amalgam dough (659 A.D.), and whitening teeth with hydrochloric acid. Acupuncture, the Chinese medical technique used to cure imbalances between yin and yang energies in the body, involves the insertion of thin needles in points along 12 meridian pathways to permits bad forces to escape and pure forces to enter the body. Of these points, 116 are believed to be aligned with the teeth and oral structures. The Chinese are also credited with creating the modern toothbrush design in the 1490s.

Excavations of Aztec, Maya, and Inca Mesoamerican civilizations, combined with the writings of early Spanish explorers and settlers, have brought to light many intriguing

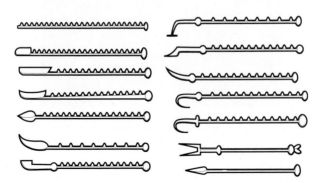

**Figure 1.4** A variety of dental scrapers used by Abu al-Qasim.

healthcare practices and beautification rituals. Oral healthcare practices among these people involved the use of herbal and botanical remedies such as chewing hot peppers or tobacco, and using coca leaves for anesthesia. Tooth restoration and wound suturing of the lips and cheeks with human hair has been documented. Widely practiced beautification rituals included filing the teeth into points or other shapes; adorning teeth with cemented inlays of gold, jade, turquoise or other minerals; and staining the teeth black. Oral cosmetic procedures included transplanting carved tooth-shaped seashells into tooth sockets—the earliest known endosseous alloplastic implants.

## MODERN HISTORY: 1600–PRESENT

### Europe and the United Kingdom

During the 17th century, France and England emerged as world powers. Englishman Francis Bacon and Frenchman René Descartes promoted analytical reasoning, which helped launch an era of advancement of scientific knowledge. Earlier, Dutchman Zacharias Janssen (1590) produced lenses that were used for the first microscopes, which opened up new areas of study. In the following century, another Dutchman, **Anton van Leeuwenhoek**, scraped the plaque from his own teeth and examined it under a magnification of 40–160×; he discovered that dentin contained microscopic tubules.

In 1728, **Pierre Fauchard** (known as the father of modern dentistry) published the two-volume *Le Chirurgien Dentiste, Oú Traité Des Dentes.* This publication covered nearly every phase of dentistry and offered a guide to modern scientific instruction. Fauchard rejected the tooth worm theory, claiming that he had never seen a worm with the eye or under a microscope. Using Fauchard's teachings, the French lead the profession for over a century in the use of silver amalgam restorative material and the manufacturing of artificial porcelain teeth.

The notable **Louis Pasteur** (1822–1895) dedicated his life to the science of microbiology and the prevention of disease and infection. As a result of his research, he was able to explain the process of fermentation. Discovering that bacterial contamination caused milk, wine, and beer to sour, Pasteur devised the method of heating liquids to kill microorganisms via the process now known as pasteurization. As an expert on bacteria, he isolated pathogenic microorganisms; discovered that microbes caused disease; and developed vaccines for cholera in fowl, anthrax in cattle, and rabies in humans.

Robert Koch (1843–1910), a physician from Germany, isolated bacteria and proved that bacteria can cause disease. He injected rats with anthrax to determine the cause and effect of the symptoms and disease. Furthermore, he isolated the bacterium in sputum that causes tuberculosis and discovered that cholera was caused by a waterborne pathogenic microorganism. He was vital in the development of clinical research methodology, which are now known as Koch's postulates.

Starting with Pasteur's and Koch's theories that bacteria cause disease, Lord Joseph Lister of Scotland (1827–1912) was able to prevent wound infection during surgery. His work in antisepsis using carbolic acid to sterilize instruments laid the foundation for modern aseptic techniques. He invented the Listerine formulation, which is still in use today as an antiseptic mouthrinse.

In 1844, **Horace Wells,** a dentist, attended a presentation on the use of nitrous oxide. The next day, he used the gas mixture for sedation to extract a tooth and subsequently used it routinely in his dental practice. Wells discussed his use of nitrous oxide with another dentist, William T. G. Morton. Morton then talked to chemist Charles Jackson, who suggested using ether, which Morton used in his dental practice for sedation beginning in 1846. Local anesthesia came into use in 1905 with the development of procaine (Novocain).

After the discovery of bacteria and development of anesthetics, the discovery of x radiation for use in diagnosis is one of the most important discoveries in modern medicine. In 1895, **Wilhelm Roentgen** (1845–1923) of Germany discovered x radiation in his laboratory at the Wurzburg Physical Institute. The radiant energy was named "x-ray," the *x* representing an unknown. The media of the day were filled with stories about the photographs Roentgen had taken with the rays that could penetrate substances. Roentgen earned the first Nobel Prize in physics in 1901.

## The Americas

Records of oral hygiene practices are available from colonial times in North America. One such practice consisted of using hard toothbrushes and abrasive toothpowders for mouth cleansing. These powders could contain pumice, emery, cream of tartar, borax, cuttlefish bone, myrrh, bark, tobacco, or ashes, and some were colored with sanguis draconis and/or flavored with camphor, as recommended in the *Treatise on Dentistry* (1794) by B. T. Longbothom of Baltimore. Longbothom discouraged the use of the powders because of their abrasiveness and recommended brushing the teeth away from the gums.

**Paul Revere**, the famous patriot and silversmith, studied dentistry under the direction of John Baker. On September 5, 1768, a notice in the *Boston Gazette* announced that Revere was offering his services to the public. He practiced dentistry for 7 years and kept records of his dental operations. His most significant contribution to the American history of dentistry is the 1776 postmortem identification of Dr. Joseph Warren, who was killed at the Battle of Bunker Hill. Revere had constructed and placed a two-unit bridge for Warren and thus was able to positively identify his remains, which were recovered from a mass burial site. This event is noted as the beginning of the science of forensics in the United States. *Box 1.1* lists other American dental first.

---

**BOX 1.1** *American Dental Firsts*

- First tooth-drawer/extractor (1636): William Dinly of the Mayflower Colony in what is now Plymouth, Massachusetts.
- First dentist (1749): French-trained surgeon dentist Sieur Roquet, who practiced in Boston.
- First African American tooth-drawer/extractor (late 1700s): Peter Hawkins of Richmond, Virginia.
- First female dentist (1854): Emeline Rubert Jones of Danielson, Connecticut, who trained and practiced with her husband and then continued his dental practice for nearly 60 years after his death.
- First dental assistant (1885): Dr. Edmund Kells hired an unnamed assistant he called the "lady in attendance" to be present during dental treatment of unescorted female patients.
- First African American female dentist (1890): Ida Gray Nelson Rollins, who studied at the University of Michigan in Ann Arbor.
- First dental hygienist (1912): Irene Newman, who practiced in Bridgeport, Connecticut.

Bostonian John Greenwood (1760–1819) moved to New York City and eventually became George Washington's dentist. He made three full and two partial sets of teeth for the president. Greenwood also invented the foot-operated drill in 1790.

One beautification practice that often proved deadly was tooth transplantation. In the late 1700s, the unfortunate practice of implanting a donor tooth from a living or dead human (or animal) into a freshly opened tooth socket of the recipient usually led to grave medical problems. Frequently, the recipient patient would slowly die from infection or from the consequences of the body's rejection of the tooth.

For a long period in American history, removable appliances were fabricated to replace missing teeth. Dentures have been constructed from a variety of materials and in several designs. In 1799, dentures were carved in ivory and riveted to a lead-based metal. Another early denture was made of hippopotamus ivory that was carved into a horseshoe-shaped base into which human or porcelain teeth were screwed into the anterior region with gold screws. The posterior teeth were carved into the ivory and generally had an occlusal pattern. The ivory base was covered with red sealing wax to simulate the gingivae. Sometimes the upper and lower dentures were held together with spiral springs. One type of denture was constructed in gold plate into which porcelain or carved ivory teeth were inserted. The base of an 1820 appliance was made of silver plate, and the replacement teeth were soldered, screwed, or riveted into the base.

One of the most remarkable Americans who made significant contributions to the practice of dentistry is **Greene Vardiman (G. V.) Black (1836–1915)**. He learned dentistry as an apprentice in his home state of Illinois and developed many dental instruments when practicing in the years before the Civil War. After the war, he taught himself chemistry, German, and cellular pathology so he could read and understand current research in his and related medical fields. He taught dental courses at the Missouri Dental College and the Chicago College of Dental Surgery, which later became Northwestern University. He authored more than 500 scholarly articles and several books. His contributions to dentistry include cavity classifications, operative dentistry techniques, and the use of fluoride as a caries-preventive agent. Near the end of his life, he was involved in the study of fluorosis. Black hoped that the practice of dentistry would eventually focus on prevention and that dental disease could be fought by systemic medication.

## Notable Women

**Juliette A. Southard,** organizer of the Education and Efficiency Society in 1921, led the way for the foundation of the national professional organization for dental assisting. She was elected as the first president of what is now called the American Dental Assistants Association (ADAA) and served for 5 years.

**Irene Newman,** dental assistant to Dr. Alfred G. Fones in Bridgeport, Connecticut, was trained on the job to examine and polish teeth above the gingival margin. Seeing the success of oral prophylaxis on his family members and patients, Fones founded the first dental hygiene educational program, called the Bridgeport Plan for Dental Public Health. He enlisted the help of fellow dentists to teach the first students in the program, which included both coursework and practice. In 1914, a total of 27 students (including Fones's wife and Newman) were graduated. Newman, the first woman licensed in dental hygiene, further contributed to the profession by joining her fellow classmates in forming the Connecticut Dental Hygienists Association (1914), and serving as its first president. Newman and the students from the class of 1917 rendered oral healthcare services to the National Guardsmen in Bridgeport, thus establishing the first organized effort to provide preventive dental services to members of the armed services.

The California Dental Hygiene Association presented a resolution to the National Dental Association (now the American Dental Association [ADA]) for the organization of the American Dental Hygienists' Association (ADHA), which was formed in 1922. The ADHA's first annual session was held the next year in Cleveland, Ohio, to form a constitution, adopt bylaws, and elect leadership. Winifred A. Hart of Bridgeport, Connecticut, was unanimously elected the association's first president. By the end of 1925, a total of 10 dental hygiene programs had been created.

## CULTURAL DIVERSITY

As this chapter demonstrates, many cultures have made significant contributions to the current practice of dentistry. Today's colleges and dental practices bring together people from a wide range of cultures, religions, and ethnicities. Individuals' attitudes toward wellness, medicine, and beauty are affected by their cultural background. The understanding and acceptance of diversity are key to positive interaction with both office personnel and patients.

Patients in almost any dental office come from a wide variety of ethnic and social backgrounds. In fact, some patients select a particular dental office based on these factors. Dental professionals must be sensitive to cultural differences when interacting with patients. The more accepting we are of those who are different from us, the better chance we have of connecting with others. Proper communication creates a positive office atmosphere while increasing productivity and profitability through mutual trust and rapport. Being able to adapt to and appreciate the uniqueness of our classmates, patients, and co-workers prepares us to succeed in today's global community.

## CONCEPT SUMMARY

- Many oral healthcare practices and beautification procedures from the past caused more physical harm than the disease processes they were meant to cure.
- The earliest written oral diagnosis from nearly 7,000 years ago was found on a Sumerian clay tablet; it notes that worms cause toothaches.
- Bronze Age cultures separated oral healthcare practices into surgery and therapies, and some groups had distinct beautification rituals.
- Religious writings and practices have defined oral healthcare practices and beautification rituals.
- Scientific practices and clinical research methodology have been developed and refined since the Middle Ages.
- Diverse cultures throughout history have added significant contributions to the collective consciousness to make dentistry what it is today.

# REVIEW QUESTIONS

1. What is the most ancient theory for the cause of toothaches, and how long did this theory persist?
2. What did the written dental records of ancient India contain?
3. What were the contributions of the Chinese to modern dental practice?
4. What is the caduceus, and what does it represent?
5. What did Galenos of Pergamon contribute to Roman medical practice?
6. Who was Apollonia and why is she known as the patron saint of dentistry?
7. What were the contributions of Abu al-Qasim to the science of dentistry?
8. What was Anton van Leeuwenhoek's contribution to science?
9. Who was Pierre Fauchard?
10. What was Paul Revere's significant contribution to American dentistry?
11. Why is G. V. Black considered one of the most remarkable U.S.-born dentists?
12. How did Juliette A. Southard affect the dental assisting profession?
13. What were Irene Newman's contributions to the dental hygiene profession?
14. Which of the early American beautification procedures proved to be the most deadly?

# General Dentistry

## LEARNING OUTCOMES

Upon mastery of the content of this chapter, the student should be able to:
- Identify the U.S. Department of Labor's recognized dental occupations.
- Determine the level of job complexity for oral healthcare occupations.
- Differentiate between licensure, registration, and certification.
- Describe the process for credentialing in each dental occupation.
- Describe mandatory continuing education.
- Describe the dental team members by job responsibilities, education, credentials, and practice settings.
- Recognize foreign dental occupations.

## KEY TERMS

certification
continuing education
credentials
dental assistant
dental hygienist
dental laboratory technicians
dental nurse
dental specialists

dental therapist
dentistry
denturist
general dentist
job titles
licensure
registration
state dental practice act

## THE DENTAL HEALTHCARE TEAM

**Dentistry** includes a group of four basic occupations focused on the examination, diagnosis, prevention, and treatment of diseases and disorders of the head, neck, and mouth. Occupational job titles in dentistry are given in *Box 2.1*. The field of dentistry is considered an interdisciplinary profession that requires advanced scientific study. Oral healthcare providers are devoted to maintaining the health of the oral cavity, including tooth function, proper speech, disease-free periodontium, and facial appearance for general health. As an oral healthcare provider, you will be involved with people in the various occupations of dentistry. There is plenty of diversity in the recognized professions of

**BOX 2.1** *U.S. Department of Labor's Occupational Titles in Dentistry*

| | | | |
|---|---|---|---|
| 072.061-010 | Oral pathologist | 712.381-018 | Dental laboratory technician |
| 072.101-010 | Dentist | 712.381-022 | Dental laboratory technician |
| 072.101-014 | Endodontist | | apprentice |
| 072.101-018 | Oral and maxillofacial surgeon | 712.381-026 | Orthodontic band maker |
| 072.101-022 | Orthodontist | 712.381-030 | Orthodontic technician |
| 072.010-026 | Pediatric dentist | 712.381-042 | Dental ceramist |
| 072.010-030 | Periodontist | 712.381-046 | Dental waxer |
| 072.010-034 | Prosthodontist | 712.381-050 | Finisher, denture |
| 072.010-038 | Public health dentist | 712.664-010 | Dental ceramist assistant |
| 072.117-010 | Director dental services | 712-684-014 | Bite-block maker |
| 078.361-010 | Dental hygienist | 712.684-030 | Opaquer |
| 079.361-018 | Dental assistant | 712.684-034 | Packer, denture |
| 712.381-014 | Contour wire specialist, denture | 712.684-046 | Denture-model maker |

Courtesy Dictionary of Occupational Titles, 1991.

dentistry, dental hygiene, dental assisting, and dental laboratory technology. With a wide variety of career options and practice settings, it is easy for an individual to find his or her niche in the workplace. *Figure 2.1* demonstrates the different levels of dental vocations organized by the knowledge required to perform the job tasks appropriately.

## ORAL HEALTHCARE PROVIDER CREDENTIALS

A common area of confusion regarding healthcare workers is the difference between a job title and credentials. **Job titles** are federally appointed occupational terms used for classification. **Credentials** are earned by individuals and allow them to perform specific duties. *Box 2.2* lists the commonly awarded credentials for professionals in the dental occupations. It can be difficult to differentiate among certification, registration, and licensure in dentistry because of the number as well as regional interpretations and definitions of these credentials. Even people in the dental professions may have difficulty differentiating among them.

**Licensure** is the legal authorization to practice an occupation in a jurisdiction, such as a state, territory, or district. Licensure requirements vary, depending on the dental occupation and the jurisdiction. There is some commonality among the licensure credentials for dentists and dental hygienists because they are required to be licensed before being legally allowed to practice in all U.S. jurisdictions. In some locations, dental assistants are also required to be licensed to perform their jobs. To become licensed, the candidate must graduate from an approved educational program and pass national written and clinical examinations. Training in cardiopulmonary resuscitation (CPR) is also a requirement in many states for licensure candidates.

Licensure is periodically renewed, for example every 3 years. To renew a licensure, the individual must pay a fee to the licensing board and may have to complete mandatory continuing education courses and current CPR instruction. Mandatory **continuing**

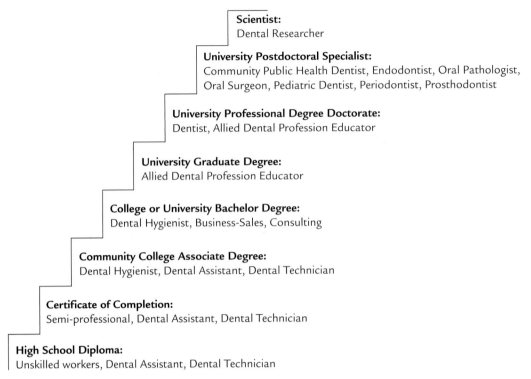

**Scientist:**
Dental Researcher

**University Postdoctoral Specialist:**
Community Public Health Dentist, Endodontist, Oral Pathologist, Oral Surgeon, Pediatric Dentist, Periodontist, Prosthodontist

**University Professional Degree Doctorate:**
Dentist, Allied Dental Profession Educator

**University Graduate Degree:**
Allied Dental Profession Educator

**College or University Bachelor Degree:**
Dental Hygienist, Business-Sales, Consulting

**Community College Associate Degree:**
Dental Hygienist, Dental Assistant, Dental Technician

**Certificate of Completion:**
Semi-professional, Dental Assistant, Dental Technician

**High School Diploma:**
Unskilled workers, Dental Assistant, Dental Technician

**Figure 2.1** Scale of dental job complexity. Adapted from Harris NC. Technical Education in the Junior College/New Programs for New Jobs. Washington, DC: American Association of Junior Colleges, 1964.

**education** is the attendance at and participation in seminars or conferences so that the professional remains up to date in the knowledge of dentistry. Continuing education is required for licensure renewal for oral healthcare professionals and covers advances in technology and techniques to safeguard the public. Generally, 12 hours of continuing education is required by the licensing authorities.

---

**BOX 2.2**  *U.S. Dental Occupation Credentials*

| | |
|---|---|
| DDS | Doctor of dental surgery |
| DMD | Doctor of dental medicine |
| RDH | Registered dental hygienist |
| CDA | Certified dental assistant |
| RDA | Registered dental assistant |
| EFDA | Expanded functions dental assistant |
| COA | Certified orthodontic assistant |
| CDPMA | Certified dental practice management assistant |
| CDT | Certified dental laboratory technologist |

## GENERAL DENTISTRY

The **general dentist** is the member of the oral healthcare team who strives to achieve the highest standards of oral healthcare delivery using skills in oral diagnosis, disease prevention, and rehabilitation. General practitioner dentists diagnose and treat disorders of the mouth and engage in patient assessment, treatment planning, patient education, disease prevention, operative dentistry, and/or surgery. Before any dental treatment is provided, oral conditions and risks are assessed for dental and systemic diseases; treatment is planned; and patients are informed regarding the need for restorations, surgery, or preventive dentistry procedures. After informed consent is given by the patient, dentists restore the teeth using a variety of dental materials, including metals, plastics, glasses, and inorganic salts (such as dental cements). Dentists also treat diseases of the supporting structures, such as gingivae and bone, in an effort to save teeth.

These dentists choose to practice general dentistry. Nearly 90% of general dentists render complete dental services in private practice. Besides private practice, these dentists may work in a group practice, share space with another dentist, or be hired by another dentist. They are required by law to refer complicated and unusual cases to dental specialists. A general dentist who completes additional education requirements to learn procedures in a discipline or dental specialty can become a dental specialist.

**Dental specialists** are general dentists who have completed additional educational and licensure requirements and generally limit their practice to a specific area of dentistry. About 80% of all dentists practice general dentistry, whereas an estimated 20% practice a particular dental specialty. Practice settings other than private practice include dental research, product development, sales, education, public service in a public or private agency or institution, and practicing in the armed services.

## Education Requirements

A person interested in becoming a dentist takes college preparatory classes in chemistry, biology, and algebra while in high school. College students need a solid background in the natural sciences, including biology and organic and inorganic chemistry. They also take psychology and business courses. The Dental Admission Test and application to dental school should be completed at least 1 year before expected admission. An education in dentistry usually takes a minimum of 6 years of college: 2–4 years of undergraduate school and 3–4 years of dental school are required to become a dentist. Most dental schools in the United States award the degree of doctor of dental surgery (DDS); some schools award the degree of doctor of dental medicine (DMD).

## Dental Licensure

To practice dentistry in the United States, the dentist must complete the licensure requirements within that jurisdiction. To become a licensed dentist, a candidate must graduate from a program approved by the American Dental Association (ADA) Council on Dental Accreditation (CODA), pass a written and clinical examination recognized by a state or region of the United States, and pay the fees. For example, if a dentist wishes to practice in the northeastern United States, he or she must take the Northeast Regional Board

Examination (NERB). A written national board examination is also required in most states. Dentists enlisted in military or other government public health service are required to have a valid dental license from any U.S. jurisdiction. Once a dentist becomes licensed to practice dentistry, he or she is required to complete the mandatory continuing dental education (CDE) or continuing education units (CEUs) each year. Beyond continuing education, the general dentist can complete further advanced study in a discipline or dental specialty to enhance his or her dental practice.

## DENTAL HYGIENIST

The **dental hygienist** is the member of the oral healthcare team who strives to achieve the highest standards of oral healthcare delivery using skills in assessment, prevention, and treatment of dental disease. Depending on the jurisdiction in which they are licensed, dental hygienists perform many job tasks and perform a wide range of oral healthcare services. Frequently working under the supervision of a dentist, dental hygienists help people maintain their oral health. They evaluate oral conditions; remove deposits, accretions, and stains from the teeth; apply anticariogenic materials; maintain patient records; educate patients about disease control; make dental radiographs and impressions; place restorations and periodontal dressings; remove sutures; polish teeth and restorations; administer local anesthesia; administer nitrous oxide sedation; and provide periodontal care and management. Dental hygienists are employed in solo dental practices (practices with one dentist), group dental practices (practices with two or more dentists), hospitals, public health agencies, clinics, schools, and various levels of government.

Dental hygienists use a variety of clinical skills to treat a diverse group of people, including the elderly, children, and the physically and mentally impaired. Because dental hygienists are in demand nationwide, there is flexibility in employment options, such as full- or part-time work, private practice, and community institutions. Dental hygienists employed by the military or other government public health service are required to have a valid license from any U.S. state, district, or territory.

### Dental Therapists

The **dental therapist** is an occupational title found outside the United States in countries such as Australia and the United Kingdom (UK). They are oral hygiene specialists who work in all sectors of dentistry to perform dental hygiene duties plus routine restorations, extractions, pulpal therapy, placement of preformed crowns on deciduous teeth, limited orthodontics, and referrals; they also provide access to care for people in need. Dental therapists may work in public dental clinics, hospitals, community health centers, mobile dental vans, private dental practices, research, management, education, and policy development. In the United States, there is a similar response to access-to-care issues, which delegates additional duties to dental hygienists to help meet the needs of underserved populations. Further discussion of dental therapists is found in Chapter 9.

### Education Requirements

Dental hygiene education programs vary from 2 to 4 years. After completion of a CODA-accredited program, one of the degrees listed in *Table 2.1* is awarded. To practice dental

| TABLE 2.1 Dental Hygiene Degrees | |
|---|---|
| **Educational Institution** | **Degrees** |
| Community college | Associates of art (AA) |
| | Associates of science (AS) |
| | Associates of art and science (AAS) |
| | Associates of applied art and science (AAAS) |
| College or university | Bachelors of art (BA) |
| | Bachelors of science (BS) |
| University | Master of science (MS) |

hygiene in a jurisdiction, the dental hygiene graduate must complete the licensure requirements within that jurisdiction. Licensure requirements involve the completion of an ADA-approved dental hygiene program; satisfactory completion of a written national board examination; and satisfactory completion of a regional board examination, which may contain written and clinical portions. After successful completion of licensing requirements, the licensed dental hygienist has earned the legal title of registered dental hygienist (RDH). To maintain licensure, CEUs and CPR are required for renewal.

## DENTAL ASSISTANT

The **dental assistant** is the member of the oral healthcare team who acts as a "second pair of hands" for the dentist. Depending on the jurisdiction in which they are employed, dental assistants undertake many job tasks and perform a wide range of oral healthcare services. Usually working under the supervision of a dentist, dental assistants combine a general education with specialized technical education in chairside assisting, radiology, dental laboratory techniques, preventive dentistry, and office procedures. Employment opportunity is variable, and the types of practice settings available include solo or group dental practices in general or specialty dentistry, public health dentistry such as county or federal dental clinics, hospitals, dental schools, insurance companies, product manufacturing, sales, and educational institutions.

### Education Requirements

Dental assistants are not required to have advanced training or earn a college degree. They can receive on-the-job training to become an on-the-job-trained (OJT) dental assistant at the entry level for employment in dentistry. The OJT dental assistant may be qualified to work in clinical procedures; however, his or her duties may be severely limited by the jurisdiction's dental practice act. The state **dental practice act** is the group of laws dental personnel must follow in the state where they work. Population growth, public awareness of oral health, and credentialing of dental assistants have created a need for formally trained dental assistants.

Dental assisting programs are found at universities, community colleges, vocational/technical schools, and private proprietary schools. The CODA-accredited educational programs for dental assisting education are 1–2 years. Formally educated dental assistants increase the efficiency of the dentist in the delivery of oral healthcare by performing expanded functions and can earn higher wages than OJT dental assistants.

## Dental Nurse

The **dental nurse** is an occupational title found in countries such as the UK. In the UK, the dental nurse performs job tasks similar to those of the dental assistant. There are no academic qualifications required to work as a student dental nurse in a dental hospital or community dental service. After 2 years of full-time surgery experience, the student dental nurse can take an examination to earn a national certificate. Dental nurses are mandated to meet these requirements before being eligible to become a dental hygienist or dental therapist.

## Certification

There are two occupations in dentistry in which professionals earn the credential of certification: dental assisting and dental laboratory technology. The national credential awarded to dental assistants is administered by the Dental Assisting National Board (DANB) located in Chicago. DANB awards the credentials of certified dental assistant (CDA), certified orthodontic assistant (COA), and certified dental practice management assistant (CDPMA). Dental assisting **certification** is a national credential that is awarded after completion of a written national board examination. It is possible for dental assistants to maintain more than one DANB credential. The board applicant must graduate from an ADA-accredited dental assisting program or be a high school graduate with at least 2 years of full-time dental office experience. In some jurisdictions, it is the legal authorization to practice dental assisting duties. DANB certifications must be renewed annually after completion of 12 hours of CEUs. The DANB also offers two additional examinations: one for radiation health and safety and the other for infection control.

## Registration

Credentials enable dental assistants to legally perform expanded functions within a specific jurisdiction. Expanded functions are a group of oral healthcare procedures that the credentialed auxiliary is allowed to perform. These additional duties are delegated by dental practice acts to be performed only by credentialed individuals. Selected examples of expanded functions are provided in Chapter 5. Individual jurisdictions have licensing or registration requirements for dental assistants, leading to the registered dental assistant (RDA) credential or, in some states, the expanded functions dental assistant (EFDA) credential. Usually, dental assisting **registration** means the professional has successfully completed a written and clinical examination, which allows him or her to perform expanded functions. The RDA has graduated from an ADA-accredited program, completed a course in expanded functions, and met other licensure requirements to legally perform the additional duties.

RDA licensure is renewed periodically with mandated current CPR and CEU course completion. In Tennessee, registration means that the professional has been approved by the state licensing authority to work as a dental assistant. This state maintains a list of people who have met the minimal requirements to practice dental assisting.

Like other highly skilled health professionals, formally trained dental assistants are in short supply, and an increase in jobs for trained assistants is expected. Many areas of the United States report a shortage of qualified dental assistants. Dental assistants earn salaries similar to other health occupations requiring 1 or 2 years of training.

## DENTAL LABORATORY TECHNICIANS

When dentures or crowns are indicated, the dentist produces laboratory cases so the dental laboratory technician can fabricate fixed or removable appliances. **Dental laboratory technicians** are members of the oral healthcare team who produce appliances such as dentures, partial dentures, bridges, crowns, orthodontic devices, and other prosthetics for dental patients. Each prosthetic device is unique and custom made to fit each patient. Technicians create the dentist's prescribed appliance in the dental laboratory setting. Such laboratories can employ from 2 to 200 people. Dental offices employ lab technicians, as do dental schools. This flexible career offers several opportunities for advancement, such as owning a laboratory, supervising others, and teaching. This profession has many job titles, because dental laboratory technicians can be trained in federal apprenticeship programs.

### Denturists

The **denturist** is a person who specializes in the preparation of removable oral prostheses in countries such as Canada. Although not an occupational title defined by the U.S. Department of Labor, denturists are found in some states. Denturists are independent practitioners who prepare removable dentures by providing oral examination, dental impressions, and jaw-relation records; by fabricating and inserting the dentures; and by instructing the patient on denture care. Adjunctive services include denture repair, relines, and adjustments of removable dentures.

### Education Requirements

There are two principal pathways for becoming a dental laboratory technician: academic programs and apprenticeship programs. Academic programs are offered by a community college, vocational school, technical institute, or dental school. Apprenticeship programs are formal education programs in which the student is paid to work while on the job. However, academic programs prepare the technician for advancement in the field more quickly. The credential earned by the laboratory technician after successful completion of a national board examination is the certified dental technician (CDT). The CDT can specialize in up to five areas: complete dentures, partial dentures, crowns and bridges, ceramics, and orthodontics. Salaries vary greatly in this field, but technicians have more opportunities than other allied dental professionals to expand their earnings by owning a laboratory and becoming self-employed.

## CONCEPT SUMMARY

- In the United States, four basic occupations are found in the field of dentistry: dentist, dental hygienist, dental assistant, and dental laboratory technician.
- The level of difficulty for performing dental occupational job tasks can be organized on a scale of job complexity.
- Each dental occupation has a unique role, educational requirement, and credentialing process.
- In other countries, the job tasks performed, educational requirements, and credentialing process are diverse.

# REVIEW QUESTIONS

1. Where can each of the following dental team members be found on the scale of job complexity?
   A. Dentist
   B. Dental hygienist
   C. Dental assistant
   D. Dental laboratory technician
2. Describe two job responsibilities for each of the following dental team members.
   A. Dentist
   B. Dental hygienist
   C. Dental assistant
   D. Dental laboratory technician
3. List the education requirements for each of the following dental team members.
   A. Dentist
   B. Dental hygienist
   C. Dental assistant
   D. Dental laboratory technician
4. List the credentials for each of the following dental team members.
   A. Dentist
   B. Dental hygienist
   C. Dental assistant
   D. Dental laboratory technician
5. What are the requirements for licensure for each of the following dental team members?
   A. Dentist
   B. Dental hygienist
   C. Dental assistant
   D. Dental laboratory technician
6. What are the requirements for certification for each of the following dental team members?
   A. Dental assistant
   B. Dental laboratory technician
7. What is a group practice? What is private practice?
8. What is on-the-job training?
9. Who is an apprentice?
10. What is the difference between an RDA and a CDA?
11. Why is mandatory continuing education a necessary requirement?
12. What additional certification may be required for the renewal of licensure?
13. Which foreign dental occupation is similar to dental assisting?
14. How is a dental therapist different from a dental hygienist?
15. Compare the dental therapist, dental nurse, and denturist to the dental hygienist, dental assistant, and dental laboratory technician, respectively.

# Dental Specialties

**Upon mastery of the content of this chapter, the student should be able to:**
- **Determine when general dentistry or specialty dentistry is performed.**
- **Describe each dental specialist's unique clinical skills and practice settings.**
- **Recognize selected diagnosis and treatment procedures in each specialty.**
- **Recognize additional areas of specialization that are not considered dental specialties.**
- **Differentiate between the disciplines and the specialties of dentistry.**

## KEY TERMS

| | |
|---|---|
| comprehensive orthodontic treatment | oral and maxillofacial pathology |
| dental public health | oral and maxillofacial radiology |
| diplomate | oral and maxillofacial surgery |
| discipline | orthodontics and dentofacial orthopedics |
| endodontics | pediatric dentistry |
| interceptive orthodontic treatment | periodontics |
| limited orthodontic treatment | prosthodontics |

## DENTAL SPECIALTIES

General dentists refer complicated or unusual cases to a dental specialist or dentist with advanced training in a concentrated subject area. The dental specialist limits his or her practice to one of nine American Dental Association (ADA)-recognized dental specialties. Dental specialists and dentists with advanced education are experts in specific disciplines of dentistry or medicine. Dental specialties are established when it has been demonstrated that a discipline advances the profession in education, practice, and research. In an effort to protect the public, the ADA considers officially recognizing a discipline only after it meets specific criteria for specialty status. The members of a new discipline organize, forming a professional association, and petition for official recognition as outlined in the ADA's "Requirements for Recognition of Dental Specialties" document.

# DENTAL SPECIALISTS

The dental specialist has completed a general dentistry degree and postgraduate training from an accredited ADA-recognized dental specialty program (*Box 3.1*). Dental specialists may work in private practice, group practice, hospitals, educational institutions, or government institutions; they may also partner or share space with, or be hired by, another dentist.

## Education Requirements

The ADA Council on Dental Accreditation (CODA) manages dental specialty education, the requirements of which vary from specialty to specialty. After graduating from dental school, the professional studies for 2–7 years in a CODA-accredited postgraduate program. Finally, the specialist must successfully pass a designated certification board examination. Once the specialist has completed his or her postgraduate work, the additional educational degree is added after the DDS or DMD degree. For example, an orthodontist's name and degrees would be written as Margaret Stone, DDS, MS, which signifies the completion of a master of science degree beyond the doctor of dental surgery program.

Upon completion of the specialty requisites, dental specialists must limit their practice to that one area of dentistry. A general dentist who receives advanced training in a subject area but does not become a specialist is able to practice all the areas of dentistry in which he or she is qualified to perform. As is true in general dentistry, completion of an advanced degree does not mean that the professional's educational process has stopped. There are academies and boards for the dental specialties and disciplines that support further academic and clinical achievement. Dentists with the title "**diplomate** of the board" are dentists who have progressed to the farthest reaches in their field of study by completing additional educational programs. Academies and boards are addressed in Chapter 4.

## Dental Public Health

**Dental public health** is the dental specialty dealing with public programs in preventive education, community treatment, and applied dental research funded by federal, state, and local government agencies. Additional funding sources include public and private grants, corporations, and companies. Funding is also available from nonprofit sources, such as religious charities, professional associations, foundations, and private trusts.

---

**BOX 3.1** *ADA-Recognized Dental Specialties*

| | |
|---|---|
| Dental public health | Orthodontics and dentofacial orthopedics |
| Endodontics | Pediatric dentistry |
| Oral and maxillofacial pathology | Periodontics |
| Oral and maxillofacial radiology | Prosthodontics |
| Oral and maxillofacial surgery | |

Because the oral health of many people, both in the United States and elsewhere, is at a deficit owing to access-to-care issues, public health personnel are needed to promote oral health, disease prevention, and education.

Two important issues in community and public health are humanitarianism and volunteerism. Many dental professionals lend their time and talents to organizations, programs, special clinics, and other outreach activities in an effort to provide oral healthcare to underserved populations. From foreign service, rural migrant clinics, urban clinics, shelters, and professional association activities to ships and/or fleets that provide relief services around the world, there are numerous ways to help, become involved, and provide charitable care to the needy.

## EDUCATION REQUIREMENTS

The general dentist completes postgraduate coursework to earn a master's degree in public and/or community health and then works in federal, state, or local public health programs. Federally funded public health programs originate in the federal Department of Health and Human Services (HHS), Department of Defense (DOD), Department of Veterans Affairs (VA), and Department of Justice (DOJ). State-funded programs may exist in rural areas, and may involve migrant farm workers or rural health initiatives. Local programs are the most prevalent public health settings for the delivery of preventive education or treatment programs in a community. Public health dentistry can be performed outside of the United States. Many times dental personnel donate time, materials, and expertise to render dental treatment in other countries. Such programs are often affiliated with a religious institution.

## ASSESSMENT

Community-based programs require planning for the delivery of dental care to populations identified as high risk. Whether the programs focus on prevention or treatment, a needs assessment of the population is performed using a variety of indices. Surveys are selected and planned, funding is obtained, and examination and recording data are collected and analyzed. Once the target population is selected, an action plan is developed and the program is implemented. After completion of the program or during the course of operations, outcomes are measured to evaluate the program's success.

## PROCEDURES

Agencies plan for the delivery of dental care after the needs assessments are completed. Resources are identified, a course of action is developed, efforts are coordinated, and prevention or treatment is delivered to the target population. Treatment procedures may include oral examination, prophylaxis, fluoride application, patient education, pit and fissure sealant placement, and nutritional counseling. After delivery of care, program performance is evaluated to measure progress, activities, accomplishments, problems, and quality of services rendered to justify the costs. A formal report is written and submitted to the funding agency to document the program's validity and necessity. *Table 3.1* lists selected procedures and insurance codes used in dental public health.

## TABLE 3.1 Selected Dental Insurance Codes

### Public Health

| | | | |
|---|---|---|---|
| D0150 | Comprehensive oral examination | D1310 | Nutritional counseling |
| D1120 | Child prophylaxis | D1330 | Oral hygiene instruction |
| D1203 | Topical fluoride application | D1351 | Pit and fissure sealant (per tooth) |

### Endodontic

| | | | |
|---|---|---|---|
| D0460 | Pulp vitality testing | D3310 | Anterior pulpectomy |
| D3220 | Therapeutic pulpotomy | D3410 | Anterior apicoectomy |
| D3221 | Pulpal débridement | | |

### Oral and Maxillofacial Pathology

| | | | |
|---|---|---|---|
| D0472 | Accession of tissue, gross examination, preparation and transmission of written report | D0474 | Accession of tissue; gross and microscopic examination, including assessment of surgical margins for presence of disease; preparation and transmission of written report |
| D0473 | Accession of tissue, gross and microscopic examination, preparation and transmission of written report | D0480 | Processing and interpretation of cytologic smears, preparation and transmission of written report |

### Oral and Maxillofacial Radiology

| | | | |
|---|---|---|---|
| D0210 | Intraoral complete series | D0330 | Panoramic film |
| D0322 | Tomographic survey | D0340 | Cephalometric film |

### Oral and Maxillofacial Surgery

| | | | |
|---|---|---|---|
| D7210 | Surgical removal of erupted tooth | D7281 | Cytology sample collection |
| D7220 | Surgical removal of soft tissue-impacted tooth | D7440 | Excision of malignant tumor |
| | | D7858 | TMJ reconstruction |
| D7286 | Biopsy of soft oral tissue | D7910 | Wound suturing |

### Orthodontic

| | | | |
|---|---|---|---|
| D8040 | Limited orthodontic treatment of the adult dentition | D8080 | Comprehensive orthodontic treatment of the adolescent dentition |
| D8050 | Interceptive orthodontic treatment of the transitional dentition | D8220 | Fixed appliance therapy for habit control |

### Pediatric

| | | | |
|---|---|---|---|
| D2330 | Resin-based composite-one surface anterior | D3230 | Pulpal therapy anterior primary tooth |
| | | D8691 | Repair of orthodontic retainer |
| D2930 | Prefabricated stainless steel crown—primary tooth | D3470 | Reimplantation of avulsed tooth |
| | | D9941 | Fabrication of athletic mouth guard |

### Periodontic

| | | | |
|---|---|---|---|
| D0415 | Bacteriologic studies for pathogenic agents | D4260 | Osseous surgery |
| | | D4263 | Bone graft |
| D4210 | Gingivectomy or gingivoplasty | D4270 | Pedicle soft tissue graft |
| D4249 | Crown lengthening | D4274 | Distal or proximal wedge |

### Prosthodontic

| | | | |
|---|---|---|---|
| D5110 | Complete maxillary denture | D6601 | Porcelain inlay |
| D5212 | Partial mandibular denture | D6720 | High noble metal crown |
| D6210 | Porcelain fused to metal pontic | | |

Excerpted from Current Dental Terminology-4. Reprinted with permission from the American Dental Association.

## Endodontics

**Endodontics** is the dental specialty dealing with the morphology, physiology, pathology, origin, diagnosis, prevention, and treatment of pulpal and periapical disease. Endodontists specialize in assessing and treating the pulpal and periapical tooth tissues, Several pulpal pathologies require endodontic therapy.

### EDUCATION REQUIREMENTS

The general dentist completes 2 years of postgraduate coursework to earn a master's degree in endodontics and then works in a variety of practice settings.

### ASSESSMENT

Endodontists use several different assessment procedures to diagnose disease, including intraoral radiographs and pulp testing. Dental radiographs allow the specialist to examine the pulp, periodontal ligament space, alveolar bone, and carious lesions. In some instances, pulpal pathology is not detectable on a dental radiograph and further testing is necessary to evaluate the vitality of the pulp. Thermal pulp testing uses extremes in temperature to assess the pulpal reaction. If the application of cold stimulates a pulpal response, it indicates the early stages of inflammation. The reaction to cold should diminish once the cold is removed. If the reaction to cold remains painful after the stimulus is removed, there is likely advanced inflammation. If the application of heat produces sharp pain but the application of cold brings relief, then the inflammation is advanced. When the dental pulp does not respond to heat or cold, it is considered nonvital.

Electric pulp testing is performed using an electric pulp tester, called a vitalometer. Several teeth are tested with electric current to assess whether pulpal necrosis has occurred and the tooth is nonvital. Percussion pulp testing and transillumination are also used to diagnose pulpal pathology. The endodontist will lightly tap several teeth to determine whether the patient feels the percussion in the tooth. Nonvital teeth will not feel the percussion, whereas inflamed teeth will hurt when tapped. A fiber optic light is used during transillumination to look for fracture or craze lines to investigate microleakage or pulpal necrosis. When comparing the color of the tooth to the adjacent teeth using the fiber optic light, dark discoloration many times indicates pulpal necrosis has occurred.

### PROCEDURES

Endodontic procedures are performed in an effort to save teeth when an advanced inflammatory state or pulpal necrosis is present. Pulpotomy is performed to remove the coronal portion of the pulpal chamber. Pulpectomy is performed to remove all of the pulpal tissues within the pulp cavity. The surgical procedure called an apicoectomy is performed to remove infected tissues around the apex of the tooth that did not heal after pulpectomy. *Table 3.1* lists selected procedures and insurance codes used in endodontics.

## Oral and Maxillofacial Pathology

**Oral and maxillofacial pathology** is the dental specialty focusing on the cause, diagnosis, management, and research of diseases that affect the maxillofacial structures. Pathology is central to the diagnosis and management of disease. Oral and maxillofacial pathologists are highly trained laboratory scientists who research the causes of disease. Pathologists work closely with dentists to help provide a diagnosis or to render a second opinion. They support other dental specialists; general dentists; oral surgeons; ear, nose, and throat physicians; personnel on military ships; and other branches of medicine. There are two main divisions in pathology: clinical pathology and anatomic pathology. In addition, there is a forensic aspect of oral pathology.

## EDUCATION REQUIREMENTS

The general dentist completes postgraduate coursework to earn a master's degree in oral and maxillofacial pathology and then works for the military; in a variety of medical arenas; or in a hospital, dental institution, or medical institution.

## ASSESSMENT

Pathologists study cell, tissue, and body fluid samples to determine if disease is present. Clinical pathology is concerned with the abnormal physiologic manifestations of disease found as a result of body fluid analysis. Anatomic pathology is concerned with the analysis of diseased tissues removed during surgery. Cytology is a division of anatomic pathology in which disease is detected within individual cells.

## PROCEDURES

Human tissue, cell, or body fluid samples arrive at the laboratory in specialized specimen jars sent through the U.S. mail, a delivery service, or interdepartmental courier within an institution or hospital. The oral pathologist working with a team of other pathologists analyzes samples to interpret test results, study tissue samples, and diagnose conditions that can be life threatening. Cellular analysis of tissue smears is used to determine the correct diagnosis of a disease condition. Tissue analysis helps the pathologist reach the correct diagnosis of a disease condition and determine whether a surgically removed biopsy or tumor is benign or malignant. Oral and maxillofacial pathologists are on the frontier of new discoveries and are most immediately affected by medical research findings. *Table 3.1* lists selected procedures and insurance codes used in oral and maxillofacial pathology.

## Oral and Maxillofacial Radiology

**Oral and maxillofacial radiology** is the dental specialty dealing with the production and interpretation of images created by radiant energy to diagnose and manage diseases that affect the maxillofacial region. Technological advances in digital imaging, tomography, magnetic resonance imaging (MRI), and other techniques have created this relatively new dental specialty. Oral and maxillofacial radiologists (OMRs) have studied radiation physics, biology, imaging technology, computed tomography (CT), MRI, subtraction radiography, arthrography, and interpretation of images. This knowledge provides the basis for understanding the correlation between clinical, histological, and radiographic findings in disease.

The OMR may teach, render imaging services to patients, or conduct clinical research. Currently, dental students learn via case studies how to interpret disease based on the various modes of image production. OMRs also serve on university committees, for example, to establish a campuswide radiation safety policy.

### EDUCATION REQUIREMENTS

The general dentist completes a 2-year postgraduate program and receives a master's degree or doctoral degree in oral and maxillofacial radiology and then works in a dental office, medical school, or hospital radiology department.

### ASSESSMENT

The OMR primarily uses assessment, diagnosis, and interpretation procedures. To be able to diagnose head and neck diseases, this specialist must complete coursework in advanced head and neck anatomy, clinical and microscopic pathology, oral medicine, and research methods, and must participate in hospital rotations. Scholarly activity by OMR faculty includes conducting research, which is based on the type of patient, the biological effects of radiant energies, the equipment available, the interests of the researcher, and funding from the National Institute for Dental and Craniofacial Research.

### PROCEDURES

Radiographic imaging, such as intraoral and extraoral radiographic surveys, and diagnostic consultations, are the standard procedures in oral and maxillofacial radiology. CT scanning is the emission of an x-ray beam from a scanner that rotates around a patient's body. Information on the x-ray absorption rate of the tissues is relayed to a computer, which converts the data into a clear image of a slice of the body.

MRI of the TMJ or an implant is a diagnostic procedure that uses nuclear magnetic resonance to generate a section image that is superior to that obtained from other technologies. The patient is placed in a cylindrical magnet and a magnetic field is created to stimulate the body with a radio wave.

The positron-emission tomography (PET) scanner works similarly to MRI and produces data on blood flow and metabolic processes. Ultrasound technology uses high-frequency sound to image the body. A computer analyzes the sound reflection to produce a moving image. Doppler is used to measure the flow of liquids. *Table 3.1* lists selected procedures and insurance codes for oral and maxillofacial radiology.

## Oral and Maxillofacial Surgery

**Oral and maxillofacial surgery** is the dental specialty dealing with the diagnosis and surgical repair of injuries, defects, and diseases of the maxillofacial region. Oral surgery is similar to medicine because it involves surgical procedures that may require the use of general anesthetics in a hospital setting. Oral surgeons treat patients in hospitals, outpatient facilities, surgery centers, and in private dental offices.

### EDUCATION REQUIREMENTS

Oral and maxillofacial surgeons (OMSs) have more advanced training than any other dental specialist. The OMS completes a hospital-based surgical residency of at least 4 years after completion of postgraduate coursework to receive advanced training in medicine, general surgery, anesthesia, and physical diagnosis. Residents learn diagnosis, treatment, and management of problems of the oral and maxillofacial region, such as trauma, tumors and cancerous lesions, surgical jaw repositioning, facial implants, cleft palate repair, cosmetic surgery, tooth extraction, and pain and anxiety control. During their residency programs, OMSs participate in hospital rotations through medical, surgical, and anesthesia services. Residents spend at least 30 months learning the reconstruction of the nose, orbits of the eye, cleft palate, and facial aesthetic surgery. In addition, the OMS must successfully complete an advanced trauma life support (ATLS) course.

## ASSESSMENT

Before a diagnosis can be made, the OMS must determine the medical history; conduct an examination; examine radiographs and other imaging; and review medical tests, laboratory reports, and the referral. A diagnosis of oral conditions, diseases, and lesions is needed before the specialist performs extractions, does surgery of the face, or manages trauma. Accurate patient information of any pathophysiology is absolutely necessary for the OMS to make a proper diagnosis.

Preoperative care instructions are told to the patient, who is also given written instructions. Written instructions regarding the use of prescription drugs, activity level, eating, operating machinery, driving, and home care must be provided before any procedure is done. Care and comfort given to allay the fears of the dental patient make the surgical experience more tolerable.

## PROCEDURES

There are many oral surgery procedures performed to repair defects, deformities, and traumatic injuries and to remove teeth, cysts, or tumors. Pain and anxiety control focuses on ambulatory anesthesia for in-office conscious sedation and local anesthetic techniques. Aesthetic surgery, such as rhinoplasty, blepharoplasty, lipectomy, facial implants, otoplasty, scar revision, cleft lip/palate, neurosensory/neuromotor deficit, and craniofacial surgeries are performed by the OMS.

Other procedures performed by the OMS relate to tumor and cancer surgery, management of malignant tumors and regional metastasis, ablative surgery, management of complications, and nutritional support. Orthognathic surgery restores jaw function by realigning the jaws and facial bones with pin or wire placement and soft tissue suturing. Temporomandibular joint disorders (TMJDs) require a diagnosis of head, neck, and facial pain as well as nonsurgical and surgical options for abnormalities. Comprehensive management of trauma, shock, fluid and electrolyte balance, resuscitation, and surgical airway management and treatment of multiple-system trauma are more complex situations in which the oral surgeon renders care. The OMS follows up on patients after surgery to remove sutures or dressings and to check healing. *Table 3.1* lists selected procedures and insurance codes used in oral and maxillofacial surgery.

## Orthodontics and Dentofacial Orthopedics

**Orthodontics and dentofacial orthopedics** is the dental specialty dealing with the correction of misaligned teeth and jaws. Orthodontic treatment is a complex dental specialty that is also the oldest and largest dental specialty. Orthodontists restore normal tooth position for proper functioning and guide facial development to improve the appearance of the dental patient.

## EDUCATION REQUIREMENTS

The general dentist completes 2–3 years of postdoctoral study in an accredited orthodontic program. Orthodontic programs cover topics in biomedical and behavioral and basic sciences to help the specialist learn complex skills in moving teeth (orthodontics) and guiding facial growth (dentofacial orthopedics). Orthodontists work in dental schools or private practice.

## ASSESSMENT

First, tooth and facial development are assessed to determine the timing for orthodontia. After the primary dentition develops and erupts, the transitional dentition phase of eruption occurs during which the deciduous molars and canines undergo exfoliation. Adolescent dentition is present after the normal loss of the primary teeth and before the halt of facial growth; adult dentition is present after the cessation of growth.

Misaligned teeth present in many variations, but a common classification system, Angle's classification (1899), is used to describe the jaw relationships. Data collected in a comprehensive oral examination aid in the orthodontic diagnosis. Data collection records made of the patient include intraoral and extraoral radiographs, consisting of cephalometric, panoramic, and bitewing radiographs. Intraoral and extraoral photographs are taken to document facial shape and symmetry and provide a visual record of tooth relationships. Diagnostic study models are made for a three-dimensional record of the patient's dentition. Clinical examination findings for swallowing, speech, jaw movement, gingival conditions, and malocclusion are used to create a treatment plan for the course of tooth movement and appointment scheduling.

## PROCEDURES

**Limited orthodontic treatment** is used to correct an existing problem with a few teeth or is directed at one aspect of a larger problem when a decision to postpone comprehensive treatment is made. Limited orthodontic treatment can be performed on the primary, transitional, adolescent, or adult dentition.

**Interceptive orthodontic treatment** is designed to guide the oral growth of a child. Some techniques that are commonly used include redirecting erupting teeth, space maintenance and space regaining, habit control, and crossbite correction. Interceptive orthodontics can be performed on the primary and transitional dentition.

**Comprehensive orthodontic treatment** improves craniofacial dysfunction and/or dentofacial deformity. Sometimes called "corrective orthodontics," it involves the use of appliances, materials, and procedures to establish proper occlusion. It takes several years of treatment to realign the teeth and for retention. Procedures used for comprehensive orthodontic treatment include extractions, maxillofacial surgery, nasopharyngeal surgery, myofunctional therapy, speech therapy, restorative care, and periodontal care. Comprehensive orthodontic treatment is used for transitional, adolescent, and adult dentition. *Table 3.1* lists selected procedures and insurance codes used in orthodontics.

# Pediatric Dentistry

**Pediatric dentistry** is the dental specialty dealing with the treatment of children. Pediatric dentists practice an advanced level of care for children in private offices, clinics, dental schools, and hospitals. They are qualified to care for patients with special needs such as those with medical, physical, or mental disabilities. The pediatric dentist specializes in children's needs in three major areas: patient management, child development, and procedures for restorative care. Patient management techniques are essential to a successful dental visit for the pediatric patient.

## EDUCATION REQUIREMENTS

The general dentist completes 2–3 years of postgraduate study in an accredited program with a concentration in child psychology, growth, and development.

## ASSESSMENT

Research into child behavior has shown that children exhibit general characteristics at different stages of growth and development. These characteristics can help guide the practitioner who deals with children. For example, 2-year-olds tend to be negative and say no when asked questions; 3-year-olds fear separation from their mother and may fear strangers. Most 4-year-olds like animals and babies but fear the unknown; they can respond to specific instructions. Typical 5-year-olds may be proud or shy and relate pain to punishment; 6-year-olds ask what, who, and why, and respond to factual explanations. By 7–8 years old, children want to be like others their age, and they enjoy past cultures. Most 9- to 11-year-olds are interested in factual information. Adolescents and teenagers may embarrass easily, may want to discuss personal problems, and generally seek peer approval.

## PROCEDURES

The same basic procedures used on adults are used for children, but there are differences. For example, rubber dam isolation is used to keep the child's mouth open, protect the soft tissues from injury by sharp instruments, and prevent aspiration of dental materials. Children often need restorative dentistry, endodontics, and orthodontics, and undergo traumatic injuries. Sports-related mouth protection is a common requirement.

Perhaps the most critical aspect of treating children is to teach them the importance of oral home care and nutrition. Brushing instructions should be reviewed at each visit and flossing should be introduced during prophylaxis. Flossing instruction is given when appropriate. Around age 11, children develop the manual dexterity to floss and their teeth have erupted with contact points. Reinforcement of flossing instruction should occur at each visit, and the various flossing aids should be introduced. Juvenile periodontal disease and caries-preventive procedures are also important to consider when treating children. *Table 3.1* lists selected procedures and insurance codes used in pediatric dentistry.

# Periodontics

**Periodontics** is the dental specialty dealing with prevention, diagnosis, treatment, and maintenance of the supporting structures of the teeth using preventive, surgical, and non-surgical techniques. These conditions threaten the integrity of the periodontium and are important because most adult patients have some degree of periodontal disease. Periodontists treat conditions that cannot be eliminated by prevention, nutrition, or oral hygiene. Patients must be receptive to the concept of maintaining general and physical health to accept periodontal treatment.

## EDUCATION REQUIREMENTS

The general dentist completes 2 years postgraduate coursework in an accredited program to earn a master's degree in periodontics. Workplaces for the periodontist include the military, dental schools, and private practice.

## ASSESSMENT

Data collection begins with the clinical examination, charting, periodontal probing, and radiographs. Additional assessment techniques are bacterial culturing and host genetic or bacterial DNA testing. The first step of bacterial assessment is to insert paper points into the gingival sulcus; these are shipped overnight to the laboratory. The periodontal pathogen complexes are then analyzed via culturing or DNA examination. Host genetic testing determines the patient's predisposition for periodontal disease; it consists of a cheek swab, which is sent to the laboratory for analysis. The specific diagnosis of the periodontal disease determines the course of treatment.

## PROCEDURES

Periodontal therapy consists of treating periodontal conditions; repairing carious teeth; providing a regimented patient education and preventive home care program; and performing professional prophylaxis of scaling, root planing, and gingival curettage. Gingivectomy, gingivoplasty, and osseous surgical procedures may be indicated to stop the process of periodontal disease. Additional surgical procedures performed by the periodontist are crown lengthening, bone tissue grafting, and distal or proximal wedges.

Prophylaxis procedures are performed by periodontists and dental hygienists, who remove deposits, polish the teeth, apply antibacterial agents, and educate the patient on disease and prevention. The periodontist and dental hygienist also render scaling and root planing procedures to remove accretions and toxins from the root surfaces and periodontal pockets. Periodontists turn to surgical procedures when prophylaxis, scaling, and root planing are ineffective to halt the disease process or to improve gingival conditions.

Gingivectomy is the surgical removal of the soft tissue to reduce pocket depth and hyperplastic tissue. Gingivoplasty is the partial removal and reshaping of the marginal gingival contour, attached gingivae, and interdental papillae when it is fibrotic, enlarged, or unaesthetic. Osseous surgery is a surgical flap procedure aimed at repositioning the gingivae to reduce pocketing and may involve osteoplasty, the recontouring of the alveolar bone to improve bony defects, or ostectomy, the removal of damaged or necrotic alveolar bone. Periodontists also perform gingival grafting and implant placement. *Table 3.1* lists selected procedures and insurance codes used in periodontics. Periodontal treatment codes for dental hygiene procedures are listed in Chapter 11.

# Prosthodontics

**Prosthodontics** is the dental specialty dealing with the replacement of lost maxillofacial structures with fixed or removable prosthetic devices. A prosthesis is an artificial substitute for a missing body part. The prompt replacement of a missing tooth structure and/or teeth prevents tooth drifting, rotation and/or tipping of adjacent teeth, and extrusion of teeth from the opposing arch. It also improves the appearance and mental health of the patient. The most common procedure in the prosthodontic office is the replacement of teeth.

A permanent replacement appliance is called a fixed prosthesis; a removable replacement appliance is called a removable prosthesis. Fixed prosthodontic devices—such as veneers, inlays, onlays, crowns, and bridges—are attached with dental cements or resins. Removable prosthodontic devices—such as partial and full dentures—can be removed from the mouth. Some patients require replacement of missing orofacial structures that were lost as a result of trauma or disease. Prompt replacement of missing orofacial structures improves the patient's appearance, function, and mental health. Fixed and removable prostheses are constructed in a dental laboratory by a dental laboratory technician.

## EDUCATION REQUIREMENTS

The general dentist completes postgraduate coursework to earn a master's degree in prosthodontics, and then works in the military, a dental school, or private practice.

## ASSESSMENT

There are few unique assessment procedures in prosthodontics. Missing tooth structures must be restored or replaced so the patient can regain form and function. Once it has been determined that a filling-type restoration cannot be placed into a tooth, a fixed appliance is constructed. When multiple teeth are missing, a removable appliance is constructed.

## PROCEDURES

Veneers are custom-fabricated appliances designed to cover the facial and incisal surfaces of teeth. They are constructed to fit prepared teeth and are composed of composite resin, porcelain, or ceramic. Inlays are custom-fabricated appliances designed to cover a tooth preparation. Onlays are custom-fabricated appliances designed to cover a tooth preparation that includes the cusps of a tooth or teeth. Crowns are custom-fabricated appliances designed to replace part of or the entire crown of a tooth. Bridges are custom-fabricated appliances designed to replace one or more missing teeth. They consist of two or more crowns that are fused together. Abutment crowns are located on either side of a space caused by missing teeth. Pontic crowns replace the missing teeth. After endodontic treatment, teeth are crowned to provide strength to the tooth.

Removable partial dentures are appliances fabricated to replace limited areas within the dental arch. Partial dentures are indicated when the patient retains enough natural teeth to support the appliance. Removable full dentures are appliances fabricated to provide a complete artificial replacement of the dental arch. Full dentures are indicated when the maxillary or mandibular arch gingivae and underlying alveolar bone can support the appliance. Extensive bone loss and the patient's refusal to accept other suggested dental treatments determine the use of dentures. Immediate dentures are placed after the tooth extractions to provide the patient with teeth and to act as a bandage during the healing process after surgery; they must be properly relined after healing has occurred to improve the fit. *Table 3.1* lists selected procedures and insurance codes used in prosthodontics.

## DENTAL DISCIPLINES

General dentists, specialists, or other oral healthcare providers may seek additional knowledge and training in subject areas known as disciplines to acquire new skills to enhance their range of service. A dental **discipline** is an area that is unique in scope and requires additional education. Dental practitioners who pursue a discipline use their knowledge to treat a particular health condition (e.g., diabetes or TMJD), manage a specific type of patient (e.g., one who is mentally, physically, or sensory challenged), or perform a certain procedure (e.g., alternative and complementary therapies). While not currently recognized as dental specialties, these subject areas may gain specialty status if practitioners fulfill the requirements for such recognition. *Box 3.2* lists the common dental disciplines.

Formal educational programs for a discipline may be in place, as in the case for oral medicine and anesthesiology. Informal continuing education programs are available for other subject areas, such as aesthetic cosmetic dentistry and the use of lasers.

### Alternative and Complementary Dentistry

Complementary and alternative therapy is the dental discipline dealing with the treatment of chronic health problems using nontraditional healthcare practices. Complementary and alternative therapy is divided into five domains of practice (*Box 3.3*). Allopathy uses antagonists to create a reaction that is different from the presenting biological condition; for example, cold may be used to reduce fever. Naturopathy is the system of restoring health to encourage the healing process. Homeopathy uses plant extracts or minerals to stimulate the body's defense mechanisms.

### Cosmetic Dentistry

Cosmetic dentistry is the dental discipline dealing with the aesthetics of dental treatment. Computer programs are available to help with the production of custom-made, tooth-colored restorations, which can be milled and precisely cut to the dimensions of the tooth preparation, eliminating impressions and reducing the number of office visits. Restorations can be delivered within an hour. Practitioners in this discipline use

---

**BOX 3.2** *Dental Disciplines*

| | |
|---|---|
| Complementary and alternative dentistry | Oral implantodontics |
| Cosmetic dentistry | Oral medicine |
| Dental anesthesiology | Special care dentistry |
| Forensic dentistry | Sports dentistry |
| Geriatric dentistry | Temporomandibular joint disorder |
| High-tech dentistry | |

voice-activated record keeping to obtain colorized periodontal, restorative, and pathology charts; services rendered; treatment plans; insurance and account information; and patient education video presentations. Intraoral videocameras, digital imaging, low-radiation radiography, and cosmetic imaging are ways in which the patient can visualize problem areas and more actively participate in aesthetic treatment decisions.

## Dental Anesthesiology

Dental anesthesiology is the dental discipline dealing with pain and anxiety control. Dental anesthesiologists have expertise in sedation, general anesthesia, and management of acute and chronic pain. They have a minimum of 2 years of full-time postgraduate training in anesthesiology, including hospital operating room anesthesiology, ambulatory anesthesia, emergency medicine, cardiology, and pain management.

In state jurisdictions in which local anesthesia is not allowed by dental hygienists, electronic anesthesia and lidocaine patch anesthesia can be used as a substitute for topical and local anesthesia. Electronic anesthesia and improved drugs and medications are advancements in oral anesthesiology. Nerve-stimulation technology to control acute, chronic, and postsurgical pain is achieved by electronic anesthesia. This patient-operated machine induces loss of sensation and is a substitute for chemical anesthetics.

## Forensic Dentistry

Forensic dentistry is the dental discipline dealing with the identification of human remains for legal purposes. This dental science uses diverse techniques to verify the identity of cadavers. Most human remains are identified by visual inspection of the body for moles, scars, tattoos, and hair and eye color. Personal effects found with the body such as clothing, jewelry, and purse and wallet contents are also used for identification. Dental comparisons, such as lip prints, teeth restorations, and alignment, are unique characteristics of individuals. Fingerprint matching further confirms identity. Finally, DNA testing positively identifies individuals that may be otherwise unidentifiable when visual recognition is not possible.

## Geriatric Dentistry

Geriatric dentistry is the dental discipline dealing with treating the elderly. In 2003, there were more than 35 million Americans aged 65 years or older, representing 12.3% of the population. This number is expected to double in the next 30 years. Thus, older adults will account for a higher percentage of practice income. The older patient's desire for good health and changing physical needs and management issues challenge the oral healthcare practitioner. Physical aspects of aging, changing socioeconomic status, and loss of independence are factors to consider when providing care to the senior citizen. Barriers that interfere with treating the older dental patient may include the complexity of dental needs, limited finances, medical complications, diminished function, misinformation, and poor attitude.

## High-Tech Dentistry

High-tech dentistry is the dental discipline dealing with incorporating the latest technological advances into dental practice. Using state-of-the-art sophisticated equipment and procedures is a nontraditional, alternative approach to dental treatment that enhances patient care, maximizes and motivates staff performance, and gives the dental practice a competitive edge in the marketplace. Lasers, computer-aided design (CAD) and modeling (CAM) of restorations, air-abrasion units, enhanced computer programs, and digital radiography are technologies being incorporated into today's dental practices.

Advances in research are extremely important in high-tech dentistry. Vaccine development for the prevention of herpes simplex virus, caries, and periodontal disease are in research. Investigation into the human immune system may have implications for dental practice. Dentistry is expected to become more like the practice of medicine, with an emphasis on prevention and lifestyle choices. Patient management and strong communication skills for motivating patients will be increasingly important as dental health becomes more closely related to general health. High-tech dentistry techniques are listed in *Box 3.4.*

## Oral Implantodontics

Oral implantodontics is the dental discipline dealing with the surgical and prosthodontic aspects of placing mechanical devices into or on the alveolar bone. These devices hold crowns, bridges, partial dentures, and full dentures in the mouth. Endosseous implants are screwed into the bone, and subperiosteal implants are placed onto the alveolar bone and under the gingivae.

Improvements in dental implants have made this a popular alternative to dentures, especially since the creation of titanium alloy. Titanium dental implant alloy is a strong biocompatible material that can be molded into tight-fitting cylinders that are screwed into the bone at the site of a missing tooth. A postoperative healing time of 3–6 months is needed for the bone and gingival tissue to grow around the implant. In the case of the screw-type implant, a temporary plastic resin crown may be attached to the implant until

---

**BOX 3.4** *High-Tech Dentistry Techniques*

| | |
|---|---|
| Lasers | CAD/CAM restoration designing |
| Air abrasion | Intraoral and digital imaging |
| Pain control procedures | Vaccines and immunology |
| Computer programs | Prevention and behavioral aspects |

healing is complete for aesthetic purposes, after which a permanent crown is fabricated. This surgical procedure is considered the standard of care for prosthetic procedures to stabilize partial and fully removable prosthetic appliances.

## Oral Medicine

Oral medicine is the dental discipline dealing with the diagnosis and treatment of oral manifestations of systemic diseases or the care of the medically compromised patient. Oral medicine specialists are concerned with the nonsurgical medical aspects of dentistry. They are involved in the primary diagnosis and treatment of oral diseases that do not respond to conventional dental or surgical procedures.

In addition, they provide consultative and supportive oral healthcare to hospitalized and nonhospitalized patients with severe, life-threatening medical disorders. Oral medicine specialists work as members of a team to provide safe and effective oral care for patients with advanced heart disease, uncontrolled diabetes, bleeding disorders, organ transplants, immune deficiencies, and cancer, and those who are suffering from the effects of chemotherapy and radiation therapy. These specialists provide consultation and oral healthcare to patients who require ongoing nonsurgical management owing to complex problems involving the mouth, jaws, and salivary glands. Salivary gland and functional disorders of the head and neck region, chronic orofacial pain, mucocutaneous lesions, and chemosensory and neurologic impairment of the oral and maxillofacial complex are also managed by the oral medicine specialist.

Oral medicine specialists receive formal and distinct advanced education of at least 2 years beyond the dental school curriculum from a CODA-accredited institution. This discipline may be among the next practice areas to be formally recognized as a specialty. Most oral medicine specialists practice within a hospital, the military, or a university-based institution. They educate the primary-care dentists in basic internal medicine and the diagnosis, treatment, and management of oral disease.

## Special Care Dentistry

Special care dentistry is the dental discipline dealing with patients who have mental, physical, or sensory disabilities. This new and emerging area is unique in its mission to care for the disabled.

## Sports Dentistry

Sports dentistry is the dental discipline dealing with the prevention and management of oral and maxillofacial sport injuries. One third of all sports injuries are dentofacial, and protecting these structures is an important aspect of sports dentistry. Trauma to the head and neck results from exposure to thermal, electrical, mechanical, or chemical energy, or from the absence of oxygen.

Examples of injuries to the head and neck are concussion, trauma to the facial bone or soft tissue, fracture of the crown of the central incisor, trauma to other fully or partially formed teeth, and tooth intrusion or extrusion. Other injuries include minor head trauma, foreign objects lodged in the body, and muscle sprains and strains. The best defense for injury and trauma is a mouthguard, which absorbs the force of a blow to the chin.

## Temporomandibular Joint Disorder

Temporomandibular joint disorder is the dental discipline dealing with the proper functioning and management of the TMJ, which is where the condyle of the mandible attaches to the glenoid fossa of the temporal bone. MRI is used to evaluate injuries to the TMJ. When the joint is dislocated, the mouth may lock open because the mandibular condyle is out of position. The patient is unable to close until the condyle is placed into the glenoid fossa of the temporal bone and is retained in position. When the patient is unable to close the mouth, a local oral surgeon or dentist with advanced training in TMJD is called to manage the case.

### CONCEPT SUMMARY

- General dentists refer complicated or unusual cases to a dental specialist or dentist with advanced training in a concentrated subject area.
- Dental specialists limit their practice to one of nine ADA-recognized specialties.
- Dental disciplines are unique subject areas relevant to the practice of dentistry that require additional education.
- Dental disciplines become dental specialties after they have been demonstrated to advance the profession in education, practice, and research.
- The ADA considers bestowing specialty status on a discipline after its practitioners have created an organized association and petition the ADA according to the "Requirements for Recognition of Dental Specialties" document.

## REVIEW QUESTIONS

1. When are general dentists required to refer patients to a dental specialist?
2. What are the requirements for becoming a dental specialist?
3. What is the difference between a specialty and a discipline?
4. What do each of the following dental specialties deal with?
   A. Dental public health
   B. Endodontics
   C. Oral and maxillofacial pathology
   D. Oral and maxillofacial radiology
   E. Oral and maxillofacial surgery
   F. Orthodontics and dentofacial orthopedics
   G. Pediatric dentistry
   H. Periodontics
   I. Prosthodontics

5. Who are diplomates?
6. Describe each of the following dental disciplines.
   A. Complementary and alternative dentistry
   B. Cosmetic dentistry
   C. Forensic dentistry
   D. Geriatric dentistry
   E. High-tech dentistry
   F. Oral anesthesiology
   G. Oral implantodontics
   H. Oral medicine
   I. Special care dentistry
   J. Sports dentistry
   K. Temporomandibular joint disorder

# Chapter
# 4

# Professional Issues

Upon mastery of the content of this chapter, the student should be able to:

- Name the professional organizations for the dental professions.
- Recognize the benefits of membership in a professional association.
- Access the websites of dental organizational hierarchies.
- Differentiate between virtues, ethics, etiquette, and protocol.
- Describe a personal and professional code of ethics.
- Recognize that the ADA, ADHA, ADAA, and NADL have a written code of ethics.
- Identify the consequences of unethical behavior.

## KEY TERMS

Academy of General Dentistry
American Board of General Dentistry
American Dental Assistants Association
American Dental Association
American Dental Hygienists' Association
diplomates of the board

ethics
peer review
personal code of ethics
philosophy
professional code of ethics
tripartite

## PROFESSIONAL ISSUES

Professional issues relate to personal ethics, the codes of ethics of associations, and membership in professional organizations. The multitude of organizations that serve the four recognized dental professions are known as associations, colleges, societies, study clubs, academies, and boards. Membership status in many professional associations offers tripartite privileges. **Tripartite** means "having three parts," and a tripartite membership indicates that the professional belongs to the national, state, and local levels of an organization. Each profession has its own particular set of professional ethics, standards, and characters related to credentialing.

# PROFESSIONAL ASSOCIATIONS AND ORGANIZATIONS

## American Dental Association

Most dentists are members of the **American Dental Association** (ADA; www.ada.org), the most widely recognized organization of dentistry in the United States. Established in 1859, the ADA (located in Chicago) provides professional interactions for its membership, represents dentists in many aspects of dentistry, and sets the ethical standards for the profession. The association also approves education programs, dental instruments, and materials; establishes councils; produces publications; and influences public health policy. Within the ADA are several hundred councils that study situations or problems relating to different aspects of the profession from dental education to products. The councils often recommend the policies of the ADA, and several important councils exist for all of the dental careers. The Commission on Dental Accreditation (CODA) periodically reviews all educational programs to determine whether they meet the standards as set by the ADA for other policy or accrediting commissions. The Council on Dental Equipment and Materials reviews products, such as restorative materials and toothpaste, for the ADA Seal of Approval program.

The ADA holds an annual national meeting and supports research. The ADA annual session meets in the fall and is held in a different city each year. At the meeting, manufacturers introduce new products, researchers present their findings in poster and table clinic sessions, and professionals take advantage of continuing education opportunities. Printed materials can be purchased from the ADA via the Internet or product catalog. The association produces display posters, pamphlets, brochures, instructional materials, and audiovisual products. The *Journal of the American Dental Association* is the association's professional periodical. The *American Dental Directory,* printed annually, contains the names and contact addresses of members, councils, officers, bureaus, publications, organizations, and many other groups affiliated with the ADA.

## Academy of General Dentistry

The **Academy of General Dentistry** (AGD; www.agd.org) is a nonprofit organization whose sole purpose is to provide education and information resources to the dental profession and the public. Dentists who opt for membership in the AGD do so for personal advancement and the opportunity, through continuing education, to earn one of two awards: fellowship or mastership. To earn fellowship status, a dentist must maintain continuous membership in the AGD for 5 years, complete 500 hours of continuing education, and pass a comprehensive written exam. To earn mastership status, a dentist must complete the fellowship requirements, another 1,100 hours of continuing dental education, and 400 hours of practicum work.

The AGD recognizes 16 disciplines of dentistry for fellowship study: aesthetics, basic sciences, endodontics, fixed and removable prosthodontics, implants, occlusion, operative dentistry, oral diagnosis/oral medicine, oral surgery, orthodontics, pediatric dentistry, periodontics, practice management, self-improvement, special patient care, and other electives. After the completion of the academy requirements, the individual earns the right to be called a fellow or master of the Academy of General Dentistry and use the acronym FAGD or MAGD to signify his or her credentials.

## The American Board of General Dentistry

Dental specialty associations establish a national board to set and review the process for certifying diplomates. **Diplomates of the board** are individuals who have completed the highest levels of education in a particular area of dentistry. The national board for certifying general dentistry diplomates is the **American Board of General Dentistry** (ABGD; www.abgd.org). After a general dentist has completed the fellowship and mastership programs of the AGD, he or she is then eligible to join the ABGD to complete additional educational and clinical requirements to earn diplomate status.

## Dental Specialty Associations

Each dental specialty has a professional association or academy and board to provide members with continuing education and the opportunity for professional advancement. These nonprofit professional associations promote their specialty by providing continuing education to the dental professional, promoting research, setting high standards of care, serving as a resource for the consumer public, conducting annual scientific meetings, and sponsoring scientific journals and/or newsletters. The specialty association sponsors the boards to certify members as diplomates. The boards conduct the certification process, maintain a list of diplomates, and audit compliance with continuing education requirements. Diplomates are certified after demonstrating the required knowledge, skills, and attributes by passing an examination administered by a panel of peers. A compilation of organizations and their websites is provided in the "Section I Summary" References and Resources list.

## American Dental Hygienists' Association

The mission of the American Dental Hygienists' Association (ADHA; www.adha.org) is to improve the public's total health by increasing awareness of and access to quality oral healthcare. Founded in 1923, the ADHA represents the majority of professional dental hygienists. Originally, the ADHA was formed as a means of communication among dental hygienists. The result of this need for communication led to the development of the *Journal of the American Dental Hygienists Association*. As the dental hygiene profession and professional association grew, a central office was necessary. Currently located in Chicago, the ADHA includes several divisions and provides many services for its members.

Dental hygienists are encouraged to join the ADHA to take advantage of the tangible benefits of membership. Prime examples of these benefits are publications, group insurance, educational opportunities, professional interactions, research funding, and the code of ethical standards. Effecting legal change can be an involved process on the state and federal levels. The legal establishment of expanded functions for professionals in many jurisdictions can be credited to efforts of ADHA members.

The professional publication *Journal of Dental Hygiene* and the news magazine *Access* contain current scientific and technical articles relating to the practice of dental hygiene, research, and education. Automobile, disability, liability, life, and medical insurance are available to ADHA members at group rates. Self-study education programs, car rental discounts, credit card programs, and professional products are additional association membership benefits.

## American Dental Assistants Association

The mission of the **American Dental Assistants Association** (ADAA; www.dentalassistant. org) is to advance the careers of dental assistants and to promote dental assisting in education, legislation, and credentialing to enhance the delivery of oral healthcare to the public. The ADAA's slogan is "education, efficiency, loyalty, and service." Founded in 1924, the ADAA is the principal organization for professional dental assistants. All dental assistants can join the ADAA, including certified dental assistants, registered dental assistants, students, insurance company employees, chairside assistants, receptionists, office managers, laboratory assistants, and dental sales representatives.

The ADAA is aligned with the AGD; the two organizations hold a joint annual national meeting each summer. Member benefits include the fellowship program for advancement in dental assisting, similar to that of the AGD. The association publishes the journal *The Dental Assistant* and newsletters, and provides professional interactions, continuing education opportunities, insurance programs with group rates, awards, scholarships, credit card options, and other discounts. Legislative representation is a major goal of the ADAA, and financial assistance is given to states for pursuit of legislative and regulatory issues.

## Dental Laboratory Technology

Most dental laboratory technicians work in commercial dental laboratories. The National Association of Dental Laboratories (NADL; www.nadl.org) provides information on voluntary certification and career opportunities in commercial laboratories. The National Board for Certification (NBC), founded by the NADL, certifies dental laboratories and technicians.

## Dental Discipline Associations

Individuals specializing in a dental discipline who seek ADA recognition of specialty status must establish an association and board to certify diplomates. Because a discipline is an emerging field, it may be some years before the practice area becomes specialized and the professional organization has enough members to form a board. *Box 4.1* provides a sampling of dental discipline associations.

## International and Other Associations

Professional associations are not limited by professions or to the United States. Many U.S. oral healthcare professionals maintain membership in groups such as the Hispanic Dental Association, the American Association of Women Dentists, and religious or international organizations that advance the art and science of dentistry throughout the

## BOX 4.1 *Dental Discipline Associations*

| | |
|---|---|
| Academy for Sports Dentistry | Sports dentistry |
| American Academy of Dental Medicine | Special care dentistry |
| American Academy of Esthetic Dentistry (AAED) | Cosmetic dentistry |
| American Academy of Forensic Sciences (AAFS) | Forensic dentistry |
| American Academy of Implant Dentistry (AAID) | Oral implantodontics |
| American Academy of Laser Dentistry | High-tech dentistry |
| American Academy of Oral Medicine (AAOM) | Oral medicine |
| American Academy of Orofacial Pain | Temporomandibular joint disorder |
| American Board of Forensic Odontology (ABFO) | Forensic dentistry |
| American Board of Oral Medicine (ABOM) | Oral medicine |
| American Board of Special Care Dentistry | Special care dentistry |
| American Dental Board of Anesthesiology | Dental anesthesiology |
| American Dental Society of Anesthesiology (ADSA) | Dental anesthesiology |
| American Society for Geriatric Dentistry (ASGD) | Geriatric dentistry |
| American Society of Dental Anesthesiologists (ASDA) | Dental anesthesiology |
| American Society of Forensic Odontology (ASFO) | Forensic dentistry |
| Holistic Dental Association (HDA) | Complementary and alternative dentistry |

world. There are more than 160 international organizations that are related to the dental professions, including the International Federation of Dental Hygienists. All members of the ADA are automatically members of the Federation Dentaire Internationale (FDI), also called the World Dental Federation. Founded in Paris in 1900, the federation is a conglomeration of international dental associations; its goal is to promote oral health and advances in dentistry worldwide. In the future, there may even be international certifying boards. A compilation of international organizations and their websites is provided in the "Section I Summary" References and Resources list.

## ETHICAL BEHAVIOR

Every day we make decisions about how to do the right thing, handle an unpleasant situation, or help or hurt someone else to make us feel happier or more secure. When interacting with other people, we use our personal code of ethics to guide our actions. **Ethics** are standards of conduct conforming to the moral principles of what is right and wrong. A **personal code of ethics** is the application of the attitudes and values we set for ourselves for interaction with others. Each individual's personal code of ethics is unique and is based on the ideas about what is right according to family beliefs, religious affiliation, and politics.

### Philosophy

Ethical codes are written rules of behavior based on virtues, which are different for each culture, civilization, and organization. Historically, these written rules have taken on a variety of overriding themes, such as do good to others, treat superiors well and inferiors poorly, and repay kindness with kindness and evil with justice. Each culture deems certain characteristics or values as being important; examples of such virtues are honesty, tolerance, patience, lawfulness, charity, responsible behavior, justice, and kindness.

A **philosophy** is a group of basic values and attitudes. One admired standard of behavior is an ancient philosophy restated in the New Testament of the Bible as "All things whatsoever ye would that men should do to you, do ye even so to them" (Matthew 7:12). Sometimes called the Golden Rule (Do unto others as you would have them do unto you), it is the basis for the code of professional conduct for the ADAA and other healthcare professions.

An organization's **professional code of ethics** recommends standards of behavior for its membership. Its purpose is to help the individual achieve high levels of ethical awareness and use ethical decision-making principles. *Box 4.2* provides an example of an ethical decision-making model. Members of a professional organization pledge to adhere to a code of ethics, and in this way, a professional organization maintains ethical members.

Etiquette is behavior related to customs and rituals, such as being courteous and dressing appropriately for a given situation. Protocol is a procedure to be followed in a certain set of circumstances, such as when filing insurance claims or what to do in case of a medical emergency.

## ADA Code of Ethics

The virtues found in the ADA Code of Ethics include self-governance, nonmaleficence, beneficence, fairness, and truthfulness. ADA members are required to comply with the code of ethics. The local dental society's peer review committee may convene an official inquiry after there is a report of a dentist in violation of these ethical principles (such as questionable conduct, poor judgment, or poor behavior). **Peer review** is an intervention by a local dental society to determine if indeed the dentist violated the ADA's ethical principles. This is the manner in which the association protects the public or the troubled dentist from harm. When a report of questionable conduct is reported to the local or state dental society, a group of local dentists meets to discuss the report and plan and implement an intervention.

For example, there may be a report that a dentist has abused drugs or alcohol. The peer review committee then meets with the dentist. If the board determines that the charges are true, the intervention plan may involve an escort to a drug or alcohol reha-

## BOX 4.2 *Ethical Decision-Making Model*

- Identify the part of the problem that is separate from legal issues.
- Determine the influences of alternative choices.
- Evaluate the long-term and short-term outcomes of the choices.
- Make your decision and implement it.

bilitation program. If the accused dentist is suffering from depression or suicidal tendencies, the intervention plan may be hospitalization. The local peer review committee then arranges for management of the dental practice during the dentist's absence.

Some states have laws for mandatory reporting of licensees to a health professional's recovery program for addiction or mental illness. If the situation is not resolved by peer review, local police action, or disciplinary actions of the regulatory boards, the dentist may lose association membership and the respect of others in the field as a result of his or her unethical or illegal behavior. Peer review is discussed further in Chapter 5.

## ADHA Code of Ethics

The dental hygiene code of ethics developed by the ADHA consists of the Standards of Professional Responsibility. This code supports the values of the ADHA and has the core values of respect, confidentiality, trust, nonmaleficence, beneficence, justice, and truth. Adopted in 1995, it is directed to "ourselves as Individuals, ourselves as Professionals, Family and Friends, Clients, Colleagues, Employees and Employers, the Dental Hygiene Profession, the Community and Society, and finally, Scientific Investigation."

## ADAA Ethics

The ADAA has three written policies on ethics. The policies are called the ADAA Statement of Professional Commitment (1988), the Principles of Ethics and Professional Conduct (1998), and the Code of Professional Conduct. Members pledge to refrain from performing job duties prohibited by state law and pledge to strive to continue learning new skills, abide by association rules, and provide quality care.

## NADL Code of Ethics

The NADL code of ethics is called the Articles of Incorporation, which include objectives for members to obtain.

## Clothing and Grooming

There are several ethical issues related to clothing and grooming. People make judgments about appearance within the first several minutes after meeting. Currently, dress codes are not statute law; but according to case law, employers have the legal right to regulate workplace dress for health or sanitation reasons. Employer policies to control clothing and grooming have held up to legal challenges under Title VII of the Civil Rights Act of 1964. The Centers for Disease Control and Prevention (CDC) establishes the standard of care for infection control. Occupational Safety and Health Administration (OSHA) regulations mandate the standards of dress for worker protection.

Traditionally, oral healthcare providers wore a white uniform, hosiery, clinic shoes, and hats. Currently, the dental staff wears personal protective equipment (PPE) clothing, which may include surgical scrubs, barrier gowns, hair bonnets, and shoe coverings.

Dental professionals often wear street clothing into the dental office and change into their work attire on site; at the end of the day, the soiled clothing is removed before leaving the building. Soiled garments are stored for laundering in a garment bag or container labeled "biohazard" to prevent the spread of infectious disease to family and friends. Slip-on clinic shoes should be left in the office after use and wiped daily with bleach. These are the standards for clothing; other standards exist for grooming.

Body odors are expected to be minimized at all times by daily bathing, and the use of fragrances should be avoided. Many patients are apprehensive about dental treatment and may find body odors particularly offensive. Fingernails should be short to prevent penetration of protective gloves. Acrylic nails and jewelry harbor microorganisms and become contaminated by contact or aerosol spray. In addition, jewelry such as earrings can become caught in ear loop-style facial masks. The professional can easily adhere to the grooming recommendations to limit fragrance use, fingernail length, and the wearing of jewelry.

## CONCEPT SUMMARY

- Each dental occupation has a professional organization to benefit its membership.
- Professional associations have a written code of ethics to which members are expected to adhere.
- Virtues, ethics, etiquette, and protocol are all aspects of ethical conduct.
- Personal behavior follows a personal and professional code of ethics, and there are consequences when unethical behavior affects society.

## REVIEW QUESTIONS

1. For each of the following dental occupations, list the name of the associated professional organization(s).
   A. Dentist
   B. Dental hygienist
   C. Dental assistant
   D. Dental laboratory technician
2. Why do professionals join organizations?
3. What are the benefits of association membership?
4. What are the ADA councils and what are their roles?
5. Name the publications of the professional organizations of dentistry.
6. Why is the Golden Rule important in dentistry?
7. What is a professional code of ethics?
8. Why do the ADA, ADHA, ADAA, and NADL have codes of ethics?
9. What are the consequences of ethical violations?
10. When does personal appearance become an ethical problem?
11. Compare ethics, etiquette, protocol, and virtues.

# CRITICAL THINKING GROUP ACTIVITY

1. Identify your personal ethics and compare your ethics with other group members.
2. Obtain and review copies of the ADA, ADHA, and ADAA codes of ethics and identify the virtues represented.
3. Apply the written rules of civilization to a code of ethics.
4. Using the ethical decision-making model (*Box 4.2*) as a guide, determine whether a professional should wear perfume or cologne in the dental office.
5. Obtain and review a copy of a mission statement from a dental discipline and compare it to a mission statement from a national professional association.
6. Compare the ethical codes from an international organization to a U.S. professional association.

## ETHICAL CASE STUDY

### Case Study Learning Outcomes

Upon mastery of the content of this scenario, the student should be able to:

- Recognize counterdependent behavior and learn ways to deal with it.
- Relate the signs and symptoms of deeper problems to behavior exhibited at work.
- Use problem solving to determine a proper course of action.
- Plan and manage confrontations.

### Discussion

The senior dental assistant is 32 years old, unmarried, and a religious individual who lives with her sister's family in her own room. After a series of confrontational episodes between you and her, office tensions have increased. She has reported you to the office manager for creating a hostile work environment.

### Background Information

The senior dental assistant has had a series of short-term-employment dental assisting jobs. As an OJT dental assistant, her knowledge and skill level are inadequate for her to perform her job according to currently established standards of care. You have seen her violate the following CDC recommendations:

- She has cut corners during instrument processing and sterilization by taking instruments out of the presoak too early.
- She has removed items from the ultrasonic cleaner before the cycle has completed.
- She has run the autoclave on the unwrapped flash setting when it was fully loaded with bagged items.
- She has reused items without allowing adequate disinfection time.
- She has used alcohol instead of an approved surface disinfectant.

In regard to dental practice act regulations you have seen her:

- Perform illegal chairside functions.
- Take radiographs without proper credentialing for your jurisdiction.
- Perform tasks on patients without adequate supervision.

In the arena of controlling inventory management, you have noted the following:

- She does not follow up on backordered dental hygiene items.
- She unpacks shipments and puts all supplies away except the dental hygiene supplies.
- She does not order hygiene supplies in a timely fashion.
- She orders items without verifying necessity and maintains a surplus of unneeded items.
- She does not purchase the specific toothbrushes that you recommend to clients, ordering the ones she likes instead.

## Case Discussion Questions

1. Does this employee have the right to report you to the office manager for creating a hostile work environment?
2. How long should you wait before making a formal complaint to the dentist regarding the senior dental assistant's infection control practices?
3. Your complaints and reports to the office manager have gone unheeded. What is your next course of action?

# CRITICAL THINKING ACTIVITY

- Develop a list of your grievances regarding this employee.
- Present the list of grievances to the office manager and dentist.
- Problem solve the infection control issue with a colleague: one person plays the role of dental assistant and the other, the dental hygienist. Involve a third person as the dentist, as needed.
- Use the ethical decision-making model (*Box 4.2*) to decide how to continue a working relationship with the dental assistant.

## Assignment: Accessing Web sites

Access the Web sites for the ADA, ADHA, ADAA, and NADL and locate each organization's code of ethics, print a copy if you have access to a printer, and determine the following:

1. What are the core values or virtues found in each document?
2. Are there any sanctions or interventions described for violation of the code?
3. How are the codes of ethics similar? How are they different?
4. Is the language clear and concise enough for association members to understand?
5. Are the codes recent and up to date?

# Legal Behavior and Risk Management

Upon mastery of the content of this chapter, the student should be able to:
- Compare and contrast ethics and jurisprudence.
- Differentiate between statutory, civil, and criminal law.
- Describe the laws and ruling bodies that affect the practice of dentistry.
- Recognize tasks delegated to allied dental personnel.
- Identify laws affecting dental practice and preventive techniques for malpractice.
- Understand the components of dental record keeping: organization, completeness, legibility, and security.
- Use public relations techniques for risk management.
- Prepare for malpractice suit and trial.
- Conceptualize the need for malpractice insurance coverage.

## KEY TERMS

| | |
|---|---|
| civil law | proximate cause |
| consent | reciprocity |
| contract law | respondeat superior |
| criminal law | risk management |
| damages | statutory laws |
| duty | supervision |
| jurisprudence | tort law |
| office manuals | |

## LEGAL BEHAVIOR AND RISK MANAGEMENT

Public opinion surveys demonstrate the high regard the public has for people in the dental professions. However, the public is much more skeptical of healthcare professionals, and trust must be earned because it can be challenged or lost. The public expects that allied dental professionals be of moral and ethical character. Dental personnel guide their actions by following personal ethics, a professional code of ethics, and jurisprudence. Yet in some locations, medical and dental malpractice is in a state of crisis owing to the willingness of the public to file lawsuits against healthcare professionals. Malpractice insurance premiums increase yearly, and some insurance companies no longer provide coverage to oral healthcare providers. With knowledge of these facts, allied dental personnel would be wise to take every precaution to avoid legal liability in a malpractice claim.

## LEGAL BEHAVIOR

The maximum level of professional conduct is achieved by adherence to ethical standards. Ethical conduct is considered a higher level of behavior than legal behavior. The minimal level of professional conduct is achieved by adherence to laws. **Jurisprudence** means "a system of laws." American law consists of federal law, state law, and judicial decisions. Federal laws apply to the whole country and regulate everyone within the United States. Dentists follow federal laws when prescribing medications and must have a federal license to write prescriptions. State laws apply within the boundaries of a state as defined in the state dental practice act, state statutes, and regulations. Judicial law (common law) is made within an area in which a judge presides. These common laws fill in the gaps of state laws and are difficult to amend. When a state enacts new legislation, it voids common law. Common law usually affects the dentist–patient relationship. A legal relationship exists between the dentist and the patient, which can be challenged in a court of law.

The legal system of the United States has three divisions of law affecting the practice of dentistry: statutory, civil, and criminal law. During the colonial era in the United States, medical practice acts were the laws enacted to protect citizens from being treated by unqualified individuals. In 1899, the U.S. Supreme Court charged states with the obligation to regulate the practice of medicine and dentistry with **statutory laws.** Presently in the United States, dental practice acts define the practice of dentistry and requirements for licensure in a jurisdiction such as a state, district, or territory. Also, a jurisdiction may have a group of general laws relating to the well-being of citizens called the public health code. Sometimes, the public health code contains laws affecting dental practice.

### Statutory Law

The need for regulation to protect the public from mistreatment and incompetent practitioners has developed over a long period of time in the United States. Dental practice acts define the legal duties of the dental team members and control the practice of dentistry. Also called administrative rules or law, dental practice acts set the requirements for licensure, duties, supervision, reprimand, suspension, and revocation of licensure. The Board of Dentistry is the state agency that enforces the dental practice act. In some states, this agency is called the State Board of Dental Examiners. In other states or jurisdictions, the enforcing agency is called the Department of Licensing and Regulation, Department of Commerce, Health Professions Bureau, Bureau of Examination Boards, Commission of Professional and Occupational Affairs, Department of Health, Department of State, or Department of Regulation and Education. These various agencies examine applicants, grant licensure, and process claims of misconduct or incompetence.

Licensure is the legal permission to operate a business or engage in a regulated occupation. The dentist and dental hygienist must be licensed; in some states, the dental assistant is also licensed to perform oral healthcare procedures. General licensure requirements for the occupational titles in dentistry include the following:

- Good moral character with no criminal convictions.
- Successful completion of an American Dental Association (ADA)-accredited educational program.
- Successful completion of written or clinical national, regional, and/or state board examinations in theory and practice.
- Cardiopulmonary resuscitation (CPR) certification.
- Payment of licensure fees.

When a licensed dental professional moves to another state, he or she is not automatically allowed to practice. The professional must obtain licensure in the new state of residence, unless there is reciprocity. **Reciprocity** or endorsement is the portability of licensure from jurisdiction to jurisdiction. Frequently, reciprocity rules prevent transfers to a new jurisdiction owing to the different requirements for licensure.

State statutes may be written in a way that requires additional certification for expanded functions, radiation exposure, and worker safety. It is extremely important that allied dental personnel be able to locate, read, and understand the regulations and requirements for the jurisdiction in which they work to protect themselves and the public. Failure to follow statutory law places the oral healthcare professional at risk for legal action.

## SUPERVISION

**Supervision** is the level of management that allows one to perform job duties. The level of supervision is defined differently in each U.S. jurisdiction. Provided that the regulatory requirements are met, the supervision conditions may be defined as follows:

- Direct supervision: the licensed dentist is in the office and evaluates the patient at the same visit.
- Indirect supervision: the licensed dentist is in the office but may evaluate the patient at a later time.
- General supervision: the licensed dentist is in the building and may be required to check the patient before the beginning and at the completion of dental tasks.
- General supervision or assignment of duties: the licensed dentist is not in the building and the client is a patient of record (someone who has been examined and accepted as a patient by the dentist).
- Undefined supervision: the licensed dentist supervises the dental auxiliary, but the supervision is not specified.
- No supervision: the licensed dentist's supervision is not specified and/or required.

## EXPANDED FUNCTIONS

Many jurisdictions list expanded function job duties that the allied dental professional may or may not perform. Some jurisdictions include a statement such as "all duties that are reversible." Some tasks delegated to the dental assistant and hygienist may be shared or divided between the two occupational job titles. *Box 5.1* provides a general list of expanded functions that allied dental professionals may be permitted to perform in the United States.

**BOX 5.1** *Examples of Expanded Functions for*
*Allied Dental Healthcare Professionals*

Administer local anesthesia
Administer nitrous oxide sedation
Apply cavity liners and bases
Apply desensitizing agents
Apply pit and fissure sealants
Apply topical anesthetic agents
Apply topical fluoride
Bend orthodontic arch wires
Bond orthodontic brackets
Counsel the patient in nutrition and/or
   tobacco cessation
Determine root and endodontic file length
Educate the patient in oral healthcare practices
Expose radiographs
Fit trial endodontic gutta percha points
Inspect the oral cavity
Make alginate impressions for study models
   or working casts
Monitor intravenous sedation

Monitor nitrous oxide sedation
Perform pulp vitality testing
Perform supragingival and subgingival scaling
Perform supragingival scaling
Place and finish restorative materials
Place and remove final impression materials
Place and remove matrices
Place and remove orthodontic arch wires, bands,
   ligatures, and separators
Place and remove periodontal dressings
Place and remove retraction cord
Place and remove rubber dams
Place and remove socket dressings
Place and remove temporary restorations and
   crowns
Polish coronal tooth surfaces
Remove excess cement supragingivally or
   subgingivally from crowns/bands
Remove sutures

## Civil Law

**Civil law** controls an offense against the private rights of a person. It is divided into contract law and tort law. Civil law requires that the preponderance of evidence indicate a 51% certainty that someone is guilty or innocent.

### CONTRACT LAW

**Contract law** is the legal agreement between two or more people to perform or not to perform a legal act in which there will be payment. Contract law controls agreements between people and is the center of the dentist–patient relationship. Three elements to a valid contract are offer, acceptance, and consideration. The offer takes place when the parties entering the agreement are legally competent. The acceptance takes place when the service covered by the agreement is lawful. The consideration is the payment of money or services for the given service.

Legally competent parties do not include children under the age of 18 years and mentally incompetent individuals. Parents or guardians must approve the care their children receive, unless the child is an emancipated minor. An emancipated minor is an individual who is no longer under the care, custody, or supervision of his or her parents. An emancipated minor should have a written order from the court as evidence of his or her legal status. Mentally incompetent people may have an appointed legal guardian, adult holding a power of attorney who is responsible for approval of care, and/or living will document of their expressed wishes. When a dentist–patient relationship is entered into with a mentally incompetent person, it is done so with the guardian, adult with a power of attorney, or according to the person's expressed wishes as indicated in the living will.

There are two types of contracts: implied and expressed. An implied contract is an agreement made by the actions of the parties concerned, even though all the facts have not been discussed. For example, when patients submit to an oral examination without discussing fees, they have implied that the dentist may perform the examination and that they will pay for the service. The dentist is not required to accept all patients for treatment. Once the dentist accepts the patient for treatment, an implied contract is made. The dentist and patient have legally defined duties, and civil action can be taken against the dentist or the patient when there is a failure of duty. Chapter 6 provides a more detailed explanation of duty.

An expressed contract is an agreement made by oral or written arrangement. For example, the patient is consulted regarding the financial arrangements used in the practice. The discussion with the patient and the dental assistant is an expressed contract. Breach of contract occurs when either party does not keep his or her part of an expressed contract; legal action may be pursued in court.

## TORT LAW

**Tort law** protects against interference with another person's right to enjoy person, property, and privacy. Violation of tort law is either unintentional (negligent) or intentional (*Box 5.2*). Unintentional tort law, commonly referred to as malpractice or negligence, protects a person against negligent injury in the course of professional duties. Intentional tort law protects a person against technical assault, technical battery, misrepresentation, deceit, breach of confidentiality, and defamation of character such as slander and libel.

Technical assault is defined as a deliberate attempt or threat to touch without the patient's permission, even without injury. Technical battery occurs when the practitioner exceeds the amount of treatment authorized by the patient. Misrepresentation is the failure to inform the patient of his or her treatment status. For example, the failure to tell the patient that a piece of a broken endodontic instrument was left in a tooth is misrepresenting the truth. Deceit is an attempt to distort information about personnel or services rendered, such as misleading the patient by allowing a noncredentialed employee to perform oral healthcare tasks that are forbidden by law.

Breach of confidentiality occurs when the confidential relationship between the patient and the dentist is violated. Information regarding the patient's medical history, treatment, or financial status is legally protected by many newly enacted and evolving laws (see Chapter 14). An example of breach of confidentiality can occur when someone overhears a discussion outside of the dental office about a patient's status and he or she tells the patient. Another example of breach of confidentiality can occur when infor-

---

**BOX 5.2**  *Civil Law and Noncompliance*

| | |
|---|---|
| Contract law | breach of contract |
| Intentional tort law | technical assault, technical battery, misrepresentation, deceit, maligning a patient (slander and libel), breach of confidentiality |
| Unintentional tort law | negligence, permitting a hazard |

mation is released to another healthcare provider or insurance company without the patient's written consent. **Consent** means "giving permission for something to be done by another person" and is discussed in detail in Chapter 6.

Defamation of character is either slander or libel. Slander is saying something about the patient that may damage his or her reputation, such as calling the patient a liar. Libel is writing something about the patient that may damage his or her reputation, such as noting in the patient's record that he or she lied.

## Criminal Law

**Criminal law** involves offenses against society, which must be proven beyond a reasonable doubt. For example, the practice of dentistry without a license is a violation of state criminal law. Dental personnel must be careful to perform only the functions that are legally allowable within the jurisdiction in which they work. Performing illegal dental procedures places the allied dental professional in the situation of practicing dentistry without a license, a serious criminal offense. If the dentist permits an auxiliary to perform illegal functions, both are held responsible in a court of law for the performance of an illegal act. Should an allied dental professional perform an illegal act and the dentist is unaware of it, the dentist may still be held responsible owing to the doctrine of **respondeat superior**, which means "let the master answer."

### PEER REVIEW

Because dentists hold a unique position of trust in society and are self-regulatory, the process of peer review may require a report to the jurisdiction's regulatory agency. The regulatory agency then decides whether to take any legal action against a dentist after peer review. Review by the state regulatory authority determines guilt or innocence and the assignment of penalties. The dentist may receive a formal reprimand that is announced to the profession via a print publication or a posting on a website. If the violation is relatively serious, licensure may be suspended temporarily or revoked permanently. Any licensed individual can be punished, including the dental assistant and dental hygienist. When a licensed individual is convicted for violation of criminal law, licensure may be revoked permanently, rendering the individual unable to practice his or her occupation.

## RISK MANAGEMENT

**Risk management** is the understanding of legal principles to prevent legal liability and responsibility. A patient may file a lawsuit against the oral healthcare professional for many reasons. Commonly, it is because of miscommunication regarding services performed, fee charges, and diagnosis. Lawsuits also result when there is a failure to diagnose or to provide adequate care. Because the dentist is respondeat superior, he or she is legally responsible for the actions of himself or herself and of employees for any breach of contract, technical assault and battery, maligning a patient, permitting a hazard in the dental office, and tort law negligence (malpractice).

Dentists must investigate the credentials of employees and verify information on résumés during the hiring procedure. Employers who fail to complete a thorough background check of newly hired employees increase their legal liability. Patient injury as a result of the action of an unqualified employee is a criminal law infraction and incurs the highest penalties. Employees lacking the appropriate credentials should not be performing unassigned clinical duties. In-service training scheduled on a regular basis is another risk management tool. The date of the in-service seminar, the principal subject matter, and the employees in attendance should be documented and maintained. The office manager usually has the responsibility for in-service training.

## Civil Contract Law: Breach of Contract

Contract law is the center of the dentist–patient relationship, and contracts are either implied or expressed. Breach of contract occurs when either party does not keep its part of an expressed contract. The dentist may choose to terminate the dentist–patient contract after the patient treatment is complete by sending a written statement of his or her intent to do so. Another way the contract is terminated is with the death of the patient or dentist. The dentist has several possible defenses against the charges of breach of contract:

- The patient withdrew by failing to return for care.
- The patient did not give the oral healthcare provider a reasonable opportunity to satisfy when satisfaction was guaranteed.
- The patient demonstrated contributory negligence by failing to follow instructions.
- The oral healthcare provider fulfilled the agreed-on requirements.

### PREVENTION

To prevent charges of abandonment, the dentist must notify the patient in writing of his or her intent to withdraw from the dentist–patient relationship. Attorneys advise that the termination of the relationship requires the use of diplomacy, with great care in attention to detail. It is not necessary to explain to the patient why the dentist has decided to terminate the relationship. A form letter should be sent by registered mail, return receipt requested. A copy of the letter is kept as a permanent part of the patient's file. The letter should contain the following information:

- A date, usually 30 days, after which the dentist will no longer care for the patient and a mandatory sentence noting the patient will be seen for any dental emergency during that time.
- A reminder to the patient to seek regular dental treatment.
- The names and phone numbers of dentists who would accept the patient for treatment or the name of a dental referral service.
- An offer to send a copy of the patient's record to the new dentist.

## Civil Tort Law—Intentional

### TECHNICAL ASSAULT AND BATTERY

Tort law protects against interference with the legitimate ability to enjoy person, property, and privacy. Violation of tort law is either unintentional (negligent) or intentional. Intentional tort law protects against technical assault and battery, misrepresentation and deceit, defamation of character (slander and libel), and breach of confidentiality.

### Prevention

Technical assault is a deliberate attempt to touch without permission. An example of technical assault is extracting the wrong tooth. The patient did not consent to have the tooth extracted; therefore, charges of technical assault can be made. Keeping the treatment plan or referral notice with the radiographs helps prevent wrong tooth extraction. Technical battery is exceeding the amount of treatment authorized by the patient. The best method of risk management for technical assault and battery is appropriate patient education followed by the completion of standardized consent forms.

There are many effective methods for teaching patients. A number of organizations produce videotapes, pamphlets, brochures, models, and computer programs for educating patients. Videotapes have higher comprehension levels and increase patient interest. The limitations of videotapes are their cost and the difficulty in customizing the information for individual use. Pamphlets and brochures are easily edited and thus can be customized to fit a particular dental office. They are inexpensive, and the patient can take them home for further reference. Pamphlets and brochures, however, lead to lower levels of patient comprehension and interest. Models, always good educational tools, can be used to demonstrate treatment to the patient. They are used to explain procedures, are inexpensive, and do not become obsolete. The use of any educational materials should be recorded in the services rendered section of the patient's file. It is recommended that customized consent forms for each commonly performed dental procedure be signed and placed in the patient's file. *Figure 5.1* shows a standardized consent form.

Many dentists concerned with proper conduct in the dental office have **office manuals** that outline office policies, job descriptions, procedure protocols, and scripts for discussions with the patient. The employer minimizes liability by creating written policies that describe certain forms of conduct or actions, such as rules prohibiting the prescription of medications by staff members. Written job descriptions eliminate confusion in regard to employee duties and responsibilities and provide the allied dental professionals with the criteria for job performance evaluation. Written outlines of procedure protocols maintained in an office manual are excellent evidence in the event of a lawsuit.

In an emergency situation, the law implies consent to administer emergency procedures. This is a valid defense in technical battery. No fewer than two staff members with current CPR certification should be present in the office when patients are being treated. Dentists who perform high-risk procedures, such as intravenous sedation, should maintain advanced cardiac life support certification. Each allied dental professional should be assigned a role in the event of an emergency; frequent practice drills should be scheduled, conducted, evaluated, and critiqued. Good Samaritan legislation protects healthcare providers from legal liability in a civil lawsuit when administering emergency care. Statutes require that emergency care be given to the best ability of the provider in a true emergency situation, with no payment expected.

## MISREPRESENTATION AND DECEIT

Misrepresentation is the failure to inform the patient of his or her treatment status, for example, leaving a piece of a broken scaler in the patient's periodontium. Fraud or deceit is an attempt to distort information about personnel or services rendered, such as the dentist misleading the patient by allowing a noncredentialed employee to perform oral healthcare tasks.

---

### Informed Consent for Dental Procedures

I, _____ , give full informed consent to Dr. Drawer/Staff for the
following procedures:

1._____
2._____
3._____
4._____

The above procedures are necessary to treat the following condition(s):

1._____
2._____
3._____
4._____

1. I also give informed consent for the administration of anesthesia (topical, local,
   analgesia, sedation) and am aware of the risks for allergic reaction, hematoma, and
   paresthesia.

2. I have been informed of all risks, benefits, and treatment alternatives for the above
   procedures by Dr. Drawer/Staff.

3. I fully understand that these risks include, but are not limited to: allergic reaction,
   bleeding, infection, postoperative discomfort, root sensitivity, gum recession, and the
   need for additional treatments in the future.

4. I understand that no guarantees have been made.

5. I have been given the opportunity to ask questions regarding the treatment and all of
   my questions have been answered to my satisfaction. I wish to proceed with the above
   procedures.

_____          _____
Signature of patient/consenting party        Print name

_____          _____
Witness                                      Date

**Figure 5.1** Informed consent form.

### Prevention

The oral healthcare provider should use properly maintained instruments and materials.
After an incident such as a broken instrument, the "reasonable" practitioner will inform
the patient, attempt to correct the incident, and, if unable to correct, refer the patient to
someone who can.

To prevent deceit, never guarantee results to the patient or create unrealistic expectations. Do not comment on the quality of care provided by another dental practitioner.
When a dentist allows a noncredentialed employee to perform oral healthcare tasks, both
are liable. Never perform procedures that you are not qualified, educated, experienced,
or licensed to perform. Keep current with changes in the laws of dental practice because
ignorance of the law is not a valid excuse.

## MALIGNING A PATIENT

Maligning a patient is considered malicious treatment. It occurs through defamation of character by slander or libel or when unnecessary dental treatment is performed. As noted earlier, slander is saying something about the patient that may damage his or her reputation, and libel is writing something about the patient that may damage his or her reputation.

### Prevention

The best course of action for a dental auxiliary to take is to never reveal information about a patient because "silence is golden." Do not discuss patients with anyone and never reveal information about a patient to an unauthorized person. Never give information about a patient over the telephone. Ask the caller to write a request for information and be sure written authorization is furnished.

### BREACH OF CONFIDENTIALITY

Breach of confidentiality occurs when the confidential relationship between the patient and the healthcare provider is violated. Every patient has a right to privacy, and the healthcare team must keep in strictest confidence information about the treatment provided. This also includes information relating to health, financial affairs, and intimate matters discussed. The dentist must have additional written consent when pictures of the patient are to be published and when observers view patient procedures.

### Prevention

Always seek the patient's permission. The most frequent opportunity for breach of confidentiality occurs when sharing patient information with insurance companies. The sharing of information regarding treatment happens when filing dental insurance claims. Patients should sign a "release of information" form or a statement on their patient registration to give consent to share information with an insurance company or clearinghouse.

## Civil Tort Law—Unintentional

### NEGLIGENCE

During the 1980s, studies were conducted to determine common reasons for malpractice lawsuits against health professionals. These studies indicated that unrealistic patient expectations accounted for some dissatisfaction. More recently, delay or error in diagnosis has emerged as a common reason for malpractice lawsuits. Unintentional tort law protects against negligent injury (malpractice) during the course of professional duties. Negligence is the breach or nonperformance of a legal duty through neglect or carelessness, resulting in damage or injury to another. There are three elements of negligence: duty and breach of duty, proximate cause, and damages.

**Duty** is the professional care owed to the patient once a dentist–patient relationship is established. The duty is measured by the standard of care by members of the profession in the same locale and the present state of science. Owing to specialization, the courts are moving toward a national standard of care to replace the local standard of care. Breach of duty is the failure to perform the professional care owed to the patient. **Proximate cause** means that there is a definite relationship between the action and the injury. It refers to the link between the breach of duty and the injury to the patient. **Damages** are awarded based on economic or noneconomic issues. Economic damages are awards of money to cover all injuries to the patient's financial interests—past, present, and future—and typically include dental bills and lost wages. Usually, there are no limits on the amount of money awarded for economic damages. Noneconomic damages include pain, suffering, mental anguish, and loss of companionship. Many states do have caps on noneconomic awards. Such limitations are often waived when:

- The patient died.
- The negligence was intentional.
- A foreign object was left in the patient's body.
- The discovery of the claim was prevented by the healthcare provider's deceit.
- A body part was wrongfully removed.
- The patient lost a body function.

### PERMIT A HAZARD

To avoid permitting a hazard in the dental office, the dentist must keep the premises safe and must warn people of any known hazards. This applies to furniture, fixtures, equipment, instruments, and the facility. Frequent injuries are slip and fall accidents. Broken instruments and faulty equipment can cause injury as well. To prevent a hazard, periodically check the facility to be sure it is safe for the public.

## Malpractice

Common target areas for dental malpractice lawsuits include the failure to diagnose and treat periodontal disease and temporomandibular joint disorder; to obtain informed consent and/or keep the patient informed; to sterilize; to refer a difficult case to a specialist; to identify medically compromised patients or drug allergies; and to take precautions to protect a patient. Claims may also arise if a foreign object is left in the body, a dental implant fails, the jaw is fractured, or dentures or bridges fit improperly.

Failure of the patient to perform his or her duty is called contributory negligence. The duties of the patient are to provide accurate information about health history and status, pay a reasonable fee for services rendered within a reasonable time, keep appointments, and cooperate in the care by following instructions.

Time limits are established in which a civil action can be filed. A statute of limitations is a law that designates the time period in which a civil action claim can be filed. These statutes vary from state to state and often don't begin until the date the patient discovers the negligent act. This could be years after the patient received the treatment. If a claim is not filed within that period of time, the patient cannot file the claim. Claims of breach of contract are limited to 6 years in most jurisdictions.

### PREVENTION PROTOCOLS

Knowledge of the law is tantamount to malpractice prevention. Defense attorneys note that accurate dental record documentation regarding patient treatment is the best defense against a malpractice claim. Good documentation is essential to patient care, plus it provides reliable information to use in comparing a patient's progress over a period of time. In the event of a malpractice lawsuit, the rationale for treatment is found in the dental record. Information gaps in the patient's chart lessen the dentist's credibility, and the plaintiff's attorney will use such gaps to attack the diagnosis and treatment decisions. The office staff must pay close attention to four aspects of record keeping: organization, completeness, legibility, and security.

### Organization

An organized patient file demonstrates the ability of the dentist to retrieve necessary information immediately, thereby making treatment decisions easier. The dental staff should also be able to find information easily. A dental chart should contain all relevant information regarding the patient's status and the treatment planned. Information to be organized includes personal history; treatment plans; medical history; anatomic charting; signed consent forms; services rendered; telephone and laboratory logs; financial records; laboratory, x-ray, referral, and consultation reports; and copies of prescriptions. Separate forms for treatment planning, medical history, and dental treatment documentation are recommended. Financial information records should not be kept with the treatment records.

### Completeness

Treatment notes must be organized in a consistent, outline format. Usually, the order in which the treatment is rendered is the order in which the information is recorded in the services rendered section (*Box 5.3*).

Services rendered entries should be in nonerasable ink, typed, and entered into a computer terminal in the operatory and then signed or initialed by the person making the entry. All conversations, cancellations, late arrivals, no shows, and change of appointments are documented as well. When informing the patient of adverse occurrences or events that take place during treatment, record that the patient was informed. Conversations held with other healthcare providers relating to the care of the patient should also be recorded. If the patient does not comply with a treatment regime, it should be documented in services rendered. Subjective evaluations not relevant to the treatment, such as opinions about the client's mental health and negative characterizations, should be avoided.

As previously stated, one of the most common allegations of malpractice is a failure to diagnose. The medical history data on which the diagnosis is made is called into question in malpractice lawsuits. On the medical history form, there should be no unanswered health question. If the question does not apply, record "not applicable" (NA)

---

**BOX 5.3** *Components of the Services Rendered Note*

| | |
|---|---|
| Treatment provided | Specific language |
| Area where treatment provided | Postoperative instructions |
| Anesthesia used | Medicaments used |
| Details of conditions present | Patient education |
| Details of conditions during treatment | Next appointment recommendation |

in the space provided. If the response is normal, write "within normal limits" (WNL). The patient's signature and the date must appear on the form to reduce the credibility problem and to make the patient responsible for providing accurate health information. Medical histories should be updated at each visit.

The failure to prescribe has been the basis for a significant number of malpractice suits. In many states, prescriptions are written in triplicate state-issued forms for schedule II prescription drugs. The dentist keeps the third copy; the original and the second copy go to the pharmacy. Keep a copy of prescriptions to help prevent later disputes as to whether the patient actually received a prescription. This also includes laboratory prescriptions for prosthetics. Telephone logs are used to document incoming and outgoing phone calls. It is important that phone calls be noted in a log to provide evidence in the event of a malpractice lawsuit.

### Legibility

Legibility of dental records is important because dental healthcare providers use them when rendering treatment. When errors occur when entering services rendered information, a single line is drawn through the entry, dated, and initialed. No attempt to black it out, erase, or white it out should be made. Any attempt to do so damages the professional's credibility; many malpractice cases have been lost owing to improper alteration of the patient record. In some states, it is a felony to alter a medical or dental record and constitutes fraud.

### Security

Attorneys recommend that patient records be kept indefinitely and heirs of the dental practice be instructed to retain records of clients. Original records should not be surrendered to anyone, except by order of the court. Copies of dental records may be sent to another dentist when a written request from the patient is received. Keep dental records in the dental office and do not allow them to be removed from the premises because a lost record cannot be replaced. It is illegal to sign a document falsely or change a document by forgery.

### Public Relations

One of the most important aspects of risk management is public relations. Public relations is defined as the promotion of goodwill between an organization or individual with the public. The quality of the relationship between the dentist and the patient has a direct bearing on malpractice claims. Patients are more likely to file malpractice lawsuits when they feel they have been overcharged, when there has been a failure to diagnose, or when adequate care is not provided. Office staff can have a positive or negative effect on clients and should attempt to pursue good public relations.

Patient surveys are one method of determining public relations in the dental office (see Chapter 20, and *Figures 20.1, 20.2,* and *20.3*). Surveys serve as a risk management tool and should be conducted periodically to assess patients' perceptions of the office.

### MALPRACTICE SUIT AND TRIAL

It is hoped that you will never be involved in a malpractice lawsuit. However, given the frequency of lawsuits against oral healthcare professionals, it is possible you will receive a summons. A summons is an official order to appear in court. The parties in a lawsuit are the plaintiff and defendant. A plaintiff is the person who files the suit, and the defendant is the person denying the action charged. Upon receipt of a summons, there are several actions to be taken (*Box 5.4*). Read about the notification requirement in your malpractice insurance policy and comply with all requirements at once. Immediately contact the liability insurance carrier by telephone to notify it of the summons. Follow-up with your malpractice insurance company by sending a copy of the summons, certified mail, return receipt requested, after receiving it. Tell the employer and employees of the suit and advise them not to speak with anyone about it without your permission. Tell your spouse and involve him or her in the process. Revise your résumé with current information for court purposes and do not communicate with the plaintiff, his or her attorney, or anyone else involved.

Cooperate with your malpractice insurance company and prepare to meet the defense attorney. Write down all the questions you have before the meeting. If you are aware of similar issues or articles, bring a copy of them with you. Determine whether you will be able to work with the attorney assigned to you by your insurance carrier. The attorney should answer all of your questions, have a list of tasks for you to do, and review the process. Maintain involvement in the lawsuit by keeping a folder of information pertaining to the case. When finding pertinent information, send it to the attorney and begin all correspondence with "Per your request." This makes the information subject to the attorney–client privilege. Notify the insurance company if you are not satisfied with the services of the lawyer assigned to your claim.

A subpoena is a written legal order to appear in court to give testimony. Your testimony is a statement of facts. You may be asked to make a deposition before appearing in court. A deposition is sworn written testimony in which a series of questions are answered under oath before the case goes to trial. Work with the lawyer to be well prepared for the deposition.

In some states, malpractice lawsuits are first submitted to a mediation panel. Mediation is the settling of differences before a case goes to trial and is an attempt to prevent frivolous lawsuits from clogging the courts. Mediation panels can consist of five members with three attorneys, one healthcare provider for the plaintiff, and one healthcare provider for the defendant. The panel makes a written evaluation of the case for each party. This evaluation is nonbinding and specifies whether there is an award and, if so, the amount of the award. Settlement of the lawsuit is a matter to be handled by the malpractice insurance company and your assigned attorney and is not an admission of guilt. Ask the defense attorney to explain mediation to be sure of the results. If one party rejects the mediation recommendation, the case goes to trial.

Pretrial review is preparation for testimony. Review all of the evidence and exhibits. Become familiar with the courtroom before trial by visiting an empty courtroom.

## BOX 5.4  *Summons Documentation*

Note the following information:

- The date and the time the papers were served.
- Who received the papers.
- How the papers were served: in person or by mail.

## MALPRACTICE INSURANCE

Allied dental professionals are not automatically covered by the dentist's malpractice insurance once employed. Attorneys recommend maintaining your own policy of malpractice insurance. Malpractice insurance is a tangible benefit of membership in professional associations, and dental professionals should purchase their own malpractice insurance coverage.

## CONCEPT SUMMARY

- Oral healthcare workers follow their own personal ethics, the professional code of ethics, and the laws of the jurisdiction.
- Patient and dental worker interactions are controlled by statutory, civil, and criminal law.
- Delegated tasks to allied dental personnel are affected by supervision rules in most jurisdictions.
- Public relations techniques are applied for risk management.
- The risk of malpractice suit and trial underscores the need for malpractice insurance coverage.

## REVIEW QUESTIONS

1. What is the difference between ethics and jurisprudence?
2. How do federal, state, and judicial law affect the practice of dentistry?
3. Name the criminal law infraction that the laws of dentistry are made to prevent?
4. What is the nature of the relationship between the dentist and the patient?
5. What are the two divisions of civil law?
6. What are the requirements for dental licensure?
7. How is supervision of allied dental personnel defined?
8. Why are expanded functions different from jurisdiction to jurisdiction?
9. What are some of the consequences of peer review?
10. What is risk management?
11. List preventive techniques for each of the following situations:
    A. Breach of contract
    B. Technical assault
    C. Technical battery
    D. Misrepresentation
    E. Deceit
    F. Maligning a patient
    G. Breach of confidentiality
    H. Permitting a hazard
    I. Negligence
12. What are the three elements of negligence?
13. List the common target areas for malpractice lawsuits.
14. Why is maintaining accurate, organized dental records a risk management technique?
15. How can good public relations be a risk management technique?
16. What should you do after receiving a summons or subpoena?
17. What is a deposition?
18. What is mediation?
19. Why is maintaining your own malpractice insurance necessary?

## CRITICAL THINKING ACTIVITY

Obtain a copy of a current dental practice act to determine the required supervision, the legally allowable tasks in that jurisdiction, and what you would like to see added based on the list of expanded duties provided in *Box 5.1*.

## CRITICAL THINKING GROUP ACTIVITY

1. Discuss the ethical and legal ramifications of cheating on an examination.

# 6

# Patient Rights

## LEARNING OUTCOMES

Upon mastery of the content of this chapter, the student should be able to:
- Recognize that dentists are not required to accept everyone as a patient.
- Describe the Patient Bill of Rights.
- Discuss implied, informed, and expressed consent.
- Identify the duties of the dentist and patient in the dentist–patient relationship.
- Discuss the Americans with Disabilities Act.
- Recognize patient rights, abuse and neglect, and reporting procedures.

## KEY TERMS

abuse

abuse of a person with a disability

Americans with Disabilities Act

clients

consent

elder abuse

emotional abuse

expressed consent

implied consent

informed consent

neglect

Patient Bill of Rights

physical abuse

sexual abuse

spousal abuse

## OVERVIEW

Rendering oral healthcare to the patient is the main reason we perform our job tasks and earn our living. We care for patients, nurture them, and educate them regarding health and disease. All dental professionals have a legal duty and responsibility to the patient once he or she has been accepted for dental treatment. Beyond our legal duty is our moral duty to the patient. When we suspect any form of abuse, we should act on our suspicion. This chapter describes the legal rights of patients and the oral healthcare provider's duty to protect them from abuse and neglect.

## PATIENT RIGHTS

Oral healthcare providers have the option of determining whom they will accept as a patient into the practice and must provide care to all accepted patients. Patients who are not accepted must be referred to an appropriate healthcare provider. Oral healthcare providers have the right to determine what types of procedures and materials to use, what their office hours will be, what to charge the patient for services rendered, and when to take a vacation. The patient has the right to change oral healthcare providers; when this occurs, a written follow-up is kept in the patient's file.

Patients are referred to as **clients** and have civil rights. The **Patient Bill of Rights** is a collection of statements based on legal duties. It is posted in public areas in many hospitals and healthcare settings for patients and family members to read (*Box 6.1*). Many of your patients will be familiar with it.

## Implied, Informed, and Expressed Consent

Consent law is constantly evolving and is a component of one of the most controversial issues in healthcare today. **Consent** is a person's right to self-determination by giving permission to someone to do something for him or her. The dentist has an obligation to obtain consent. There are three types of consent: implied, informed, and expressed. **Implied consent** is assumed by the actions of the patient. When the patient enters the dental office, implied consent is given to the physical contact necessary for an oral examination, diagnosis, and consultation. After the examination, diagnosis, and consultation, the patient or guardian must give expressed consent before any treatment is rendered. The patient gives **informed consent** to the healthcare provider when information has been given to allow him or her to make an intelligent choice. **Expressed consent** is informed consent given orally or in writing for a procedure to be performed. Standardized consent forms are used in dental offices for permanent records of written consent, and a copy is given to the patient as well because an educated and informed patient is less likely to file a legal complaint (*Box 6.2*). Patients who refuse treatment must be informed of risks and may be asked to sign an informed refusal form.

**BOX 6.1** *Patient Bill of Rights*

1. The patient has a right to prompt attention without excuse.
2. The patient has the right to be informed of all decisions and contemplated actions with complete and accurate information concerning the rationale, prognosis, risks, and side effects.
3. The informed consent should encompass consent in writing with competent information on and comprehending awareness of the contemplated procedures so that the patient will not be subjected to regimens without first understanding and agreeing to have the right of refusal.
4. Patients have a right to knowledge of treatment and have the right to know their status and progress.
5. Patients have a right to strict privacy with no recognizable discussion or publication of their case without prior permission.
6. Patients have a right to know about their discharge and can question the desirability as planned.
7. Respect for the Patient Bill of Rights can help solidify the relationship between patients and their doctors. These are the rights of patients. With rights come responsibilities. Patients must respect the fact that doctors too have rights, and the behavior of patients must reflect the civility and courtesy so essential to our harmonious relationship.

**BOX 6.2**  *Guidelines for Informed Consent*

1. A fair explanation of the nature of the procedure in simple language.
2. A discussion of who will perform the procedure.
3. A description of the discomfort and risks.
4. A description of the benefits.
5. A discussion of any alternatives to the recommended procedure.
6. A discussion of no guarantee of success.
7. A discussion of the ramifications of refusing treatment.
8. An explanation of the option to seek a second opinion.
9. An offer to discuss any questions pertaining to the procedure.
10. Instructions that the patient is free to withdraw consent and stop treatment at any time.

## Duties in the Dentist–Patient Relationship

Dentists have many duties to their patients that are implied by law. Patients have fewer duties to their dentists implied by law. Failure to perform any of these duties can become the basis for a lawsuit. The dental assistant and hygienist act as agents for the dentist and follow the dentist's direction. The dentist is responsible for any treatment given to the patient by any allied dental professional because of the doctrine of respondeat superior. The employer-dentist is held responsible for the acts of employees when an injury occurs within the course of employment. Allied dental personnel are not automatically relieved of responsibility when they commit a negligent, unintentional act. The one exception to the doctrine of respondeat superior occurs when an employee acts outside the scope of employment. Civil court action can be brought against the dental office staff when there is a failure of duty (negligence). The implied duties of allied dental professionals are given in *Box 6.3*, and the duties of the patient or client are given in *Box 6.4*.

**BOX 6.3**  *Implied Duties of Allied Dental Professionals*

1. The oral healthcare provider must be licensed and meet all legal requirements to engage in the practice of dentistry.
2. The dentist must use reasonable care and skill in diagnosis and treatment by using standard drugs, materials, and techniques. Experimental procedures and those outside the standard of care, such as laser dentistry, require written informed consent.
3. Patient treatment must be completed within a reasonable length of time.
4. The provider must not abandon patients and is obligated to care for all the needs of the patient. Care for the patient must be arranged in case of an emergency when the dentist is unavailable.
5. The dental team member must do only those services consented to by the patient.
6. The provider must refer unusual cases to a specialist.
7. The dental team member must provide adequate patient instructions.
8. The provider must charge a reasonable fee for services rendered.
9. The dental team member must achieve a reasonable result.
10. The dental team member must maintain the client's right to privacy and confidentiality.

**BOX 6.4** *Duties of the Patient/Client*

1. The patient must provide accurate information about his or her health history and status.
2. The patient must pay a reasonable fee for services rendered within a reasonable time.
3. The patient must keep appointments.
4. The patient must cooperate in his or her care and follow the oral healthcare providers' instructions.

## Americans with Disabilities Act

The **Americans with Disabilities Act** became effective in January 1992 and has significantly affected the dental office. Title III of the act prohibits discrimination against disabled people in places of public accommodation. Physical barriers in existing facilities must be removed or alternative methods of providing services must be offered, such as wheelchair ramps for physically challenged clients and auxiliary aids and services for sensory impaired clients. Auxiliary aids can include interpreters, lifts for vans, directional signs, and Braille elevator boards. All new construction of public facilities must be accessible by disabled clients.

Three simple things must be remembered when evaluating compliance: awareness, access, and accommodation. Awareness means becoming familiar with the different types of disabilities. Access means looking at your present facility for any additional improvements. Accommodation means making the modifications necessary to enable disabled persons to use the facility. Private individuals and the U.S. Department of Justice can file lawsuits to stop discriminatory practices, and monetary penalties can be recovered by the government.

More information about the Americans with Disabilities Act can be obtained from the U.S. Department of Justice.

## PATIENT ABUSE AND NEGLECT

Patients may arrive in the office for treatment with evidence of family violence, including abuse. **Abuse** includes physical and emotional battering, sexual misconduct, and neglect. Approximately 65% of physical violence is aimed at the head and neck. Patients who are at higher risk for family violence are children, spouses, the elderly, and the patient with a disability.

## Child Abuse and Neglect

Child abuse has been inflicted on children since the dawn of civilization. Both men and women abuse children. Statistically, the child abuser has a median age of 25 years, is experiencing marital problems, or was abused himself or herself as a child. Abuse can also occur when children are away from home in day care or with a baby-sitter; sometimes, the child is abused by a friend of the baby-sitter. Currently, this phenomenon is legally defined and its pathology has been researched. The first prosecuted case of child abuse in the

United States was in 1875 and was pursued under the laws for the prevention of cruelty to animals. In the early 1960s, the traumatization of children was termed the *battered child syndrome;* and in 1962, federal laws were enacted to make it mandatory to report child abuse. Today the term *child abuse* encompasses neglect as well as physical, emotional, and sexual abuse.

Individual states have laws to protect children; those laws require certain adults to report suspected abuse of people younger than 18 years of age. A physician, dentist or other oral healthcare provider, teacher, or duly regulated childcare provider must file a written report within 72 hours of discovery. In some states, the dental hygienist and dental assistant are required to report. Reports can be made via a telephone call to the state's Department of Social Services office located in the jurisdiction where the suspected child abuse is found. After the telephone report is made, a written report with a detailed description is made. Reports made in good faith by a healthcare professional are confidential and exempt from prosecution. A healthcare worker who is mandated to report suspected abuse or neglect and who fails to do so may be liable in a civil suit for the damages proximately caused by the failure to report. Currently, dental professionals report less than 1% of child abuse cases.

Several national organizations provide statistics on child abuse and neglect in the United States, what you can do to recognize and alleviate the problem, and local resources. They include Prevent Child Abuse America (www.preventchildabuse.org), the Child Welfare League of America (www.cwla.org), and the Children's Defense Fund (www.childrensdefense.org).

## PHYSICAL ABUSE

**Physical abuse** is the nonaccidental physical injury of a child from beatings, burns, strangulation, human bites, and other causes. Signs of physical abuse include:

- Unexplained lacerations, bruises, and welts (in various stages of healing).
- Unexplained burns, such as a cigarette or patterned burns.
- Unexplained fractured bones.
- Fear of parents or of going home from school at the end of the day.
- Wariness of adult contacts or inquiries.
- Inconsistency in the report of how an injury occurred when asked open-ended questions.

## EMOTIONAL ABUSE

**Emotional abuse** is the criticizing, belittling, insulting, and rejecting of a child. It also includes lack of love, support, and guidance. Indicators of emotional abuse are:

- Speech disorders.
- Failure to thrive.
- Lagging physical development.
- Habit disorders (rocking, sucking, biting).
- Neurotic behaviors (hysteria, obsession, phobias).
- Extreme behaviors (passive or aggressive).
- Suicide attempts.

### SEXUAL ABUSE

**Sexual abuse** is the exploitation of the child by an adult for sexual gratification, such as incest, molestation, rape, fondling, and exhibitionism. Oral indicators of sexual abuse are:

- Bruising of the palate.
- Unexplained sores around the lips.
- Oral signs of venereal disease.

### NEGLECT

**Neglect** is the failure to provide the basic necessities of life, including food, shelter, medical care, education, and supervision. Signs of child neglect are:

- Hunger, poor hygiene, constant fatigue, filthy clothing, or clothing improper for the weather.
- Untreated physical conditions, such as caries, abscesses, and oral pain.
- Lack of supervision for long periods of time.
- Alcohol or drug abuse.
- Abandonment.

## Family Violence

### SPOUSAL ABUSE

An estimated 95% of spousal abuse is directed toward women. Many women feel embarrassed, afraid, guilty, or ashamed about abuse. **Spousal abuse** is the misuse of power and control. Physical abuse enforces the cycle of violence, which has two phases. During the tension-building phase, stress and pressure increase and end in an explosion of violence. The honeymoon phase occurs after the violence and may be characterized by gift giving. The violence usually escalates over time. When questioning the patient about spousal abuse, it is appropriate to ask "Are you afraid?" or "Are you safe?" The dental office can be a source of information for battered women. For example, brochures that include the telephone number of a shelter for battered women can be placed in the women's restroom in the dental office.

### ELDER ABUSE

**Elder abuse** is any act or omission that causes injury to people age 60 years or older. Between 1 and 2 million elderly people are abused and exploited each year. An elderly person may fear abandonment or be ashamed that his or her family would behave in such a way. Both men and women abuse the elderly, and spouses reportedly perpetrate about half of elder abuse. Sometimes the cycle of abuse is reversed. The abused spouse becomes the abuser when the spouse becomes disabled. Children may abuse their elderly parents for financial gain. Elder abuse is less likely to be reported than other abuse. Suspected abuse is reported to the local Office of Elder Affairs, and a caseworker is assigned to investigate.

Examples of physical abuse are slapping, pushing down, tying to a chair, and breaking the person's dentures. Sexual abuse can range from fondling to nonconsensual sex and rape. Emotional abuse includes screaming or the threat of institutionalizing. Neglect can be the withholding of food or medical service as a form of punishment. Watch for missed or canceled dental appointments because it may be a sign that someone else is exerting power over the elderly patient.

## Abuse of a Person with a Disability

**Abuse of a person with a disability** involves people ages 18–59 years. Abuse to individuals younger than age 18 is considered child abuse; abuse to those older than age 60 is considered elder abuse. Disabled people fail to report abuse because they are afraid that their needs will then no longer be met. Abuse of a person with a disability is reported to the local Disabled Persons Protection Agency.

A person with a disability may have a number of oral health problems, such as inadequate dental care, poor oral hygiene, or bruxism. He or she may exhibit a fear of dental equipment, rubber dams, impressions, or the smell of latex. Empower the patient by telling him or her to communicate by raising a hand to stop treatment. Patient empowerment and understanding are vital to the successful treatment of a patient who has a history of being abused.

### CONCEPT SUMMARY

- Oral healthcare providers are not required to accept everyone as a patient.
- The Patient Bill of Rights is an example of a philosophical statement related to protecting the public.
- Implied, informed, and expressed consent are the three types of consent.
- The duties of the oral healthcare provider exceed the duties of the patient in the provider–patient relationship.
- The Americans with Disabilities Act was enacted to ease restrictions for people with a disability.
- Abuse and neglect have a variety of signs that must be reported by oral healthcare providers.

## REVIEW QUESTIONS

1. What are the requirements for oral healthcare providers in regard to accepting everyone as a patient?
2. What is another term for patient?
3. Why is the Patient Bill of Rights a good thing to have posted in the office?
4. What is the difference between implied, informed, and expressed consent?
5. Identify the duties of the dentist in the dentist–patient relationship.
6. Identify the duties of the patient in the dentist–patient relationship.
7. How does the Americans with Disabilities Act affect the practice of dentistry?
8. How was the first child abuse case in the United States prosecuted?
9. List the signs of physical abuse of children.
10. List the signs of emotional abuse of children.
11. List the signs of sexual abuse of children.
12. List the signs of neglect of children.
13. What is spousal abuse?
14. What is elder abuse?
15. How is the abuse of the physically disabled detected by the dental office staff?

## CASE STUDY

### Learning Outcomes

Upon mastery of the content of this scenario, the student should be able to:

- Assess client characteristics.
- Recognize the relationship between the client and the caregiver.
- Relate the oral signs and symptoms of elder abuse to the proper authority.
- Plan and manage dental hygiene care.
- Select the appropriate dental hygiene procedure for treatment.

### Discussion

Darrell is an active senior citizen who lives on Social Security and pension retirement benefits. He suffered a series of ischemic episodes from which he recovered, and reports enjoying retirement. He presents to the dental office for routine periodontal maintenance prophylaxis.

### Client Information

Darrell's current vital statistics are as follows:

| | |
|---|---|
| Age | 82 years |
| Sex | male |
| Height/Weight | 5′6″/160 lb. |
| Blood Pressure | 154/92 mm Hg |
| Pulse Rate | 70 bpm |
| Respiration Rate | 14 rpm |

### Medical History

Darrel is under the care of a physician after hospitalization several years earlier for ischemia. He has high blood pressure and is taking Cardizem (diltiazem hydrochloride). He reports a slowing down in activity level owing to effects from the ischemia but views his health as good. Osteoarthritis in his hands and fingers causes mild to moderate pain during small motor skill activities, for which he takes ibuprofen. He wears trifocal glasses.

### Dental History

Darrell keeps his regular periodontal maintenance appointments. When taking his blood pressure, the dental professional notices several bruises consistent with forceful grasping on his left arm. He reports that he fell down and broke his teeth. When questioned about the fall, he says he doesn't remember much. Darrell is satisfied with the appearance of his teeth and proud that he has most of them, even if they are chipped and broken. He reports brushing twice daily and never flossing.

## Social History

Darrell is a widower, and his 30-year-old, unemployed youngest son lives with him. Darrell maintains a garden plot in the community garden, where he grows vegetables for himself and his neighbors. His son drives Darrell's car to the dental appointment and appears falsely concerned with his father's oral status.

Darrell's current oral hygiene status is as follows:

- Chipped and broken teeth.
- Generalized bleeding on probing.
- Healing lip sores that appear to be lacerated.
- Moderate xerostomia.

## Client's Human Needs Deficits

The dental professionals note that some of Darrell's needs are not being met. Darrel may need protection from a variety of health risks:

General health
  Due to: High blood pressure medication
  Evidenced by: Client's self-report
Biologically sound and functional dentition
  Due to: Recent fall
  Evidenced by: Broken teeth
Skin and mucous membrane integrity of the head and neck
  Due to: Presence of plaque
  Evidenced by: Bleeding on probing and periodontal disease
Responsibility for oral health
  Due to: Lack of daily home care
  Evidenced by: Periodontal disease and caries
Freedom from anxiety or stress
  Due to: Suspected elder abuse
  Evidenced by: Chipped, broken teeth; lip sores; bruises on left arm
Conceptualization and understanding
  Due to: Lack of awareness of need for more frequent brushing and interproximal removal of plaque
  Evidenced by: Client's self-report brushing twice a day and not flossing

## Case Study Questions

1. Darrell's chipped teeth and lip sores are the result of his advanced age. His gingival recession is related to his present periodontal condition. [Assessment of client characteristics]
   A. The first statement is true, and the second statement is false.
   B. The first statement is false, and the second statement is true.
   C. Both statements are true.
   D. Both statements are false.

2. Which of the following would be the best recommendation for Darrell's oral self-care program? [Using preventive agents]
   A. Powered toothbrush
   B. Interproximal brushes
   C. Home fluoride rinse
   D. Oral irrigation device
   E. Flossing

## Case Discussion Questions

1. List your concerns for this patient.
2. How would you present your suspicions to the dentist?
3. To whom do you report your suspicions in your locale?
4. Is it appropriate for you to discuss family violence in the form of elder abuse with Darrell?
5. Is it appropriate for you to discuss your suspicions with the son?
6. Should the dental office pursue any further action?

# Basics of Dentistry and Dental Law

*Dental Hygiene Domain Competencies*[1]

## PROFESSIONALISM AND ETHICS

### Professional Behavior

- Assume responsibility for dental hygiene services.
- Provide accurate documentation when serving in professional roles.

### Ethical Behavior

- Integrate the American Dental Hygienists' Association (ADHA) code of ethics in all professional endeavors.
- Adhere to federal, state, and local laws.
- Appreciate the cultural diversity of the patient.
- Apply principles of risk management to prevent legal liability.

### Professional Commitment

- Advance the values of the profession by affiliation with professional and public organizations.
- Assume the role of clinician, educator, researcher, change agent, consumer advocate, and administrator as defined by the ADHA.
- Assume responsibility for lifelong learning.

## ORAL HEALTH PROMOTION AND COMMUNITY HEALTH

- Assess community oral healthcare needs, risks, and resources and evaluate outcomes to access the healthcare system.
- Screen, educate, and refer services that allow patients to access the resources of the healthcare system.
- Facilitate patient access to oral healthcare services through a variety of healthcare settings as a member of a multidisciplinary team.

---

[1]Adapted from American Dental Education Association. Competencies for Entry into the Profession of Dental Hygiene (as approved by the 2003 House of Delegates). J Dent Educ 2004,68:745–749.

# DENTAL HYGIENE PROCESS OF CARE

## Patient Diagnosis

- Analyze and interpret data to formulate a dental hygiene diagnosis.
- Obtain consultations as appropriate.
- Refer clients to other healthcare providers as needed.

## Implementation

- Provide adjunct dental hygiene services as legally allowed in the jurisdiction of practice.

## Evaluation and Maintenance

- Determine client satisfaction with care received and oral health status achieved.

## REFERENCES & RESOURCES

**Organizations**
Academy for Sports Dentistry (www.sportsdentistry-asd.org)
Academy of Cosmetic Dentistry (www.aacd.com)
Academy of General Dentistry (www.agd.org)
Academy of Laser Dentistry (www.laserdentistry.org)
American Academy of Esthetic Dentistry (www.estheticacademy.org)
American Academy of Forensic Sciences (www.aafs.org)
American Academy of Implant Dentistry (www.aaid-implant.cnchost.org)
American Academy of Oral & Maxillofacial Pathology (www.aaomp.org)
American Academy of Oral and Maxillofacial Radiology (www.aaomr.org)
American Academy of Oral Medicine (www.aaom.com)
American Academy of Orofacial Pain (www.aaop.org)
American Academy of Pediatric Dentistry (www.aapd.org)
American Academy of Periodontology (www.perio.org)
American Association of Endodontists (www.aae.org)
American Association of Oral and Maxillofacial Surgeons (www.aaoms.org)
American Association of Orthodontists (www.aaortho.org)
American Association of Public Health Dentistry (www.aaphd.org)
American Board of Forensic Odontology (www.abfo.org)
American Board of General Dentistry (www.abgd.org)
American Board of Oral Implantology/Implant Dentistry (www.aboi.org)
American College of Prosthodontists (www.prosthodontics.org)
American Dental Association (www.ada.org)
American Dental Society of Anesthesiology (www.adsahome.org)
American Society of Dentists Anesthesiologists (www.asdahq.org)
American Society of Forensic Odontology (www.asfo.org)
College of American Pathologists (www.cap.org)
Denturist Association of Canada (www.denturist.org)
FDI World Dental Federation (www.fdiworlddental.org)
Hispanic Dental Association (www.hdassoc.org)
Holistic Dental Association (www.holisticdental.org)
International Academy of Periodontology (www.perioiap.org)
International Association for Disability and Oral Health (www.iadh.org)
International Association of Dento-Maxillo-Facial Radiology (www.iadmfr.org)
International Association of Oral and Maxillofacial Surgeons (www.iaoms.org)
International Association of Oral Pathologists (www.iaop.com)
International Association of Paediatric Dentistry (www.iapdworld.org)
International Federation of Dental Hygienists (www.ifdh.org)
International Federation of Endodontic Associations (www.ifeaendo.org)
National Dental Association (www.ndaonline.org)
Online Sports Dentistry (www.sportsdentistry.com)
Special Care Dentistry (www.scdonline.org)
TMJ Association (www.tmj.org)
U.S. Department of Health and Human Services (www.hhs.gov)
Victorian Government Health Information: Dental Therapists (www.health.vic.gov.au/dentistry/careers/therapy.htm)

World Federation of Orthodontists (www.wfo.org)

World Health Organization, Oral Health Organization (www.who.int/oral_health/en)

### Online Resources

American Dental Hygienists' Association government affairs information (www.adha.org/governmental_affairs/index.html)

American with Disabilities Act (www.ada.gov)

Ancient Egyptian medicine and herbal remedies (www.crystalinks.com/egyptmedicine.html)

Ayurved and homeopathy (gujhealth.gov.in/ayurvedhomeopathy/index.htm)

Child Welfare League of America (www.cwla.org)

Children's Defense Fund (www.childrensdefense.org)

Dental careers (www.ada.org/public/education/careers/index.asp; www.ada.org/public/education/careers/dentistry_careers_powerpoint.pdf)

*Dental Cosmos* (www.hti.umich.edu/d/dencos)

Dental Law Group (www.dentalaw.com)

Dental Nurse ( www.nhscareers.nhs.uk//nhs-knowledge_base/data/4671.html )

Dental Therapist (www.nhscareers.nhs.uk//nhs-knowledge_base/data/5250.html)

Family Violence Prevention Fund (www.endabuse.org)

History of dentistry (www.goodteeth.com/museum.htm)

Images from the history of dentistry (www.ihm.nlm.nih.gov/cgi-bin/gw_44_3/chameleon?skin=nlm&lng=en)

Occupational titles (www.doleta.gov/Programs/onet)

Prevent Child Abuse America (www.preventchildabuse.org)

Public health (www.osophs.dhhs.gov )

U.S. Department of Heath and Human Services: statistics on aging (www.hhs.gov/aging/index.shtml#data)

Volunteering (www.ada.org/ada/international/volunteer/index.asp; www.ihs.gov; www.redcross.org)

### Pamphlets, Dissertations, Papers

Fales MJH. History of dental hygiene (doctoral dissertation). Ann Arbor, MI: University of Michigan, 1975.

Hamilton J. Lasers: A decade of progress. Paper presented at the 127th midwinter meeting of the Chicago Dental Society, February 1992.

National Dental Assistants Association. Working together for continued growth and continuity. July 1992.

U.S. Department of Justice, Civil Rights Division, Coordination and Review Service. Americans with Disabilities Act requirements fact sheet.

Prevent Child Abuse America. Recognizing Child Abuse: What Parents Should Know. Available at www.preventchildabuse.org/publications/parents/index.shtml. Accessed April 25, 2006.

### Articles

American Dental Assistants Association. The changing look of dental assisting. Dent Assist J 1984;23.

Bednarch H, Eklund K. TB prevention calls for a national standard. Access 1994.

Collins RJ, Dugoni AA, Formicola AJ, et al. A glimpse into the 21st century. J Am Dent Assoc 1992;123:59–64.

Darby, ML, Connelly IM, Thomson EM, Magee KW. Cultural adaptability of dental hygiene students in the United States: A pilot study. J Dent Hyg 2004;78.

Dental hygiene: 75 and going strong. Dent Teamwork 1988.

Elsea, Blitz. Building a solid foundation of trust. RDH 1993.

Fultz O. New-age dentistry. Popular Mechanics February 1991.

Harris JB. Michigan's black dental heritage. J Mich Dent Assoc 1992.

Hoewisch C. Relaxation and imagery for the fearful patient. Access 1993.

Is alternative medicine right for you? [Personally Speaking]. NEA Today November 1993.

Jameson C. 10 barriers to quality staff meetings. Dent Teamwork 1992.

King L. Treating the anxious patient. Access 1991.

Lally J. Diversity: Looking for a place to bloom in dental hygiene. Access 1995.

Majeski J. Phobias: Facts on fear. Access 1993.

McCarthy P. Don't be fooled by nutrition misinformation. Dentalhygienistnews 1993.

Novak D. Dental auxiliary evolution: A historical perspective, the dental assistant. J Am Dent Assist Assoc 1984.

Sagan C. A new way to think about rules to live by. Parade Magazine, November 28, 1993:12–14.

Sklar B. Hypnosis as an alternative in dentistry. Access 1993.

Sreebny LM. Salivary flow in health and disease. Compend Contin Educ Dent 1989;(Suppl 13).

Tennant D. Mind over matter. Virginian-Pilot and Ledger Star, March 13, 1994.

The Merits of Siwaak. Al Jumuah Magazine 8:20–21.

Waldman HB. The economics of dentistry for the elderly. Compend Contin Educ Dent 14(2).

### Books

Ash MM, Ward ML. Oral Pathology: An Introduction to General and Oral Pathology for Hygienists (6th ed.). Philadelphia: Lea & Febiger, 1992.

Auerbach L. The Babylonian Talmud in Selection. New York: Philosophical Library, 1944.

Bassett M. Achieving Excellence. Rockville, MD: Aspen, 1986.

Boyett JH, Boyet JT. Beyond Workplace 2000. New York: Penguin, 1995.

Bremner MDK. The Story of Dentistry from the Dawn of Civilization to the Present . . . with Special Emphasis on the American Scene (3rd ed. rev.). Brooklyn, NY: Dental Items of Interest, 1964.

Chasteen JE. Essentials of Clinical Dental Assisting (2nd ed.). St. Louis: Mosby, 1980.

Dental Assisting National Board. DANB Task Analysis (9th ed.). Order at www.danb.org/main/publications.asp.).

Dental Assisting National Board. Issue 22. Chicago: Certified Press, 1992.

Douglas M. Purity and Danger: An Analysis of the Concepts of Pollution and Taboo (rpt. ed.). London: Ark, 1989.

Edge G. The Ethics of Health Care: A Guide for Clinical Practice. Albany, NY: Delmar, 1994.

Ehrlich A. Fundamentals of Dental Ethics and Jurisprudence. Colwell Systems, 1985.

Flight M. Law. Liability and Ethics for Medical Office Personnel (2nd ed.). Albany, NY: Delmar, 1993.

Foley GPH. Foley's Footnotes: A Treasury of Dentistry. Wallingford, PA: Washington Square East, 1972.

Guerini V. A History of Dentistry. Pound Ridge, NY: Milford House, 1969.

Harris NC. Technical Education in the Junior College/New Programs for New Jobs. Washington, DC: American Association of Junior Colleges, 1964.

History of the American Dental Assistants Association. Chicago: American Dental Assistants Association, 1970.

Hoffmann-Axthelm W. History of Dentistry. Chicago: Quintessence, 1981.

Ibsen P. Oral Pathology for the Dental Hygienist. Saunders, 1992.

Ingersol B. Behavioral Aspects in Dentistry. Appleton-Century-Crofts, 1982.

Ingersol B. Patient Management Skills for Dental Assistants and Hygienists. Appleton-Century-Crofts, 1986.

Johnson DW, Johnson RT, Holubec E. Cooperation in the Classroom. Edna, MN: Interactive Book Co., 1991.

Jong A. Community Dental Health (2nd ed.). Mosby, 1988.

Keir L, Wise BA, Krebs C. Medical Assisting, Administrative and Clinical Competencies (3rd ed.). Albany, NY: Delmar, 1993.

Kidder RM. How Good People Make Tough Choices. New York: Morrow, 1995.

Lieber JG, Levine RE, Dervitz HL. Management Principles for Health Professionals. Rockville, MD: Aspen, 1984.

Marzano RJ, Arredondo DE. Tactics for Thinking. Aurora, CO: Mid-Continent Regional Education Laboratory, 1986.

Mordecai S. Richmond in By-Gone Days—Being Reminiscences of an Old Citizen. Philadelphia: King & Baird Printers, 1856, p. 205.

Occupational Outlook Handbook. 2006-2007 edition. Available at www.bls.gov/oco.

Ring M. Dentistry: An Illustrated History. St. Louis: Mosby, 1985.

Robinson D, Bird D. Ehrlich and Torres Essentials of Dental Assisting (3rd ed.) Philadelphia: Saunders, 2001.

Schwartzrock J. Effective Dental Assisting (4th ed.). Dubuque, IA: Brown, 1974.

Simmers L. Diversified Health Occupations (3rd ed.). Albany, NY: Delmar, 1993.

Steele PF. Dental Specialties for the Dental Hygienist (2nd ed.). Philadelphia: Lea & Febiger, 1978.

The Professional Difference. Chicago: American Dental Assistants Association, 1990

U.S. Department of Labor, Employment and Training Administration. Dictionary of Occupational Titles (vols. 1–2; 4th rev. ed.), 1991, pp. 57–58, 66, 71, 706–707.

Umiker W. Management Skills for the New Health Care Supervisor. Rockville, MD: Aspen, 1988.

Weinberger BW. An Introduction to the History of Dentistry in America. St. Louis: Mosby, 1948.

Weinstein BD. Dental Ethics. Philadelphia: Lea & Febiger, 1993.

Wilkins E. Clinical Practice of the Dental Hygienist (6th ed.). Philadelphia: Lea & Febiger, 1989.

Woodall I. Comprehensive Dental Hygiene Care (4th ed.). St. Louis: Mosby, 1993.

Woodall I. Legal, Ethical and Management Aspects of the Dental Care System (3rd ed.). St. Louis: Mosby, 1987.

Wynbrandt J. The Excruciating History of Dentistry: Toothsome Tales and Oral Oddities from Babylon to Braces. New York: St. Martin's Griffin, 1998.

# Office Management

# The Business of Dentistry

## LEARNING OUTCOMES

Upon mastery of the content of this chapter, the student should be able to:
- Differentiate between a sole proprietorship, partnership, and corporation.
- Write a business plan.
- Describe the general layout of the dental office, the reception area, business office, dental treatment operatories, central sterilization, dental laboratory, conference room, darkroom, staff lounge, storage room, and private office.
- List the tasks performed by the business dental assistant and office manager.
- Identify the components of patient reception.
- Recognize the characteristics of a staff meeting.

## KEY TERMS

business plans
corporation
ergonomic

partnership
patient reception
sole proprietorship

## THE BUSINESS OF DENTISTRY

Dental and dental hygiene practices are places of business where oral healthcare is provided. Most dentists provide general dentistry procedures in a private practice setting using skills in oral diagnosis, disease prevention, and rehabilitation. Successful dentists rely on allied dental personnel working together as a team for oral healthcare delivery. Dental hygienists who own an independent practice or are in an alternative practice or collaborative partnership also rely on allied dental personnel to assist in oral healthcare delivery. Because of rapidly changing technology, dental professionals are constantly upgrading skills, equipment, and office decor to show that they are up to date and maintain the dental industry standard of care.

Dental offices have a basic layout and floor plan. The design of the modern dental office should reflect the ergonomic needs of the dental team. **Ergonomic** means the "application of engineering and biology principles to the work environment so that the worker has a physically comfortable workstation." Dental assistants perform business office functions common to many small businesses, such as bookkeeping and operating business machines.

## THE DENTAL PRACTICE

Dental practices are generally privately owned businesses. There are several basic business entities on which a dental practice can be modeled: a proprietorship, partnership, or corporation. Business taxes are processed based on the type of business the owner operates. **Sole proprietorship** is the type of business in which one dentist or dental hygienist owns the business; as the owner, he or she is called a proprietor. Sole proprietorships are easy businesses to initiate, name, and sell. **Partnership** is the type of business in which two or more people own the business, share the responsibility, and are called partners. Partnerships are usually set up with a legal agreement describing the rights and responsibilities of each partner. General partnerships are business entities in which both partners make the major business decisions. Limited partnerships are business entities in which one partner makes the major decisions and the other partners are not active in decision making.

A **corporation** is a business entity in which the dentist or hygienist is an employee of his or her own business. Corporations have shareholders, a board of directors to manage the business, and officers to manage the daily operations. A corporation is a business choice that makes the professional eligible for corporate benefits, tax breaks, and retirement accounts. In addition, the corporation protects the shareholders, board of directors, and officers from debts and legal liability to reduce the risks associated with business ownership.

A corporation may own and manage a single practice or multiple dental practices, and all members of the dental staff are employees of the corporation. Dentists and/or dental hygienists use the abbreviation PC (for professional corporation) when they have incorporated—for example, John Doe, DDS, PC, or Jane Doe, RDH, PC—and are frequently the president of the corporation. The organization may be made up of nondental business people who own the company.

## THE BUSINESS PLAN

**Business plans** are written documents, 30–40 pages in length, that describe the business, offer a means for measuring performance over time, and make projections about growth potential. They are presented to grantors, lenders, or investors when the owner wishes to obtain money for investment in the business. A business plan helps define the scope, strengths, and weaknesses of the organization and keeps the owner focused on making the business a financial success. *Box 7.1* lists the components of a business plan.

---

**BOX 7.1** *Components of a Business Plan*

| | |
|---|---|
| Cover page | Management and personnel plan |
| Table of contents | Competition |
| Business Description | Future Trends |
| Products and Services | Sources of Funding |
| Résumé and financial statement | Appendices |
| Public relations marketing plan | |

Money is needed to start a business, and many budding entrepreneurs look for creative sources to raise it, including personal funds; friends, family, and business associates; lending institutions; investors; and grant and development institutions.

## DENTAL OFFICE LAYOUT

An important aspect of running a business is whether to rent or own the space. Owning the actual building in which the practice is located has many benefits, such as tax breaks. Furthermore, the building will probably appreciate in value and the professional is free of landlord issues and thus has the ability to make improvements as desired. All entrepreneurs should seriously consider purchasing the building space. Many dental professionals who start out in a rented space eventually move into their own building after the practice has been established and the initial startup costs have been paid.

Many dental offices have a theme or personality, which usually reflects the personality of the dentist or dental hygienist (*Fig. 7.1*). Oral healthcare providers with an interest in photography may display some of their framed photographs of landscapes or people. The provider who likes to fish may decorate the office with fishing gear and artifacts. The partners who share an activity such as sailing may have yachting memorabilia exhibited for the public to see. Furthermore, dental practices may be adapted

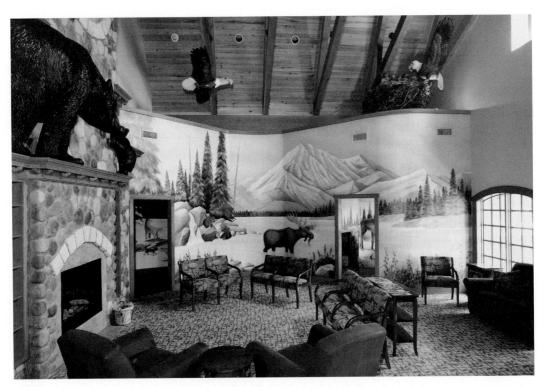

**Figure 7.1** This office has been decorated in an Alaskan wilderness theme. Courtesy of Dr. Lee Baker and Jeff Barnes, Augusta, GA.

to a theme based on their location, such as a forest, river, lake, or urban center. Some dental offices are designed so the reception area is separate from the business office.

## Patient Reception Area

Deliveries, salespeople, and the general public are received in the reception area or business office. Usually, the first person the client meets is the dental assistant working in the business area. The patient has called previously to schedule an appointment and enters the dental office through the reception area. The reception area is an extension of the business office, and it is the first contact the patient has with the entire office.

**Patient reception** is the meeting and greeting of patients and informing the staff of the patient's arrival using a communication system. There are many different technologies to choose from when selecting a communication system. For example, a closed-circuit television system includes a stationary camera mounted to capture the patient sign-in board; the image is then broadcast to viewing screens in several locations throughout the office. This allows staff to monitor patient arrivals without being present in the reception area. Other technologies use colored lights, written messages, and/or sounds (with or without display panels) to communicate among staff.

It is a human characteristic to make judgments based on appearance within the first minute of the encounter. Therefore, the appearance of the reception area requires careful consideration—from the selection of magazines to the color scheme, lighting, music, and furniture—to create an aesthetically pleasing and welcoming environment for patients. Current magazines containing appropriate family content should be available for waiting clients to read. Outdated magazines do not reflect the state-of-the-art atmosphere desired for modern practices. Color affects our emotions in both positive and negative ways, and the colors used in the dental office should create a positive atmosphere. Lighting is also important for the creation of a positive atmosphere. Professionals may want to consult with an interior designer when planning or redecorating the office, ensuring appropriate color and lighting selections.

Background music creates a mood to help patients relax and to minimize their fear and anxiety. The staff may pick entertaining music to make the waiting time more enjoyable. Many businesses pay a fee for a music service, which can provide the background music. Some offices play CDs on an office stereo system, and others tune in to the local radio station. Whatever the delivery system used, music plays an important role in the business day in most dental offices.

Furniture, rugs, plants, pictures, reading material, and televisions are found in many dental offices. Plants should be healthy and attractive looking to further promote the practice as having an upscale and current atmosphere. The furniture in the reception area should provide suitable seating arrangements for waiting patients and be in good repair. Children and adults should be accommodated with seating. A dental office may use chairs and/or couches for patient seating and smaller seating areas for children. Children need activities to keep them busy while waiting. Children's areas may have a bulletin board for showing photos of young patients in the "no-cavity club" and may include informational books about a visit to the dentist, age-appropriate magazines, building blocks, stuffed animals, or coloring books and crayons.

Air quality is a concern for many individuals, and patients with allergies need a dust- and mold-free environment. Air purifiers or filtration systems may be in use to improve the air quality. Aromatherapy and filtered fresh air are found in dental offices as a way to improve the air quality and remove the "dental office smell" frequently associated with practices. Temperature control is another way to provide patient comfort. It is one of the best ways to maintain a comfortable environment for patients and office staff. However, temperature can be an area of debate among dental team members. Thus, the temperature settings should be agreed on and set for everyone's comfort. A small fan is frequently found in all rooms of the dental office to ensure air flow.

## Treatment Operatories

Oral diagnosis, disease prevention, and patient care are rendered in the dental operatory. The oral healthcare provider works from an operatory with a dental assistant for improved efficiency. Time and motion studies influence equipment design, and equipment should be selected with ergonomic factors in mind so the dental operatory is physically comfortable. All dental operatories contain basic equipment: dental unit, dental light, operating dental chair, two operating stools, cabinets, sink, and waste receptacle.

The dental unit may be fixed or mobile, with room for the provider and dental assistant to work comfortably. The dental unit contains attachments for the handpieces and air/water syringe, with adjustment knobs to mix the air and water. Handpieces and air/water syringes require a central air compressor. This noisy piece of equipment is outside of the operatory and requires regular maintenance. Suction equipment—either a high-volume evacuator or saliva ejector—may be attached separately. The central vacuum system is located near the air compressor and contains a solid debris collector, which requires regular maintenance per the manufacturer's maintenance instructions.

The dental light is either suspended from the ceiling or attached to the dental chair. Patient positioning is different for different procedures; therefore, the dental chair is contoured to fit the body comfortably and to accommodate many body sizes and positions. Operating stools are used by the provider and the dental assistant; the stools adjust via a hydraulic lever, which raises and lowers the padded seat.

Cabinetry comes in many different designs and provides a variety of work surfaces and storage space. Sinks for hand washing in view of the patient are extremely important for patient treatment and may have foot controls or electronic controls for water and soap. Lined waste receptacles hold most solid waste generated during patient treatment. They are emptied at the end of the day and are labeled "biohazardous waste" to be discarded as mandated by state health and safety laws.

## Central Sterilization

Central sterilization is the area in the dental office where instruments and materials are cleaned, sterilized, prepared for the next procedure, and stored. The contaminated side holds the used trays and instruments for cleaning and disposable of solid waste items. The clean side holds the sterile instruments and materials needed to set up for dental procedures. Specific details concerning the required protocols and techniques of sterilization and worker safety issues are found in comprehensive dental hygiene textbooks.

## Dental Laboratory

The dental laboratory is the area in the dental office where laboratory procedures are performed. The dental laboratory contains a counter work station, laboratory handpiece and attachments, a vibrator, a model trimmer, a dental lathe, a vacuum former, and various dental materials used in the construction of custom-made products.

## Conference Room

The conference room is the area in the dental office where a dental team member conducts a patient conference. It provides privacy for discussing financial arrangements, patient education, case presentation, or private conversations. Conference rooms contain a large table or desk and chairs, a computer, DVD player, videotape player and monitor, x-ray view boxes, patient education brochures/pamphlets, videotapes and DVDs, and models.

## Darkroom

The darkroom is the area in the dental office where dental film is processed into dental radiographs. Usually it contains an automatic processor and/or dip tanks, a safe light, white light, film mounts, labels, and other miscellaneous equipment such as a film duplicator. In offices that use digital radiography, the film processor is replaced by electronic equipment to send the images to the computer system.

## Staff Lounge

The staff lounge is the area of the dental office where employees may change into their uniforms, take breaks, eat snacks and meals, or make personal phone calls. Food storage areas should be separate from any dental products, according to health and safety laws.

## Storage Room

Stored inventory items are kept in storage rooms. New instruments, equipment, supplies, and materials may also be kept in a storage room. Nitrous equipment is usually stored in a lock-out secured storage room that requires a key or electronic code for entrance.

## Private Office

The practice owner, partners, and/or office manager may each have a private office to conduct business, such as treatment planning. Often, these areas are restricted, and privacy is to be respected. Some dental offices do not have conference rooms, and the private office may be used for client consultation.

## THE BUSINESS OFFICE

The business office is the area of the dental office in which business transactions are managed, such as patient exiting procedures, appointment scheduling, financial transactions, records management, and business correspondence. Clients are managed using business office systems outlined in policy and procedures manuals (discussed further in Chapter 23). Communication and productivity are key components for the financial success of the practice; to meet this requirement, the dental assistant performs many business tasks.

## Business Tasks of the Dental Assistant

The dental assistant reinforces the practice image in the business office using skills in public relations, client management, records management, accounting, and operating office equipment. Recall from Chapter 2 that the recognized occupational job title of dental assistant notes that the individual will perform business tasks. The title of the dental assistant who concentrates on business tasks varies among practices; this person may be referred to as the administrative assistant, receptionist, insurance clerk, records manager, appointment coordinator, financial coordinator, bookkeeper, or collections clerk. A basic knowledge of dentistry when performing dental office functions and using interpersonal communication skills enables the dental assistant to be organized and effective. Other personal qualities that are particularly important for the business dental assistant to possess are a good personal appearance, integrity, dependability, and a positive attitude. *Box* 7.2 lists the job tasks performed by the business dental assistant.

## Reception Procedures

Because first impressions are lasting ones, the reception area must be kept tidy throughout the business day. Magazines and daily newspapers are kept in an orderly fashion and made easily accessible to clients. Some dental offices have coffee, tea, juice, or water available for waiting patients. The reception area requires daily housekeeping such as vacuuming, dusting, and general cleanup, and live plants need weekly watering. If the room contains a children's area, games and toys should be stored within reach and picked up during the day.

Each person who enters the reception area of the dental office should receive immediate attention. The daily schedule is followed to greet patients by name as they enter the reception area. Respect is given to all guests to the office via friendly and polite personal attention. The dental staff is informed of patient arrival promptly to maintain the appointment schedule. Clients are treated as individuals by using their names in formal greetings—for example, "Good morning, Mrs. Newton." Immediately inform the patient of any anticipated wait and the estimated time involved. Most people become angry when their personal time is not considered to be valuable. Children are greeted with a smile and formal greeting using their name. Show them where to find books, games, toys, or coloring materials in the event of a waiting time.

Visitors and new patients are given tours of the dental office but should not be allowed in treatment areas because of patients' legal rights to privacy. Any visitor, such as a student performing an observation, must obtain permission from each patient to be present in the operatory.

Unfortunately, any business open to the public can be a setting for crime to occur. Dental offices must be prepared for such an eventuality; therefore, it is prudent to be alert for criminal activity. The presence of a stranger is always investigated for security reasons, and when a stranger enters the office, immediate attention is given to him or her so staff can determine the purpose of the visit. An emergency protocol should be in place and practiced so all are prepared for a dangerous and/or potentially violent situation. The local police department will be willing to visit the office to note any security weaknesses and can make recommendations to improve safety measures. Commonly

**BOX 7.2**  *Dental Assistant Business Tasks*

**Public relations**

Produce written materials, such as newsletters, media releases, and brochures

Mail welcome packets to new patients, greeting cards, and direct mail advertising

Distribute business cards and free samples to
clients

Keep the dentist on schedule

Thank patients for referrals

Sponsor athletic teams

Volunteer for community functions

**Client management**

Treat clients as individuals

Develop client trust

Use formal greetings

Educate patients

Recognize client stress

Schedule appointments

Call patients after treatment

Maintain patient records

Negotiate financial arrangements

**Records management**

Type charts, forms, and letters

Process dental insurance

Write prescriptions

Use records-management systems

Transfers records by mail, fax, electronic filing,
or in person

Prepare tax statements

**Accounts receivable**

Keep accurate financial records

Post monthly statements

Prepare aged account analysis

Make bank deposits

Negotiate credit and collections

**Accounts payable**

Check writing

Maintain petty cash

Maintain inventory control

Banking

**Operate office equipment**

Telecommunications equipment—computer
e-mail, fax, telephone, messaging center,
answering service or machine

Computer network, website, software
programs, automated appointment-
confirmation software

Postage equipment

Photocopying equipment

used security systems include video monitoring, locked entrances with a buzzer to allow entrance, and a burglar alarm system.

## Office Manager

Usually, a dental assistant with the job description of office manager directs the employees, participates in staffing procedures, handles difficult business office functions, and plans for the future. Sometimes called the practice administrator, his or her job tasks are focused on the dental practice as a whole, not on just one department. *Box 7.3* lists the tasks of the office manager. One special task performed by the office manager is conducting meetings. Morning meetings and staff meetings are essential components of a well-managed dental practice. They allow the dental office staff to come together in a joint meeting to discuss daily operations. Effective communication in a forum provides

## BOX 7.3 *Dental Office Manager Tasks*

**Direct employees**

Issue instructions

Determine job descriptions

Schedule work hours

Train new employees

Orient temporary workers

**Staffing procedures**

Recruit employees

Hire employees

Terminate employees

Mediate staff disputes

**Planning**

In-service education programs

Staff meetings

Monitor inventory and overhead expenses

Meet federal and state regulations

Develop procedures protocol

Market dental practice

**Office functions**

Intervene to process difficult insurance claims

Process payroll

Maintain accounts payable

Handle patient complaints

Run computer backup procedures

Operate equipment

an opportunity for input from everyone. Morning meetings are held before seeing patients to discuss the day. Monthly staff meetings should be held during working hours at peak energy time such as morning or lunchtime to discuss the practice and to help maintain an efficiently managed dental office.

Typically, agenda items—the information to be discussed at staff meetings—are submitted, prioritized, and presented to staff by the office manager. Reports on production, collection, new patients, and projects are examples of agenda items. The open forum setting allows all employees to provide input when problems and concerns of staff and management arise. The staff uses problem-solving techniques, listening skills, and brainstorming during the meetings to resolve problems. Announcements regarding new procedures, policies, or government regulations to be instituted by the practice owner are made at staff meetings. Staff meetings are an excellent time to conduct in-service activities; update staff on new trends, legislation, or technology advances; and renew CPR certification.

## CONCEPT SUMMARY

- The proprietorship, partnership, professional corporation, and business corporation are business entities in the dental industry.
- The general layout of the dental office uses basic design theory and a decor that personalizes the business.
- Patient reception should be prompt and courteous and performed as soon as the person enters the practice.
- Dental assistants perform business office tasks.
- Office managers are needed for a well-managed practice and have unique job tasks.
- Staff meetings are held each morning and at least once a month.

# REVIEW QUESTIONS

1. What is the difference between a sole proprietorship, partnership, and corporation?
2. Why are corporations a business choice for dentists and dental hygienists?
3. Why is it necessary to formulate a business plan?
4. How can dental office design be unique for each business while maintaining a universal layout?
5. How are the client's sense of sight, smell, sound, and touch affected by the dental office environment?
6. List the categories of business tasks performed in the dental business office.
7. What are the personal qualities needed by the business dental assistant?
8. List the tasks performed by the business dental assistant.
9. What are the components of patient reception?
10. Why are reception procedures so important?
11. List the categories of tasks performed by the dental office manager.
12. What are the characteristics of a staff conference?
13. How do ergonomic designs influence the dental operatory?
14. How is a conference room used?
15. Why is the private office area restricted to some employees?

# CRITICAL THINKING ACTIVITY

- Perform a web search to locate dental office designs.
- Describe your ideas for the perfect dental operatory and the necessary elements needed.
- If you were planning to open your own independent or collaborative practice, what elements of decor do you think are mandatory?
- Discuss in a group the elements that you have observed to be good or poor in dental practices.
- How would the dental specialty office differ from a general dental practice in terms of design layout and decor?

## Assignment: Create a Business Plan

Develop a brief business plan incorporating the items in *Box 7.1.*

# Telecommunications

## TELECOMMUNICATIONS

**Telecommunication** systems involve the transmission of words, sounds, or images in the form of electronic signals via devices such as landline or mobile telephones, facsimile (fax), computer, web cameras (webcams), radio, television, microwave, or satellite. Telecommunication services used by the dental office are public or private businesses such as telephone companies, Internet service provider companies, and insurance clearing-houses used for electronically filing insurance claims. The telephone plays a major role in virtually every business in the United States. It is estimated that more than 95% of the dental office's business is received from telephone calls. With this in mind, first impressions over the telephone are quite important. Computers are used for a large variety of small business tasks and operations. Dental offices and insurance companies have websites and email to help patients select an oral healthcare provider. Daily business transactions are performed using integrated dental software programs.

Communication does not take place until the information in one person's mind is accurately transmitted to another person's mind. Communicating by telephone, facsimile, and computer can be more difficult than communicating face to face because only a small part of communication involves the use of words. Humans communicate more through nonverbal gestures and facial expressions.

## TELEPHONE

The successful dental practice uses specific telephone techniques to promote effective communication. Because a telephone call is the first contact a new patient has with the office, it is vital for the caller to have a positive experience. The image portrayed by your telephone voice can be courteous and friendly, or hurried and mechanical. First impressions are made from telephone calls, so it is important to use telephone techniques that have been proven effective.

**Telephone techniques** refer to telephone etiquette, rate of speech, voice clarity, and voice volume, as well as listening skills and questioning strategies. There is a proper way to speak into a telephone mouthpiece, a correct time to answer the ringing phone, and proven ways to greet and question the patient. **Telephone etiquette** is the proper use of the telephone. Answer the telephone before the end of the second ring. If you answer too quickly, you may surprise the caller; but if you take too long to answer, you may anger the caller. When speaking into the telephone mouthpiece, your lips should be ½–1 inch from the receiver. Be sure to speak directly into the mouthpiece and use the dental office's script. Ask open-ended questions to find out who the caller is and the reason for the call. *Box 8.1* lists two scripts for answering the telephone.

One of the most important telephone techniques is the ability to listen to the caller. Listening is affected by the tone of voice, rate of speech, voice volume, and background noise. The caller judges the office by listening to the tone and inflection of your voice, which can telegraph and reflect your emotions. When a person smiles, it relaxes the vocal cords and affects the sound of the voice; therefore, many dental offices have a mirror next to the telephone as a reminder to smile. Although the caller may have never met you, he or she should feel warmly welcomed by your voice.

The rate of your speech affects the caller's ability to understand what you are saying. If you speak too quickly, he or she may be confused; but if you speak too slowly, the caller may become annoyed. The volume of your voice is also important. If you speak too loudly on the telephone, the listener may be forced to hold the phone away from his or her ear, creating a psychological distance between the two of you. If you speak too

**BOX 8.1** *Scripts for Answering the Dental Office Telephone*

- "Good morning, This is Mary from Dental Hygiene Associates. How can I help you?"
- "Dental Hygiene Associates; this is Mary. How can I help you?"

softly, the listener has difficulty paying attention. To achieve a comfortable volume, speak into the phone as if you were talking to a person sitting across the desk from you.

## Questioning Strategies

**Questioning strategies** involve asking the correct types of questions to gather information from the caller so you can evaluate the information received. Closed questions require short responses, and open questions require an explanation. Closed questions are used for information gathering (e.g., name, address, and age of the caller), and should be asked as soon as possible in the conversation. Open questions are used to collect information regarding a chief complaint or past dental experiences. It is helpful to take accurate notes for each call, writing on a scrap piece of paper, message form, telephone conversation recording form, or telephone log.

## Telephone Communication Documentation

Documentation of telephone use involves taking telephone messages, using a telephone conversation recording form, or completing a telephone log. Telephone message forms are used to document information gathered from a caller when the person being called is unable to answer the phone. Whether it is a telephone log, conversation recording form, or message, the information gathered must be accurate. Request the correct spelling of the caller's name and use the name several times during the conversation. Everyone likes to hear the sound of his or her name, and it makes the caller feel valued. Restating information after listening to the caller's message verifies that the correct information was received. Use questioning strategies to check that an accurate message transfer has occurred. If you are familiar with the problem the caller is describing, maintain your level of attention until he or she has finished talking before responding. Once you are certain you understand the caller's request, suggest a course of action. To end the call, explain the office procedure regarding appointment scheduling, financial arrangements, and other pertinent information.

Telephone conversation recording forms are questionnaires used to document the information gathered from a phone conversation regarding a patient's description of his or her current health situation (*Box 8.2*). Determining the reason the patient is calling helps you focus on his or her need for care and comfort in a potentially stressful situation.

---

**BOX 8.2** *Telephone Conversation Recording Form*

Time and date of call: _____

Name: _____

Address: _____

Home phone number: _____

Cell phone number: _____

Work phone number: _____

Patient's description of the problem: _____

The questions on the conversation recording form help you assess whether the caller is having a true dental emergency. Patients in an emergency situation will have specific answers to questions about discomfort, the location of the discomfort, the length of time in discomfort, and the presence of swelling. Emergency dental patients complaining of pain, swelling, or bleeding are usually seen by the dentist as soon as possible.

A **telephone log** is a written record kept in a journal of all telephone calls placed and received each day. It is maintained as a legal record of business performed and is helpful in determining telephone use.

## Incoming and Outgoing Telephone Calls

The dental office receives many incoming calls during business hours. Calls are received for office personnel and for conducting business. There are many outgoing calls made during business hours, and it helps to know the person's name and telephone number before dialing. Organize your thoughts beforehand—for example, have a written list of supplies to be ordered or questions to ask. Dial the number, greet the person, and identify yourself before stating the reason for the call; be sure to end the conversation politely.

Frequently called names and phone numbers are located near the telephone to save time and the inconvenience of having to look up the number. Automatic dialing buttons on programmable telephones help with frequently dialed numbers. Automated computer software programs, such as *TeleVox*, make patient appointment confirmation calls and then document whether someone listened to the whole message, the message was left on a recorder, or no one answered. A report can be printed from the service via a secure Internet website. Although confirmation calls are made as a courtesy service for patients, the patients are still responsible for keeping their scheduled appointments.

## FACSIMILE

**Facsimile** machines, commonly called fax machines, offer a form of electronic communication that transmits a digital or photocopy image via telephone lines. A fax machine scans typed, handwritten, and graphic material and converts it into electrical impulses to produce a copy on the receiver's machine. Usually, a separate telephone line is dedicated for the use of a fax machine. Examples of faxed transmissions are privacy information, prescriptions to a pharmacy, supply orders, insurance company information, and product sales information.

## COMPUTERS

Computers are an integral part of the dental office, and the number of computerized dental practices is increasing dramatically. Computers are used for telecommunications via Internet advertising, the practice website, and email communication with clients. Although email communication with clients is becoming more common, the telephone is still the most vital telecommunication tool. Computers are also used to manage the clinical and business aspects of the practice. An estimated 7 out of 10 dental offices use a computer for business management procedures, recording clinical treatment data, and internal/external marketing techniques. Successful use of a computerized business office system depends on the practice needs and the staff's ability.

## Computer Software

Software programs implement specific tasks or applications. **Application programs** perform specific functions, such as word processing, accounting procedures, graphics, appointment scheduling, treatment planning and diagnosis, insurance claims processing, and recording assessment findings.

Software selection depends on reliability, technical support, and ease of use. User-friendly programs are available for a number of functions and in a variety of designs; however, they should enhance the production and management of the dental practice and improve oral healthcare delivery, helping the practice attain its long- and short-term goals. Firewall and virus-protection software programs are essential to prevent attempts to destroy data, overload the office's computers, or even crash the computer system.

Internet access is useful in the operatory to find medical, drug, product, and other information to inform the patient. Many dental practices have a website to promote the practice, post surveys, provide information, educate the public, post newsletters, and interest new residents. Web cam video capability allows the public to view the practice operation. Email provides another method of written communication with patients and allows the office to send newsletters, statements, and patient education materials directly to patients, reducing the use of paper and postage costs. Digital radiographs can be shared via email with other healthcare providers, once client permission is given. Caution should be used in transmitting material electronically, in accessing online resources or discussions, and in posting any materials, because of the risk of viruses, hackers, and security breaches.

## Business Administration Applications

Computerized business systems reduce administrative procedures and allow staff more time for other tasks. The dental software program should follow established procedures for efficient processing of patient accounts during exiting procedures. Dental software programs allow dental and medical insurance claims processing. *Box 8.3* lists a typical sce-

---

**BOX 8.3** *Patient Exiting Procedures*

Inputting treatment descriptions and dental/medical insurance codes
Posting charges
Collecting and posting payments
Producing a walk-out statement and insurance claim
Updating recare status
Appointment scheduling

nario of patient exiting procedures. Related dental business tasks performed by a computer system are given in *Box 8.4*.

### ACCOUNTS RECEIVABLE AND PAYABLE

The **accounts receivable** program generates the unpaid patient balances for services rendered. The patient account, amount owed, and account age (30, 60, 90 days) are itemized on an accounts receivable report. The **accounts payable** program allows for the payment of dental office bills and for check writing. Payroll processing and the calculation of quarterly tax data are usually found within this program.

### INSURANCE CLAIMS PROCESSING

**Insurance claims processing** is the preparation of dental and medical insurance forms. It encompasses the following tasks:

- Inputting pending or completed treatment information for single or multiple insurance carriers.
- Printing claims for each patient or in batch processing.
- Filing claims by mail or electronically.
- Tracking the payment status of claims.

Electronically filed claims are transmitted from the dental office computers to those of the insurance carrier or clearinghouse. This method of filing claims saves up to 80% of processing time and reduces paperwork. An aged insurance receivable report tracks the payment status of unpaid insurance claims and how long they have been outstanding.

### PRETREATMENT ESTIMATES AND TREATMENT NARRATIVES

Pretreatment estimate reports track when and to which insurance carrier pretreatment estimates were submitted. Insurance companies require pretreatment estimates when more expensive treatment is proposed. Not all dental treatment is posted to the account at the initial appointment (for example, prosthetics). These procedures can be posted when a completion date is available.

   Treatment narratives are written reports that detail treatment rendered to facilitate claim payment of specialized procedures. Treatment narratives are found in many software programs and are generated from a word-processing program.

---

**BOX 8.4** *Dental Software Program Tasks*

| | |
|---|---|
| Accounts payable | Patient financial accounts |
| Accounts receivable | Practice production analysis reports |
| Appointment scheduling | Prescription writing |
| Insurance claims processing | Pretreatment estimates |
| Letter writing | Recare/preventative management |
| Patient billing and financial management | |

## APPOINTMENT SCHEDULING

Appointment scheduling programs help the office deliver oral healthcare services in a reasonable amount of time and in an efficient, financially productive manner. They can keep track of multiple office locations, treatment rooms, and oral healthcare providers (dentist, specialist, hygienist, expanded function assistant). Production planning reports estimate the expected daily, weekly, monthly, or yearly income based on currently scheduled appointments. **Production goals** are income-planning strategies. Short-term production goals focus on daily or weekly planning, whereas long-term goals take a monthly or yearly approach. Production goals are discussed further in Chapter 12.

## RECARE/PREVENTATIVE MANAGEMENT

Recare programs are extremely significant for a productive dental practice. Effective recare/preventative systems result in more efficiency and increased practice production. A weak or mismanaged recare system will have negative effects in the areas of diagnosis, accepted dental treatment, and accounts receivable. A comprehensive computer program enables patient tracking and updating of the patient's current recare status. Computer-generated production goals and the tracking of missed appointments are essential for maintaining an effective recare/preventative system. Recare reports can generate a list of all patients with outstanding unscheduled recare appointments and can even create mailing labels. Recare systems are discussed in greater detail in Chapter 16.

## PATIENT RECORDS

The patient record database is the heart of any dental practice management system. A **database** is a group of related files. It is imperative that the records are accurate and updated regularly. Patient records consist of financial account data and patient health information. Insurance coverage information is found in the financial account. Basic account information should include the first and last name of the responsible party, along with the patient's name (and nickname), address, telephone numbers, birth date, Social Security number, employer information, referral source, and current balance status. Computer programs assign an account number and indicate the account type (cash, insurance, payment plan) for each patient.

Computerized patient records are accessed by entering the account number, by conducting an alphabetical search of first or last name, or by searching for the Social Security number. Patient account data are entered and updated at each visit.

## PATIENT BILLING AND FINANCIAL MANAGEMENT

Patient billing and financial management directly affect the condition of the accounts receivable. Mismanaged patient billing procedures do not allow for a productive cash flow situation. The staff member enters the insurance procedure codes that define which comprehensive services were performed, and the computer generates insurance claims and walk-out statements. Patient billing begins after treatment when a routing slip or superbill is generated. The form serves as a billing and treatment record. Billing information notes the current balance, fees for services rendered, insurance codes, and posted payments. The treatment record indicates recare status, procedures performed, next appointment procedures, and procedure descriptions. The routing slip/superbill can be used as a walk-out statement for the patient or can be attached to an insurance claim for payment processing.

Monthly billing statements are generated and mailed to patients as a demand for payment of services rendered. This system can be done on a selected date, once a month, or cyclically. Accounts are aged at the beginning of each month before statements are printed to determine length of time for carryover balances. Assessment of finance charges or the printing of customized messages are performed at billing time.

Financial management, as it applies to patient billing, may include installment plans to allow monthly payments. Installment coupons can be computer generated and used as an effective collection tool.

## PRACTICE PRODUCTION ANALYSIS REPORTS

Practice production analysis reports provide vital information when the offices wants to assess the practice's growth and stability. Productivity and production goals can be monitored and analyzed on an as-needed basis. Although reports may vary in format, they generally include an analysis of production, collection, accounts receivable, new patient totals, referral sources, treatment provider summaries, and treatment pending summaries.

- Daily reports: transaction listing, personnel production summary (one per provider), charges and payments (day sheet), insurance claims filed, summary of procedures performed, new patients added, new/modified recalls, bank deposit slip, transferred to installments.
- Monthly: purged recalls report, purged insurance claims, purged installments, account activity detail report, cash receivables aged trial balance (by provider), insurance claims status report (by provider), installment accounts receivable aged trail balance (by provider), monthly provider summary, monthly practice summary, practice management reports (combined and individual).
- Yearly: account history detail report, accounts receivable reports, superbill/MTD statement/YTD statement, account history (2 years), monthly statement (mailer or standard), accounts receivable aged trial balance, accounts receivable past due listing.

## PRACTICE MARKETING APPLICATIONS

Promoting the dental practice is a marketing tool to increase production, patient referrals, and treatment acceptance. Correspondence generated from a word-processing program can be merged with information from patient and treatment records. More information regarding public relations can be found in Chapter 20.

## CLINICAL APPLICATIONS

Computer systems are also used when diagnosing and recording clinical data. Many dental operatories are equipped with a computer station with a keyboard or other input device to allow for the entering of patient data. These data may include dental charting, periodontal examination, restorative treatment, appointment scheduling, and preoperative and postoperative treatment instructional aids and handouts. A hard copy of this information can be printed for the patient or oral healthcare provider to use in the development of case presentations. Practices that employ a computer system in this manner develop better interaction and rapport with their patients.

Inventory control management can also be performed using computer programs. These allow the practice to monitor inventory stock, use, and expenses. Inventory purchasing application programs, online purchasing, and access to websites for product recommendations are additional systems managed by the computer.

## CONCEPT SUMMARY

- Telecommunication systems in the dental office include landline and mobile telephones, facsimile (fax) machines, computers, webcams, radio, television, microwave, and satellite.
- The telephone is one of the most important and monitored office systems; more than 95% of the dental office's business is received via the telephone.
- Business administration, practice promotion, and the clinical applications of a dental practice can be managed via computer programs.
- Dental office management reports include those related to patient data, accounts payable and receivable, insurance, and inventory.

## REVIEW QUESTIONS

1. What is telecommunications?
2. Why is the role of the telephone so vital in the dental office?
3. How quickly should the telephone be answered?
4. What is the difference between open and closed questions?
5. Why is it necessary to restate directions over the telephone?
6. What information do you expect to obtain from a patient in the case of an emergency?
7. Why are messages taken, conversations recorded, and telephone logs maintained?
8. How does a facsimile machine affect daily business operation?
9. How are computerized dental systems used in the practice setting?
10. List nine business administrative applications that can be managed on a computer system.
11. Describe the three parts of computerized patient records.
12. What are the functions of a routing slip or superbill?
13. List examples of daily reports, monthly reports, and yearly reports.
14. How is a dental office's computer used for public relations and clinical management of patients?

# CRITICAL THINKING ACTIVITY

- Search the Internet for dental practice websites in your area and evaluate one site based on the information provided, appearance, and office promotion.
- Write an email message to the practice to tell it your thoughts about its website.
- Search the Internet for patient information on the topics of xerostomia products, toothpaste allergy, and sonic toothbrushes.

## Group Assignment: Role-Playing

Using role-playing, work out a script for each of the following situations.

- Take a call to schedule an appointment with a patient who is difficult to satisfy.
- Make a call to request an overdue financial account payment.
- Make a call to reschedule an appointment because of the healthcare provider's absence.
- Make a call to confirm an appointment with a patient.
- Make a call to order supplies.
- Make a call to schedule an appointment for a patient on the wait list.
- Take a call from a patient shopping for dental procedure prices.
- Take a call from a patient who wants to talk to the dentist to schedule an appointment.
- Take a call from a patient who wants to speak personally to the dentist.
- Take a call from a patient who is upset about his or her account balance.

# Dental Hygiene Treatment

## LEARNING OUTCOMES

**Upon mastery of the content of this chapter, the student should be able to:**
- Differentiate between the dental hygienist and the advanced dental hygiene practitioner.
- Recognize the minimal intervention philosophy in minimally invasive therapy.
- Describe the dental hygiene process of care in assessment, planning, and implementation of dental hygiene comprehensive services associated with dental practice management.
- Determine the opportunities available in alternative forms of practice.
- Conceptualize the notion of treating the patient's care and comfort needs as a customer service.
- Characterize the services delivered in the dental spa.

## KEY TERMS

| | |
|---|---|
| advanced dental hygiene practitioner | implementation |
| alternative practice | independent practice |
| collaborative practice | minimal intervention |
| dental hygiene diagnosis | minimally invasive therapy |
| dental spas | oral risk assessment |
| evidence-based care | treatment planning |

## DENTAL HYGIENE TREATMENT

The careful assessment, planning, and implementation of dental hygiene care and the opportunity to work in various settings have made practice management skills vitally important. Dental hygienists are becoming entrepreneurs by opening independent practices and entering collaborative partnerships that require knowledge of practice management systems. Although most dental hygienists work in the dental hygiene department of a private dental practice owned by a dentist, ongoing changes in supervision, technology, and healthcare philosophy are turning the dental hygiene profession into an expanding field of healthcare practice that uses a variety of interventions and therapies. These advances in the dental hygiene profession are the result of a global transformation. The practice of dental hygiene is beginning to resemble other healthcare fields because professionals are able to open their own businesses as supervision and practice restrictions are moderated. Today's dental hygienists must be able to locate and critically review new technologies and clinical research findings that affect the way in which they treat their clients. The competitive edge is in treating patients' care and comfort needs in a business environment that takes advantage of all available technology.

In the United States, dental hygiene practice evolved to the point at which the licensed dental hygienist performed comprehensive oral healthcare services under the direct supervision of a dentist. This traditional standard of care is still the norm in a little over half of the states; in the remaining U.S. jurisdictions, the mode of practice supervision has changed. There is a current trend in dental hygiene for the easing of restrictions in supervision and care. General supervision and/or unsupervised practice are allowable in 19 states (*Table 9.1*). Fewer restrictions on supervision allow dental hygienists to work independently of a dentist, to own their own business, to work in collaborative or alternative practices, and to bill for services rendered as providers to the federal government's Medicaid reimbursement program and other insurance carriers. With the freedom to practice in a variety of situations, dental hygienists help more people receive oral healthcare services.

## ADVANCED DENTAL HYGIENE PRACTITIONER

Practice restrictions in oral healthcare delivery are changing to permit licensed dental hygienists to perform additional dental procedures, such as administering local anesthesia (*Table 9.2*). The current emphasis on expanding legally allowable duties through advanced education enables dental hygienists to continue this evolution of their practice. As noted in Chapter 2, dental therapists practicing in Australia and the UK are oral hygiene specialists who perform advanced duties, such as routine restorations and extractions (*Box 9.1*). In New Zealand, Scandinavia, and Canada, citizens have access to care from dental hygienists, nurses, and therapists in public dental settings.

### TABLE 9.1 Extended Supervision by State

| State | Year | Supervision | State | Year | Supervision |
|-------|------|-------------|-------|------|-------------|
| CA | 1998 | General | MO | 2001 | Unsupervised |
| CO | 1987 | Unsupervised | MT | 2003 | General |
| CT | 1999 | Unsupervised | NH | 1993 | General |
| IA | 2004 | General | NM | 1999 | General |
| IL | 2004 | General | NV | 1998 | Unsupervised |
| IN | 1992 | Unsupervised | OK | 2003 | General |
| KS | 2003 | General | OR | 1997 | Unsupervised |
| ME | 2001 | General | TX | 2001 | Unsupervised |
| MI | 1991 | Assignment (general) | WA | 1984 | Unsupervised |
| MN | 2001 | General | | | |

Reprinted from Ring T. Trends in dental hygiene supervision. With permission from the American Dental Hygienists' Association publication *Access* (2004).

## TABLE 9.2 Local Anesthesia Administration by State

| State | Year | Supervision | State | Year | Supervision |
|-------|------|-------------|-------|------|-------------|
| AK | 1981 | Direct | MT | 1985 | Direct |
| AR | 1995 | Direct | ND | 2003 | Direct |
| AZ | 1976 | Direct | NE | 1995 | Direct |
| CA | 1976 | Direct | NH | 2002 | Direct |
| CO | 1977 | Direct | NM | 1972 | Direct |
| CT | 2005 | Indirect | NV | 1972 | Direct* |
| DC | 2004 | Direct | NY | 2001 | Direct |
| HI | 1987 | Direct | OK | 1980 | Direct |
| IA | 1998 | Direct | OR | 1975 | General |
| ID | 1975 | General | RI | 2005 | Pending |
| IL | 2000 | Direct | SC | 1995 | Direct |
| KS | 1993 | Direct | SD | 1992 | Direct |
| KY | 2002 | Direct | TN | 2004 | Direct |
| LA | 1998 | Direct | UT | 1983 | Direct |
| MA | 2004 | Direct | VT | 1993 | Direct |
| ME | 1997 | Direct | WA | 1971 | Direct |
| MI | 2002 | Direct | WI | 1998 | Direct |
| MN | 1995 | Indirect | WV | 2003 | Direct |
| MO | 1973 | Direct | WY | 1991 | Direct |

*General in some institutions.

Reprinted from www.adha.org/governmental_affairs/downloads/LocalAnthsiachart.pdf. With permission from the American Dental Hygienists' Association.

In the United States, the **advanced dental hygiene practitioner** (ADHP) is a new practice standard for which dental hygienists earn an additional credential after completing an advanced curriculum in diagnostic, preventative, restorative, and therapeutic services. It is thought that the ADHP will perform additional procedural regimens. The American Dental Hygienists' Association (ADHA) created the ADHP in response to needs expressed in the first-ever dental report from the U.S. surgeon general, titled *Oral*

**BOX 9.1** *Advanced Practitioner Procedures*

Advise on oral healthcare
Consult and refer when necessary to another healthcare provider
Extract deciduous teeth
Intraoral and extraoral assessment and care plan development
Perform pulpal therapy and place preformed crowns on deciduous teeth
Prepare temporary crown and filling replacements
Provide limited orthodontic procedures
Restore deciduous and permanent teeth
Take impressions
Use dental materials

*Healthcare in America.* This 2000 report identified access-to-care issues in underserved populations. Current trends in dental education are for increased numbers of dental hygiene graduates and decreased numbers of dental school graduates. These trends have lead to a decline in the availability of oral healthcare professionals overall and especially for low-income, uninsured, and geographically underserved citizens in urban and rural settings.

## Minimally Invasive Therapy

The dental therapist practicing in other countries may follow the principle of minimal intervention. **Minimal intervention** (MI) is a philosophy that uses the medical model to treat disease therapeutically. The MI philosophy separates dentistry into two main segments, similar to medicine: surgical and nonsurgical interventions for the treatment of microbial-based infections, such as caries and periodontal diseases. Currently, dental hygienists perform **minimally invasive therapy,** which is the nonsurgical approach to oral healthcare delivery using therapeutic agents and regimens. Caries removal involves the surgical amputation of the tooth structure, which is replaced with a biocompatible dental material. Caries therapy is a nonsurgical method of treating tooth infection using toothpastes, nutritional counseling, nutritional supplements, prescriptions such as fluoride and chlorhexidine gluconate, and other processes and products to improve saliva quality. Caries therapeutics and regimens are billable dental hygiene procedures performed within the dental hygienist's scope of practice.

Periodontal diseases are treated using therapies and regimens to stop the infection process. Nonsurgical periodontal treatment is at the heart of soft tissue management programs administered by dental hygienists. The basic categories of comprehensive oral healthcare services are preventive, periodontal, and adjunct procedures. These are the major billable procedure code services performed by dental hygienists during nonsurgical periodontal therapy. When these interventions are not successful, referral to the periodontist becomes necessary for the surgical aspect of periodontal care.

## DENTAL HYGIENE PROCESS OF CARE

Basic dental treatment follows a planned sequence that includes immediate care, assessment/diagnostic procedures, nonsurgical therapy, surgical therapy, and maintenance. Comprehensive patient care is based on dental hygiene diagnosis and a care plan that is a progression of procedures performed after informed consent has been obtained. Consultation with the patient's medical doctor, a dental specialist, or a healthcare provider who is an expert in a discipline may be required to identify all treatment options and technologies available for patient care. *Box 9.2* offers a guideline for patient care procedures.

### Assessment

Assessment procedures identify thousands of dollars' worth of dental needs, yet the average dental patient spends less than $200 per year for oral healthcare services. Attention to detail during data-collection procedures is a valuable service given to patients. Patient-centered total care requires the completion and review of the personal, medical, and

> **BOX 9.2**  *Summary of Data Collection and Care Implementation*
>
> Assessment information, including personal and dental history; financial, medical, and dental insurance information; and oral risk assessment
> Radiographic and photographic, periodontal, and clinical examination plus diagnostic testing
> Treatment planning, case presentation, informed consent, and financial arrangements
> Treatment scheduling and implementation, documentation of services rendered, routing slips, and narrative reports
> Recare appointment scheduling

dental histories; a risk assessment survey; and clinical, periodontal, and radiographic examinations performed during the comprehensive oral examination appointment. By interviewing the patient and reviewing the completed forms with him or her, the professional will be able to discover any areas of noncompliance with prescribed medications, any omissions in treatment, and any fears the patient may have. This process also builds trust and develops rapport, especially with patients who have nonphysical concerns. Office forms used to document patient information are covered in Chapter 22.

Personal history screening forms document information about residency, financial status, and insurance coverage, and are further evidence of the patient's status. Medical history screening forms document information about medical conditions reported by the client. The dental hygienist does not make a medical diagnosis; the client reports a diagnosis that has already been made. Dental history screening forms document signs and symptoms of dental disease and/or disorders reported by the patient.

### ORAL RISK ASSESSMENT

Risk assessment is a method of data collection in which the patient completes a document referred to as an oral risk assessment survey. The **oral risk assessment** survey is used to assist in making an accurate diagnosis by identifying patient factors that increase the risk of oral disease from environmental, behavioral, or biological conditions. Factors reported by the patient that adversely affect oral health, such as smoking, certain medications, and some systemic diseases, may identify treatment interventions within the scope of practice for dental hygiene. Early intervention and treatment are based on the findings of the oral risk assessment survey along with all other data collected.

## Diagnosis

Diagnosis is a key component for adequate treatment of dental diseases. Dental hygienists are educated to perform comprehensive oral examinations as a requirement for licensure; however, the dental insurance procedural code for the comprehensive examination is defined as "performed by a dentist or dental specialist" and thus excludes the dental hygienist. The jurisdiction may define who performs examinations and further legislative change may be necessary to allow dental hygienists to perform comprehensive oral examinations and to permit more access to care. The dental insurance code definitions do not specify the dentist as the provider of the periodic examination, problem-focused examination, or periodontal examination. The periodic examination is performed routinely on the patient who has been accepted for treatment. An example of a problem-focused examination appointment is evaluating periodontal conditions in a specific quadrant to determine whether retreatment is necessary during periodontal antibiotic chemotherapy. Periodontal examination is the evaluation of periodontal conditions and may be performed during a periodontal maintenance appointment.

## Planning

Planning is a reflection of the provider's mission or philosophy of care and allows the focus of treatment to be the pursuit of measurable results. Planning directs behavior, establishes activities to be performed, and increases accountability; in other words, without a plan, you will not know where you are going. A dental hygiene diagnosis determines the limits of oral healthcare services. There are many definitions for the dental hygiene diagnosis, and an ongoing debate regarding this issue exists as a result of state statutes and practice parameters. The **dental hygiene diagnosis** can be based on human needs deficits, client oral hygiene needs, statements regarding necessary care but not diagnostic statements, or the identification of conditions that are treated by the dental hygienist. Dental hygiene treatment interventions can then be planned and implemented because the diagnosis is made from the factual assessment of evidence.

**Treatment planning** is an organized sequence of appointments intended to control, eliminate, prevent, and stabilize disease by phases, and each phase includes a reevaluation to assess disease management. There are many ways to document treatment plans using a variety of paper forms and computer programs. A universal sequence or protocol can be followed, depending on patient needs, the plans used by the practice, and the standard of care (*Box 9.3*). The premium treatment plan is recommended first, then alternative therapies and regimens are made available from which the patient can choose when he or she does not accept the best care plan. The optimum treatment is not necessarily the most difficult or expensive. If the patient chooses a no-treatment option, the risks associated with continued disease and systemic illness must be fully explained.

### EVIDENTIAL RESEARCH

The association between oral infection and physical health has changed the focus of dental hygiene treatment to patient-centered, evidence-based care. **Evidence-based care (EBC)** is a treatment approach that integrates a variety of patient information to make an assessment of the treatment needs and then offers the patient choices. Successful treat-

---

**BOX 9.3** *Basic Treatment Plan Sequence*

1. Urgent, immediate care
2. Diagnostic procedures
3. Nonsurgical therapy and regimens
4. Surgical therapy, including reconstruction
5. Maintenance

ment outcomes using EBC affect the patient psychologically, physiologically, and economically. The written plans associated with rehabilitation, effective therapies, and alternative treatments have outcomes that can be measured. Influential factors in clinical decision making include success and failure rate and proven and possible risks. For example, a patient with type III adult chronic periodontitis who smokes one pack of cigarettes per day has a risk factor that may affect the outcome of a nonsurgical periodontal therapy plan.

An Internet search for scientific information is considered the most effective way to get proven evidence regarding possible treatment outcomes. Using electronic searches also enables the clinician to access current treatment recommendations and therapeutics. It is important to find supporting information and documentation of evidence from a variety of Internet sources because no one website can provide access to all oral healthcare information. Databases that can help the dental hygienist locate oral healthcare information include the Cochrane Group (www.cochrane-oral.man.ac.uk), PubMed (www.ncbi.nlm.nih.gov), Agency for Healthcare Policy and Research (www.ahcpr.gov/clinic/index.html), National Guideline Clearinghouse (www.guideline.gov), and university and professional association websites.

## CASE PRESENTATION

The dental hygienist does not "make up" or decide on treatment for the patient; treatment is based on assessment and planning procedures. Dental hygiene services have real value for the patient. Unfortunately, dental treatment is considered by many to be an optional use of discretionary income and agreeing to begin treatment for diseases of the mouth is frequently based on the patient's economic priorities. It is easy for the client to devalue his or her mouth with the multitude of choices on which to spend one's money, such as cell phones, portable computers, cosmetic and plastic surgery, casinos, vacations, and designer clothing items. Perhaps this explains why the average patient has thousands of dollars of need yet spends less than $200 per year on dental care.

Patients need to be continually educated about the value of oral healthcare for their well-being. Creating value using patient education helps clients understand and want the services they need. Education should use a multimedia approach, such as an intraoral camera to photograph the appearance of the oral conditions; cosmetic imaging; and CD-ROM educational programs that include photos, graphics, animation, and sound to appeal to all levels of learning. Once the patient has the perception of value for oral healthcare, he or she will be more eager to purchase the care required. Additional tips on case presentation are found in Chapter 19.

## Implementation

After all of the preliminary procedures are performed, the treatment is presented, and informed consent is obtained, financial arrangements are made with the patient before work begins. Financial arrangements depend on the choices and plans available from the practice and are discussed in Chapter 13. It is vitally important to have the patient begin treatment as soon as possible once consent and financial arrangements are negotiated. Once the consent is obtained and financial arrangements are made, schedule the client as soon as possible to increase the likelihood of treatment completion.

**Implementation** is the delivery of dental hygiene comprehensive services. Several factors related to practice management are important for the delivery of a high level of customer service to the patient. Dental hygienists need excellent clinical skills plus people and business skills. Clinical excellence must be communicated; patients should understand that they are receiving current treatment modalities and appropriate and up-to-date technology, and that the dental professional is following government regulations for the standard of care.

However, patients will not necessarily return for continued care, even if clinical excellence was delivered, if they believe they were given inadequate customer service. Office appearance is one criterion clients use to make judgments about their service. The patient's overall experience must be pleasant in addition to being delivered via state-of-the-art procedures and materials to instill a sense of value for the care received. This level of customer service entails giving the patient undivided attention during communication and establishing a rapport by being a trustworthy people person. Satisfied patients who have had a positive experience, and who feel valued and liked, will become devoted customers who recommend the practice to family and friends.

Once the patient arrives for a scheduled appointment, avoid making him or her wait for treatment. A waiting patient quickly becomes disgruntled. When the patient must wait because of scheduling delays, make sure he or she is told about the waiting time. One method to make amends for being more than 10 minutes behind schedule is to offer to reschedule with a monetary credit applied to the patient's account (for example, $25), if he or she agrees to reappoint. This may make the patient slightly less aggravated by the situation.

## Exiting Procedures

After each dental appointment, the dental care delivered is documented on a paper form referred to as the routing slip or superbill, which is given to the person in the front office, who performs the exiting procedures. The routing slip identifies procedures completed by the insurance code or office code number to be charged to the patient. Exiting procedures allow for discussion of care, any perceived discrepancies between oral healthcare procedures delivered and account charges, account payments, appointment scheduling, insurance transactions, purchasing of additional goods or services, and enjoyment of refreshments such as bottled water or coffee. Document all services rendered by either insurance code or office procedure code, even when there is no fee attached to the service. Entering a "no charge" after the treatment name will reinforce to the patient that more care was delivered than what was paid for, giving the perception of added value.

## INDEPENDENT PRACTICE ENTREPRENEURS

**Independent practice** is the right of a dental hygienist to own a practice in the same way as other healthcare providers. Dental hygienists in Colorado, New Mexico, and California have the option to own a dental hygiene practice. A limited number of dental hygienists practice independently in Colorado and face the entrepreneurial challenges of working under contract, renting office space, working as independent contractors, and starting a practice. A limited number of dental hygienists are participating Medicaid providers, treating underserved populations. In Oregon and Washington, dental hygienists practice without supervision and own dental hygiene businesses. Dental hygiene entrepreneurs are motivated risk takers who want to own a business for many reasons, including job security, personal advancement, financial incentives, and fewer restrictions on practice because in the traditional workplace the dentist delegates time and procedures. These restrictions may result in a philosophical dilemma for the dental hygiene practitioner wishing to provide comprehensive services.

Office systems must be in place for business operations to calculate and capitalize on resources to ensure quality of care (*Box 9.4*). As is true for all healthcare settings, a clearly defined mission statement helps set the tone and parameters of the practice. Some independent practices have a defined mission to perform outreach work with portable equipment for use in areas without oral healthcare providers.

Limitations to owning a dental hygiene practice include supervision issues, establishing dental supply accounts, and insurance company acceptance to become a provider. As previously noted, most jurisdictions require direct supervision for the administration of local anesthesia (see *Table 9.2*); therefore, the independent practice requires the presence of a dentist for supervision when anesthesia is administered for scaling and root planing. Dental supply companies have accounts established for dentists with prescription drug identification numbers, thus excluding the dental hygienist from purchasing power. The exception is Oregon, which is the first jurisdiction in the United States to permit dental hygienists to prescribe and dispense fluoride, fluoride varnish, antimicrobial rinses, and resorbable antimicrobial agents. Another exclusionary hurdle in some states is a specific type of insurance law that mandates payment of services be made to licensed dentists. A limitation of dental hygiene practice may be attracting and hiring employees to assist in oral healthcare delivery and the management of office systems. This occurs when the dental hygiene practice is experiencing growth and needs dental assistants. There is a nationwide shortage of dental assistants, and trained assistants are a premium commodity.

## Alternative Practice

**Alternative practice** is a licensure category in California. Candidates with a current California RDH license, a minimum of 2,000 hours of clinical practice during the pre-

---

**BOX 9.4** *Practice Management Systems*

| | |
|---|---|
| Accounting | Production |
| Appointment scheduling | Public relations |
| Communications | Recare/continued care |
| Credit and collections | Records management |
| Insurance | Staffing |
| Inventory | Taxation |
| Payroll | Telecommunications |
| Policy and procedures manual | |

ceding 36 months, a bachelor's degree or its equivalent, and 150 hours of an approved educational program, and who have passed a written examination, become a registered dental hygienist in alternative practice (RDHAP). An RDHAP practices as an employee of a dentist, an employee of another registered dental hygienist in alternative practice, an independent contractor, a sole proprietor of an alternative dental hygiene practice, an employee of a primary care clinic or specialty clinic, or an employee of a clinic owned or operated by a public hospital or health system. The RDHAP must provide documentation of an existing relationship with at least one dentist with a current license. RDHAP services require a written prescription valid for 15 months from issuance by a dentist, physician, or surgeon after a physical examination and diagnosis.

## Collaborative Practice

**Collaborative practice,** administered in Minnesota and New Mexico, allows dental hygienists to practice under general supervision with one or more consulting dentists after receiving standing orders for established treatment protocols and any additional procedures that require authorization to perform. Consultations may be provided via teledentistry, which is the use of electronic technology to transmit information such as digital x-rays, images, and patient information to a dentist.

## EVALUATION/CONTINUING CARE

Communication is important throughout the course of treatment to emphasize the need for continuing care. Many people have the misconception that after completion of their current course of treatment, their treatment is finished and continuing care is not necessary. The patient must be educated regarding the necessity of recare to follow the profession's standard of care protocols. It is not just your office policy but the industry standard that dictates the recare continuum. Choose words such as *recare, reevaluation,* and *continuing care* instead of *recall.* The word *recall* has negative connotations because it is often used to describe defective merchandise and services. Evaluation procedures are performed during examinations, consultations, recare, and office visits.

## PATIENT CARE AND COMFORT NEEDS

In many geographical locations, the public has plenty of choice when selecting a dental practice. The economic climate and job market conditions dictate the decision regarding choice. This makes the competition for patients in the dental service industry fairly intense in some locales. Patients may postpone elective procedures, making it necessary to keep a loyal client base by providing first-class customer service. Clinical excellence plus patient satisfaction, individualized care, and comfort are becoming important aspects of the dental visit experience. In addition, many clients have less personal time in which to pamper themselves, and meeting these perceived needs for care and comfort can be accomplished in many ways. Certainly seeing the patient on time and valuing his or her time cannot be overemphasized. Time is everyone's greatest commodity and it needs to be treated respectfully.

## THE DENTAL SPA

More people are interested in the appearance of their smile, such as having whiter, straighter teeth, and in having fresh breath. A beautiful smile is more than a fashion accessory; it demonstrates good physical health and beauty and boosts mental health. One emerging trend to meet patient demands for service is the dental spa. **Dental spas** are dental practices that offer a blend of medicine with dentistry plus any number of services, such as hair, skin, hand, and foot care plus hair removal, massage, makeup, and/or fashion advice.

The association between a visit to the dental office and pain makes some clients avoid seeking dental care because of their fear. Human needs and deficits, Maslow's hierarchy of needs, and other methods explain the basics of what humans need and want. The dental office spa takes into account that care and comfort are primary needs. Amenities to meet these needs take into consideration all the senses—touch, smell, sight, sound, and taste.

It is recommended that the dental treatment areas be separate from the spa areas. To evoke serenity, the entry of the dental spa may have an upscale personality to help create favorable first impressions. The entry may be fashioned like a living room, with large overstuffed chairs and couches, or be similar to a hotel lobby, with plenty of space to give the impression of openness. The reception desk may resemble a hotel/business lobby or a concierge workstation from which greetings and office tours are handled. Serene color schemes, lighting, music, temperature, and air quality continue to create this welcoming environment. Refreshment bars offering beverages and fresh baked goods may be available for waiting patients. Colored lights and written messages from the communication system should not detract from the restful waiting experience. The area reserved for exiting procedures should be set apart from the business space to allow for private financial discussion and transactions with the client.

### Dental Operatory Spa

In the operatory, spa care begins with modern equipment as well as ergonomic chair designs for comfort to accommodate many body sizes and positions. Warm towels and blankets, pillows, and posttreatment washcloths are given as needed. Oral cancer screenings with an emphasis on head and neck massage further address the sense of touch. Aromatherapy is used to induce serenity using the sense of smell via air fragrance and scented gloves. The room lights are dimmed and objects are placed around the room in regard to feng shui and to allow open air space. Entertainment systems, such as satellite or cable television, CD/DVD players, movies, and music delivered via earphones or headsets provide distraction to make the time more pleasant and seem to go by faster. Flavored gloves, dental unit water, and rinses appeal to the patient's sense of taste. Any room with equipment that generates loud noise or smells, such as the staff lounge, sterilization room, and dental laboratory, should be placed away from patient care areas to complete the attention to detail.

## PRIVATE DISCUSSIONS

By focusing attention on care and comfort, the dental hygienist helps to put the patient at ease and strives to make him or her comfortable in the dental operatory. In addition to the intimacy of the contact made with patients and the level of trust that develops is the intimate relationship the professional builds with them. Dental hygienists frequently are the healthcare provider that an individual visits more often than any other. This allows for private discussions with patients. Patients may want to discuss their grief over the loss of a loved one, family situation or dynamics, fears, or abuse and neglect. Many times being a listener is all that is required. But just as the hygienist refers the patient to other healthcare providers, he or she may make referrals to domestic violence programs, suicide hotlines, or the local department of social services. Keep simple notes in the chart regarding these discussions, such as "patient reports mother's recent death." These notes of the patient's special needs serve as a reminder of the conversation and allows the professional to sincerely ask a patient how he or she is feeling about a recent life event. This level of total patient care embodies the holistic view of health as the integration of the mind, spirit, and body.

## CONCEPT SUMMARY

- The dental hygiene profession is evolving, which has led to the development of the advanced dental hygiene practitioner.
- The minimal intervention philosophy medical model has affected dentistry in a similar way as medicine by delineating practice into surgical and nonsurgical interventions for the treatment of microbial-based infections.
- Minimally invasive therapy is the nonsurgical use of therapeutic agents and regimens.
- The dental hygiene process of care uses dental practice management systems.
- Alternative forms of dental hygiene practice are enabling dental hygienists to become entrepreneurs.
- Attention to the care and comfort needs of clients is an important component of quality customer service.
- Dental spas offer additional services, such as hair, skin, hand, and foot care, and hair removal, massage, and makeup and/or fashion advice.

# REVIEW QUESTIONS

1. What is the difference between the dental hygienist and an advanced dental hygiene practitioner?
2. What are the attributes of the minimal intervention philosophy?
3. How are comprehensive dental hygiene services minimally invasive therapies?
4. Which practice management systems are used for the following aspects of patient care?
   A. Assessment
   B. Diagnosis
   C. Treatment planning and case presentation
   D. Implementation of dental hygiene services
   E. Evaluation of care
5. What is the difference between independent, collaborative, and alternative practice?
6. How are less restrictive forms of practice making oral healthcare available to underserved populations?
7. What are the variations in the dental hygiene diagnosis?

8. What types of services may be delivered at a dental spa?

9. Why are the five senses addressed at the dental spa?

10. When should you write notes about private conversations in the patient's chart?

## CRITICAL THINKING ACTIVITY

- Select a patient variable—such as complex medical history, systemic disorder, or oral risk factor—and search for EBC protocols on the websites provided in this chapter.
- Create a business plan for your own dental hygiene independent, alternative, or collaborative practice incorporating the dental spa philosophy of first-class customer service and appealing to the patient's care and comfort needs. (Perhaps you have some acquaintances that perform baking/culinary arts, cosmetology procedures, certified massage therapy, or hair removal; determine how you could incorporate their services into your business.)
- Identify ways in which a dental assistant can help in the dental hygiene independent, alternative, or collaborative practice.

# Accounting Principles

Upon mastery of the content of this chapter, the student should be able to:

- Differentiate between the accounting systems of accounts receivable, accounts payable, petty cash control, and barter exchanges.
- Describe accounts receivable bookkeeping transactions using a computer software program and accounting board system.
- Recognize accounts receivable activities: transactions, posting, payments, adjustments, daily summaries, accounts receivable, proof of posting, cash control, and bank deposit.
- Recognize accounts payable activities: check writing, completing check stubs, recording disbursements in journals, and performing monthly summaries.
- Recognize cash control and banking activities.
- Describe the internal controls needed to safeguard office assets.

accounting board system
accounts payable
accounts receivable
barter services
disbursement journal
monthly disbursement summary sheets

petty cash control
posting
proof of posting
transactions
walk-out statements

## ACCOUNTING PRINCIPLES

Dentistry is a service industry. All business transactions have a financial value and are documented according to labor, business, corporate, and tax laws. **Transactions** are any account activity, including fees charged, payments received, exchange of goods and services, and account adjustments. Comprehensive oral healthcare procedures are performed to generate an income and all business transactions are documented and monitored. The well-managed dental practice or independent dental hygiene practice has a minimum of three accounting systems: accounts receivable, accounts payable, and petty cash control.

Some oral healthcare providers render dental care using the barter system in which dental services are exchanged for services provided by the patient.

To collect fees for services rendered, the accounts receivable system is implemented. The **accounts receivable** office system is the management of production fees that are owed to the dental practice, payment or credits received, and the summation of unpaid monies due to the dental office. To provide the oral healthcare services that generate office income, an accounts payable system must be in place to pay overhead expenses, employee salaries, dental supply bills, and taxes. The **accounts payable** system is the recording of check and cash disbursements from the dental practice or independent practice bank account. Cash transactions for goods and services, such as postage due or the occasional pizza for lunch, are made from the petty cash fund. The **petty cash control** system is used for recording small cash transactions from the petty cash fund. **Barter services** are organized for trading services in lieu of monetary transactions. Members of barter service organizations provide their service in exchange for a needed service. An example of a barter exchange of services is when an independent dental hygienist performs scaling and root planing services on a carpenter in exchange for the installation of new cabinetry by that carpenter. These business exchanges must be documented similarly to all other transactions.

## ACCOUNTS RECEIVABLE

Accounts receivable can be performed using one of two methods: entering financial data into a dental office computer software program or manually entering data in an account board bookkeeping accounting system. Entering any data into a bookkeeping system is called **posting**. Posting transactions documents the exchange of goods and services and informs the patient about the status of his or her financial obligations. Posting also lets the practice keep track of income generated and monies collected and owed.

Computer software programs facilitate account postings, generate routing slips, and print walk-out statements to document transactions related to daily services rendered. Routing slips are financial accounting forms used by the oral healthcare provider to communicate to the front office staff the charges incurred by the office or insurance procedure code number. This form is completed in addition to the services rendered form, which is found in the patient's file and is used to document treatment details. Account postings of treatment charges are entered into the computer accounting system based on the data recorded on the routing slip, and the form is destroyed during check-out procedures. **Walk-out statements** are financial accounting paper forms similar to receipts; they are generated by the computer software accounting system to serve as an acknowledgment of services performed and monies exchanged.

At the end of each business day, a daily transaction summary report is generated by the dental software system to determine any errors in posting. Account entries made in error are never deleted but just adjusted to remove the error; an electronic note is attached to explain why the adjustment was made. All of the day's transactions are listed alphabetically. The independent dental hygiene practitioner or dentist should monitor the bookkeeping system for errors, fraud, and embezzlement (the theft of office money). Auditing and the use of internal controls help the staff keep an eye on accounting errors.

## Accounting Board System

The **accounting board system** is used to document daily transactions manually on a day sheet. Data include the patient's name, services rendered for that day, previous balance on the patient's account, cash or check payments, adjustments, and new balance. An accounting board system generates routing slips for account postings and receipts to post services rendered; it also registers payment onto the patient's account ledger card. The components of the system consist of a board with pegs or a clamping device along the left side, which is used as a base for the insertion and alignment of several paper forms. The forms inserted onto the board are the day sheet/daily journal page, charge/receipt slip, and patient account ledger card (*Fig. 10.1*).

Each account payment made by cash, check, or credit card at patient check-out, from walk-ins, and from delivered mail is posted. Adjustments, or deductions in the amount due, are discounts given to certain patients. An office may offer a discount to patients who pay in full before treatment begins; to senior citizens; and to friends, family members, and business associates. Other types of adjustments include insurance research and development fees, Medicaid write-offs, nonsufficient funds checks, and client accounts that are sent to a collection agency.

### DAILY SUMMARIES

The total accounts receivable of all services rendered, cash and checks received, and outstanding balances is calculated each day (called a daily summary) to determine the cur-

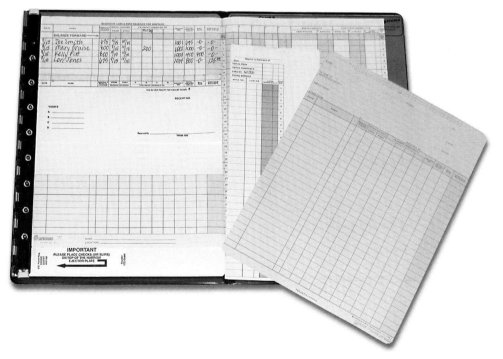

Figure 10.1 An accounting board system. System provided courtesy of Safeguard.

rent balance (*Box 10.1*). Summaries verify the accuracy of entries and help the staff find accounting errors. The calculation of the daily accounts receivable is performed in a specially designed section of the day sheet called "daily accounts receivable control," which is a summary procedure performed to check the accuracy of entries and to find errors in math, transaction postings, and bank deposit amounts.

Another section of the day sheet is **proof of posting**, which is a summary procedure performed to add the day's receivables to the previous day's balance to determine the total accounts receivable balance; the result represents all money due to the practice. The steps for computing total accounts receivable are given in *Box 10.2*. The office also calculates a cash control daily summary. Found on the day sheet, this summarizes the bank deposit information from cash, currency, and checks received that day.

## Account Billing Statements

Billing statements are demands for payment mailed to patients to inform them of their financial status with the dental office. Often, they are sent at the same time each month—typically the 1st, 15th, or 30th—unless the office uses a bimonthly or quarterly billing cycle. Statements show current account charges for each family member, payments received, previous balance, and current account balance. Statements are itemized for each transaction or may be nonitemized, typed, photocopied from an account ledger card, or electronically generated from the dental office software program. A return envelope is frequently included for remittance. Some statements allow for abbreviations with explanations at the bottom of the statement or a computer-generated message. Dental offices may hire an outside private firm or service to prepare statements. Statements are produced, folded, and placed in envelopes; stamped; and bundled by ZIP code.

## ACCOUNTS PAYABLE

Calculations and formulas related to supplies, overhead, and payroll expenses are used to keep spending aligned with income for a healthy private practice. The average total overhead for dental practices is generally 73%. Check disbursements, banking functions, payroll, overhead, and other expenses are documented to track how office funds are spent. The accounts payable system consists of office checks, a disbursement journal containing a monthly summary sheet, and ledger sheets/cards (*Figure 10.2*).

A **disbursement journal** is a special ledger book designed to reflect the dental practice's business transactions related to operational costs. It is maintained similarly to an accounts receivable daily journal page, except that it contains a monthly sheet to register a month of transactions. Disbursement journals allow for the insertion of monthly disbursement summary sheets, ledger control sheets, and office checks.

**Monthly disbursement summary sheets** are paper forms used to record itemized totals (*Box 10.3*). The monthly disbursement summary sheet is divided into columns that provide space for recording the expenses of the office. Yearly summary totals of expenses, quarterly payroll totals for taxation, and a check registry are further uses of the disbursement summary. It is advised that personal checking accounts be kept separate from the office account.

Ledger control sheets are paper forms used for banking, payroll, and other expenses. Banking ledger control sheets record the bank balance and all deposits and checks written for office expenses. Office checks are used to pay for office expenses, and a journal/check register is used to document all checks written.

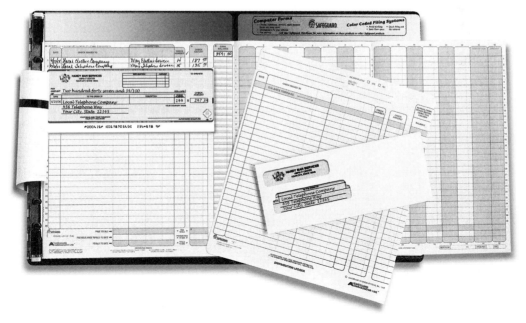

**Figure 10.2** An accounts payable system. System provided courtesy of Safeguard.

## BANKING

Monies received are accounted for and are deposited daily into the practice's account at the bank to reduce the risk for missing funds. A copy of the deposit slip is attached to the daily summary of transactions to validate the proper handling of funds. Daily accounts receivable deposits reduce the chances of office checks being returned for nonsufficient funds. All check payments made related to office operation, including salaries of auxiliary personnel, are documented. Careful and complete record keeping is essential for reducing legal liability of tax fraud by documenting proof that funds are handled properly. Bank statements sent for the office account list previous balance, current balance, checks written, and deposits, similar to the statement of a personal checking account (*Box 10.4*).

### Reconcile Bank Statement

All banking procedures must be monitored. Bank accounts are reconciled monthly as an internal control to protect office assets. There are basically five steps to follow to reconcile a banking account. A worksheet is usually provided on the bank statement for the office accountant to use for completing reconciliation. First, enter the current balance listed on the statement on the worksheet. Second, deposit slips are verified with the amount listed on the bank statement. Any uncredited deposit amounts are listed separately by date in the appropriate area of the worksheet and totaled. Third, canceled check amounts listed on the bank statement are verified with the amount recorded in the disbursement journal check register. Fourth, outstanding checks are listed on the worksheet and totaled. Finally, the necessary calculations are tabulated on the worksheet.

## CASH CONTROL JOURNALS

A petty cash fund is kept on hand for incidental purchases and usually contains $50 to $100. The proper monitoring of cash and cash receipts prevents lost or unaccounted cash. Cash control journals contain a control sheet for recording cash disbursements and cash vouchers from the petty cash fund. Cash control journal sheets itemize cash-in and cash-out transactions. Cash vouchers are numbered receipt forms completed for each transaction. A daily reconciliation of the petty cash fund is recorded onto the day sheet. Proofing the cash control journal page is like completing a proof of posting of accounts receivable.

## INTERNAL CONTROL SYSTEMS

Internal controls are a series of office processes used to safeguard assets and the reliability of financial records when handling cash and patient receivables. Embezzlement occurs when a staff member is dishonest or has a personal value system that allows him or her to rationalize such behavior. The stealing of office funds costs the industry millions of dollars a year and can be eliminated with control systems and monitoring to make it difficult to steal money. It is recommended that all personnel be bonded and that their bonding coverage be reviewed yearly. New employees should have references, and their financial stability should be evaluated before bonding.

Several people should have the ability to perform transactions as a way of preserving the integrity of the accounting system; thus control is removed from just one office member. Conversely, cash transactions should be handled by one individual to lessen the likelihood of cash shortages. This places accountability on one individual. Transactions that do not generate a walk-out statement, an account receipt, or a cash voucher should be recorded in a book containing numbered receipts that are written in duplicate. The top copy is given to the payee, the second copy remains in the receipt book. Any missing duplicate copies are suspect for cash mishandling. All monies received, especially cash, are deposited into the office account each day to reduce the opportunity for missing funds.

To prevent misappropriation of funds, the bank should have a standing order not to cash checks payable to the payer on the office account (dentist, independent dental hygienist practitioner), and a blank check should never be signed. The payer on the office account should review the daily summary and deposit slip each day and sign off when finished. All accounts payable should be made by numbered office account checks signed by the payer.

Daily summaries should be reviewed by the provider each day to verify all patient visits were documented and charges were entered into accounts receivable. The business owner must follow the accounts receivable and proof of posting to be sure daily totals and running balances are accurate. Careful monitoring makes it less likely that someone will manipulate numbers.

## CONCEPT SUMMARY

- The four types of dental business transactions are accounts receivable, accounts payable, petty cash, and bartering.
- Accounts receivable is an accounting system that monitors production, incoming payments, and outstanding money.
- Accounts payable is an accounting system that monitors outgoing payments.
- Petty cash control is an accounting system that monitors small cash disbursements.
- Bartering is an exchange of goods and services between two individuals.
- Internal control systems and the monitoring of financial records help prevent embezzlement.

# REVIEW QUESTIONS

1. List four types of business transactions used in dentistry.
2. What is the difference between accounts receivable and accounts payable?
3. Why is it important to have monitored accounting systems?
4. What is the difference between a walk-out statement and a routing slip?
5. What is a transaction?
6. Why are daily transaction summary reports generated?
7. What is proof of posting?
8. What is a disbursement journal?
9. How often should money be deposited?
10. What is a monthly disbursement summary sheet?
11. When are ledger control sheets used?
12. How should the petty cash fund and the cash control journal be used?
13. Which monetary internal control in the office gives responsibility to just one person?
14. Which monetary internal control in the office gives responsibility to more than one person?
15. How does embezzlement affect dental practices?

# Insurance Programs

## LEARNING OUTCOMES

Upon mastery of the content of this chapter, the student should be able to:
- Describe insurance protocols, regulatory agencies, program characteristics, and prevention of fraudulent procedures.
- Determine dental hygiene procedures to be submitted to insurance companies.
- Recognize how insurance eligibility verification procedures are performed.
- Distinguish between the American Dental Association's attending dentist's statement and the Centers for Medicare and Medicaid Services standardized insurance claim form.
- Recall how dental procedures can be coded for dental and medical insurance submissions.
- Discuss the processing and monitoring of insurance claims for reimbursement.
- Complete a narrative report based on supporting information.

## KEY TERMS

ADA attending dentist's statement dental
   insurance form
bundling
CMS-1500 medical insurance form
coordination of benefits
co-payment
cross-coding
explanation of benefits

fee for service
insurance fraud
narrative report
preauthorization
schedule of benefits
subrogation
usual, customary, and reasonable (UCR)
   plans

## INSURANCE PROGRAMS

Evidence collected during the oral risk assessment and diagnostic procedures is used for treatment planning, for case presentation, and as supporting information submitted with insurance claims. Documentation must support the need for treatment because comprehensive dental hygiene procedures are medical and dental in nature, allowing patients to use medical and dental insurance benefits. Accurately reporting comprehensive dental hygiene treatment to medical and dental insurance companies maximizes patients' use of their insurance benefits, which ultimately affects the amount of oral healthcare delivered.

Case acceptance is frequently based on economics, and submitting insurance forms on behalf of the patient allows patients to obtain the care they need. Patients are more likely to accept necessary treatment when a thorough explanation of and utilization of their insurance benefits are available. Dental practices follow office systems to manage insurance claim submissions, which reduces legal liability, prevents problems in accounting, and minimizes delays in payments. Dental insurance claims are commonly filed in dental practices, whereas medical insurance claims are frequently ignored because most people have the misconception that only dental insurance will cover the cost of dental care. Medical insurance **cross-coding** is the filing of medical insurance claims for dental procedures.

Experienced business dental assistants are able to file insurance claims using the correct procedure codes, can determine reasons to accept insurance plans, and understand insurance claim processing and how to proceed with unpaid claims. Dental hygienists need to have a general understanding of insurance protocols to complete treatment plans for case presentations, routing slips, superbills, narrative reports, and letters to insurance companies regarding the need for treatment when filing claims and claim rejection. A narrative report and a letter to an insurance company are given in Chapter 22.

Employers usually offer insurance programs as a benefit of employment. Individuals involved in insurance are the employee (first party), the oral healthcare provider (second party), the insurance company (third party), and the employer. Accepting any insurance as a form of payment allows the patient to have more access to dental care at a reduced out-of-pocket cost. Patients usually do not want to pay out-of-pocket expenses for dental care and insist that insurance pay for all of their treatment costs. This is usually not the case for most dental insurances, and the situation must be thoroughly explained, in great detail, to patients. Most patients who have dental insurance have to meet a deductible and are responsible for office visit fees and a percentage (such as 50%) of the treatment cost, called the **co-payment.** Medical insurance policies may require patients to pay an office visit fee, but deductibles and percentages are not as common as they are for dental procedures.

Using third-party payment increases the patient base, oral healthcare services delivery, patient referrals and rapport, public relations, and cash flow, which are major advantages for accepting insurance. Submission of insurance claims to insurance companies depends on many variables. In the United States, federal and state law heavily regulate the insurance industry because of the large sums of money involved and the possibility of unscrupulous activity. It is essential to file accurate claims to avoid engaging in any action that may appear fraudulent.

Frequently, patients request only the treatment that is covered by their insurance rather than what is recommended by the oral healthcare provider. It is the oral healthcare provider's responsibility to make recommendations based on patient need, regardless of insurance coverage. Patient education regarding costs and coverage from the providers and the business staff is crucial for good public relations, a healthy accounts receivable, and a satisfied customer.

## INSURANCE REGULATORY ENTITIES

Federal and state regulations in the United States protect public interests in healthcare delivery and reimbursement. Therefore, insurance processing must conform to federal and state laws. Legal advice should be obtained before establishing an insurance reimbursement system to decrease the risk of legal liability.

### Dental Insurance Organizations

The American Dental Association's (ADA's) Council on Dental Benefit Programs (CDBPs) determines and implements new national dental insurance policy. The ADA and CDBP developed the lists of procedure codes and descriptions, the Code on Dental Procedures and Nomenclature, found in the *Current Dental Terminology (CDT)* handbook available from the ADA. The CDBP and insurance carrier representatives regularly revise the *CDT* handbook, update code descriptors, work to standardize insurance practices, and develop standardized dental insurance forms. The *CDT* revisions add new codes and procedure descriptions and delete outdated and obsolete codes; updates are published periodically in the *Journal of the American Dental Association.*

### Medical Insurance Organizations

The U.S. Department of Health and Human Services (DHHS) oversees healthcare in the United States. The Centers for Medicare and Medicaid Services (CMS) provide government healthcare programs and compile data on medical insurance. The United Nations World Health Organization (WHO) develops and revises medical diagnostic codes published in the *International Classification of Diseases*, 9th revised edition, *Clinical Modification Codes* (ICD-9-CM). The American Medical Association (AMA) develops and revises the procedure codes yearly and publishes them in the *Current Procedural Terminology (CPT)*.

## DENTAL INSURANCE PROGRAMS

Dental insurance programs include traditional fee-for-service and alternative dental plans. There are two types of traditional fee-for-service (indemnity) plans and several alternative dental plans. The two types of traditional fee-for-service plans—**usual, customary, and reasonable (UCR) plans** and **schedule of benefits**—are determined by dental practices in different geographical areas. UCR plans are fee schedules determined by the insurance carrier, which pays a set amount for each procedure code number. *Usual* is defined as the fee charged by the dentist for a single procedure. *Customary* is defined as the range of usual fees charged by dentists in a particular geographical area. *Reasonable* is defined as the fee determined by the insurance carrier when a procedure charge is above the usual amount.

The schedule of benefits, table of allowances, or schedule of allowances is a fee schedule determined by the insurance carrier, who pays a specified amount for each procedure number, leaving the patient financially responsible for any remaining fee. Alternative dental insurance plans are given in *Box 11.1.*

## MEDICAL INSURANCE PROGRAMS

A select number of dental hygiene procedures can be billed to medical insurance carriers. Medical claims are filed with the diagnosis, modifying, and procedure codes after coverage is verified. In addition, when the dental condition is related to a medical condition (such as with diabetes or trauma), medical claims can be filed. It is important to note that medical insurance may allow up to $1 million in benefits yearly, whereas dental insurance carriers typically have yearly caps between $1,000 and $5,000. Cross-coding office systems provide for increased case acceptance, improved office revenue, a higher level of expertise among business dental assistants, and practice marketing opportunities. Some dental software programs are capable of filing medical insurance claims and of preparing computer-generated claims. Medical insurance programs encompass hospitalization and major medical policies, managed care agreements, Medicaid and Medicare, personal injury protection (automobile policies), and worker's compensation (employment-related injuries). Hospitalization and major medical insurance policies pay for hospital care and will not cover dental hygiene procedures performed in a dental office. Preferred provider organizations (PPOs) are more likely than other managed care insurers to accept out-of-network providers.

## DENTAL HYGIENE REIMBURSEMENT

Dental hygienists perform a variety of comprehensive oral healthcare services that are delegated duties and thus differ from office to office, person to person, and jurisdiction to jurisdiction. Factual evidence from the medical and dental histories; clinical, periodontal, and radiographic examinations; and an oral risk assessment survey assist in planning procedures.

### Procedures for Dental Reimbursement

The first step in reimbursement from dental insurance companies is to determine which dental hygiene procedures were performed. Dental hygiene procedure codes fall into

## TABLE 11.1 ADA Procedure Codes for Comprehensive Dental Hygiene Services

**Preventive**

| | | | |
|---|---|---|---|
| D0170 | Reevaluation—limited problem, focused | D0470 | Diagnostic casts |
| D0180 | Comprehensive periodontal evaluation | D1100 | Prophylaxis |
| D0200 | Radiographs | D1200 | Topical application of fluoride |
| D0350 | Intraoral imaging | D1310 | Nutritional counseling |
| D0415 | Bacteriologic studies | D1320 | Tobacco cessation |
| D0425 | Caries susceptibility tests | D1330 | Oral hygiene instruction |
| D0460 | Pulp vitality testing | D1351 | Sealant per tooth |

**Periodontal**

| | | | |
|---|---|---|---|
| D4341 | Scaling and root planing, 4 or more teeth per quadrant | D4910 | Periodontal maintenance |
| | | D4920 | Unscheduled dressing change |
| D4342 | Scaling and root planing, 1–3 teeth per quadrant | D4999 | Unspecified periodontal procedure, by report |
| D4355 | Full mouth débridement | | |
| D4381 | Localized delivery of chemotherapeutic agents | | |

**Adjunct Services**

| | | | |
|---|---|---|---|
| D7281 | Cytologic sample collection (brush biopsy) | D9910 | Desensitizer application |
| D9230 | Analgesia inhalation of nitrous oxide–oxygen | D9911 | Resin desensitization |
| D9430 | Office visit for observation | D9940 | Occlusal guard |
| D9450 | Case presentation | D9941 | Mouthguard |
| D9630 | Dispensing medicaments (fluoride, antibiotics, analgesics, mouth rinses) | D9972 | External bleaching per arch |

Excerpted from Current Dental Terminology–4. Reprinted with permission from the American Dental Association.

three basic categories: preventive services, periodontal services, and adjunct services (*Table 11.1*).

## Procedures for Medical Reimbursement

Filing medical insurance claims requires a higher level of expertise by the business office staff. The practice owner who decides to initiate a medical reimbursement office system delegates medical claim processing to a business dental assistant, who verifies, files, and monitors insurance claims. Comprehensive dental hygiene procedures that can be billed to medical insurance carriers are listed in *Box 11.2*.

### BOX 11.2 *Comprehensive Dental Hygiene Services That May Be Billed to Medical Insurance*

Brush biopsy
Occlusal guards and stents
Office visits
Pathology and laboratory reports

Periodontal scaling and root planing
Prescription drugs and locally applied chemotherapeutic agents
Radiographs and imaging

## VERIFICATION OF PATIENT INSURANCE COVERAGE

Before any treatment, the business office staff determines patient insurance eligibility, procedure coverage, co-payments, deductibles, maximum benefit amounts, exclusions, subrogation, and limitations using verification procedures. **Subrogation** is the communication process between two insurance carriers when the patient has two dental insurance plans (dual coverage) or dental and medical insurance coverage. Verification procedures are similar for both dental and medical insurance programs. Because there are thousands of insurance plans, each with its own set of detailed requirements, it is impossible to know everything; but a general understanding of insurance claims processing is necessary. Coverage is documented and verified using each plan's benefit summary booklet, or via telephone, fax, email, or the Internet, before treatment is started.

### Medical Insurance Verification

Patients may have both dental and medical insurance policies; therefore both coverages must be verified. The business dental assistant calls, faxes, or sends an email to the medical insurance carrier to ask about patient eligibility, coverage of procedures by specific medical code number, and deductibles. Then, a telephone call is made to notify the medical insurance company of the procedures to be performed.

## THE ADA ATTENDING DENTIST'S STATEMENT INSURANCE FORM

The **ADA attending dentist's statement insurance form** is the standardized dental insurance claim form used to submit dental insurance claims for payment or preauthorization for services to be performed (*Figure 11.1*). It documents the patient's personal and insurance information, diagnosis codes, and treatment codes. The patient signs an original to be kept on file, and subsequent submissions note "signature on file." The attending dentist's statement is divided into six sections.

### Dental Procedure Codes

The *CDT* procedure codes are divided into 12 categories, based on the type of dental service—from diagnosis to adjunct services. Five-digit procedure codes begin with the letter *D* to identify them as dental codes; then each number has a specific meaning. The first number is 0, the second number describes the category (such as preventive or periodontics), and the third through fifth numbers describe the dental service.

Dental insurance submissions for dental hygiene comprehensive services can be bundled. Insurance code **bundling** is the grouping of related procedure codes based on multiple appointments (*Box 11.3*). Following the American Academy of Periodontology (AAP) descriptions of periodontal case type diagnoses, sequenced nonsurgical treatment procedures are grouped together for a total case fee. The expected insurance reimbursement and the patient's out-of-pocket expenses are calculated to help with the financial arrangements for these necessary procedures.

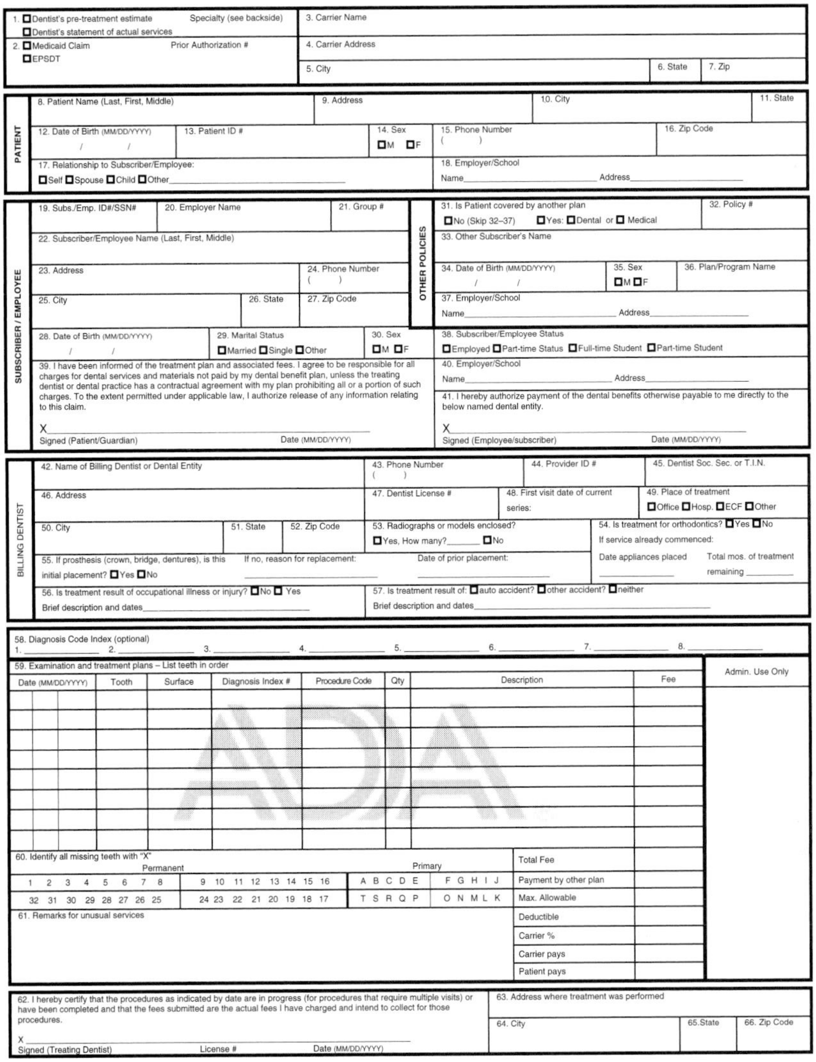

**Figure 11.1** ADA attending dentist's statement insurance claim form. © American Dental Association, 1999.

## THE CMS-1500 MEDICAL INSURANCE FORM

The appropriate staff member calls the patient's medical insurance company to inform it that a procedure will be performed. Then the medical insurance claim form is filed. The **CMS-1500 medical insurance form** is the standardized form used to submit medical insurance claims (*Fig. 11.2*). It documents the patient's personal and insurance information, diagnosis codes, V and E codes (discussed later in this chapter), modifier codes, and treatment codes. Narrative reports that provide information on diagnosis and treatment are required when filing medical insurance claims.

---

**BOX 11.3** *Dental Hygiene Insurance Code Bundle: Gingivitis Case Type I*

**Appointment 1**
| | |
|---|---|
| D01330 | Oral hygiene instruction |
| D04355 | Full mouth débridement |
| D09630 | Dispensing medicaments (e.g., home fluoride) |

**Appointment 2**
| | |
|---|---|
| D01330 | Oral hygiene instruction |
| D01110 | Adult prophylaxis |
| D09630 | Dispensing medicaments (e.g., automated toothbrush) |

---

## Medical Insurance Diagnosis Codes

As noted, diagnosis codes are published in the ICD-9-CM. This diagnosis codebook is published by the CMS, under the auspices of the DHHS. It comes in three volumes, and volumes 2 and 3 are needed to report dental procedures. Diagnosis codes associated with dental hygiene are found in Chapter 9, "Diseases of the Digestive System." The diagnosis codes for periodontal conditions are between 520.3 and 524.6, bruxism is 306.8, sleep apnea is 780.57, and temporomandibular joint disease has multiple codes related to pain, muscles, and bone.

## Medical Insurance Procedure Codes

The 7000 medical procedure codes are also published in the *CPT* handbook (compared to the 500 dental procedure codes). The codes are divided into six sections: evaluation and management, anesthesiology, surgery, radiology, pathology and laboratory, and medicine. Supplemental informational codes, called V and E codes, are four digits preceded by the letter *V* or *E*. The V codes are "factors influencing health status and contact with health services" and describe the history of the illness, injury, or systemic condition. The E codes classify external causes of injury and poisonings, such as accidents involving transportation and machinery and other injury circumstances. Modifying codes are added to treatment codes to further describe the condition, such as LT (left side) or RT (right side).

## NARRATIVE REPORTS

Occasionally, the dental hygienist may be asked to write a narrative report. A **narrative report** is a documentation of information provided to insurance carriers, other healthcare professionals, attorneys, the court system, and the client records. It provides supporting documentation that is submitted to avoid delays in claim processing or after a claim rejection as a means to expedite resolution. A narrative report must be sent with the dental insurance claims when a code descriptor states "by report." Dental insurance procedure codes for which the third through fifth numbers are designated 999 are unspecified and are used when there is no code for a particular service. For example, code 4999 indicates an unspecified periodontal procedure, so a narrative report describing

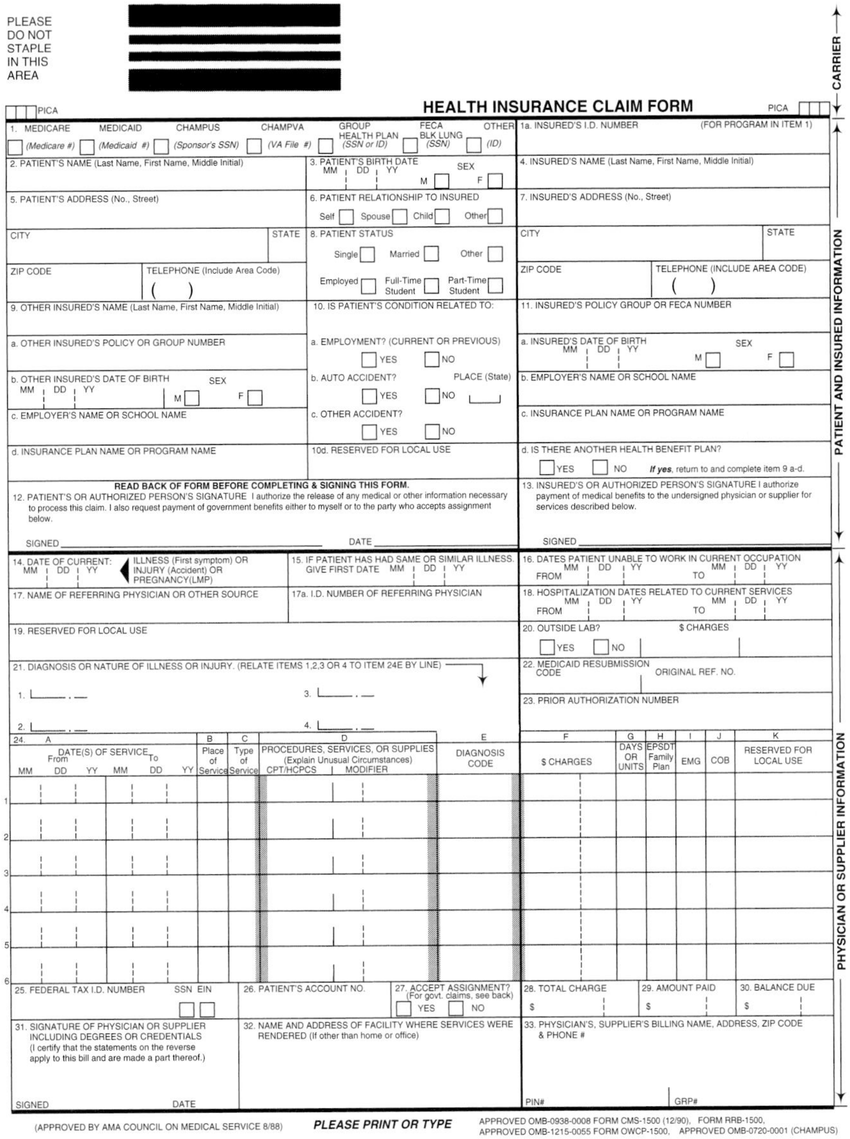

PLEASE DO NOT STAPLE IN THIS AREA

PICA **HEALTH INSURANCE CLAIM FORM** PICA

CARRIER

1. MEDICARE (Medicare #) MEDICAID (Medicaid #) CHAMPUS (Sponsor's SSN) CHAMPVA (VA File #) GROUP HEALTH PLAN (SSN or ID) FECA BLK LUNG (SSN) OTHER (ID)
1a. INSURED'S I.D. NUMBER (FOR PROGRAM IN ITEM 1)
2. PATIENT'S NAME (Last Name, First Name, Middle Initial)
3. PATIENT'S BIRTH DATE MM DD YY SEX M F
4. INSURED'S NAME (Last Name, First Name, Middle Initial)
5. PATIENT'S ADDRESS (No., Street)
6. PATIENT RELATIONSHIP TO INSURED Self Spouse Child Other
7. INSURED'S ADDRESS (No., Street)
CITY STATE
8. PATIENT STATUS Single Married Other; Employed Full-Time Student Part-Time Student
CITY STATE
ZIP CODE TELEPHONE (Include Area Code) ( )
ZIP CODE TELEPHONE (INCLUDE AREA CODE) ( )
9. OTHER INSURED'S NAME (Last Name, First Name, Middle Initial)
10. IS PATIENT'S CONDITION RELATED TO:
11. INSURED'S POLICY GROUP OR FECA NUMBER
a. OTHER INSURED'S POLICY OR GROUP NUMBER
a. EMPLOYMENT? (CURRENT OR PREVIOUS) YES NO
a. INSURED'S DATE OF BIRTH MM DD YY SEX M F
b. OTHER INSURED'S DATE OF BIRTH MM DD YY SEX M F
b. AUTO ACCIDENT? PLACE (State) YES NO
b. EMPLOYER'S NAME OR SCHOOL NAME
c. EMPLOYER'S NAME OR SCHOOL NAME
c. OTHER ACCIDENT? YES NO
c. INSURANCE PLAN NAME OR PROGRAM NAME
d. INSURANCE PLAN NAME OR PROGRAM NAME
10d. RESERVED FOR LOCAL USE
d. IS THERE ANOTHER HEALTH BENEFIT PLAN? YES NO *If yes*, return to and complete item 9 a-d.
READ BACK OF FORM BEFORE COMPLETING & SIGNING THIS FORM.
12. PATIENT'S OR AUTHORIZED PERSON'S SIGNATURE I authorize the release of any medical or other information necessary to process this claim. I also request payment of government benefits either to myself or to the party who accepts assignment below.
SIGNED DATE
13. INSURED'S OR AUTHORIZED PERSON'S SIGNATURE I authorize payment of medical benefits to the undersigned physician or supplier for services described below.
SIGNED

PATIENT AND INSURED INFORMATION

14. DATE OF CURRENT: MM DD YY ILLNESS (First symptom) OR INJURY (Accident) OR PREGNANCY(LMP)
15. IF PATIENT HAS HAD SAME OR SIMILAR ILLNESS. GIVE FIRST DATE MM DD YY
16. DATES PATIENT UNABLE TO WORK IN CURRENT OCCUPATION FROM MM DD YY TO MM DD YY
17. NAME OF REFERRING PHYSICIAN OR OTHER SOURCE
17a. I.D. NUMBER OF REFERRING PHYSICIAN
18. HOSPITALIZATION DATES RELATED TO CURRENT SERVICES FROM MM DD YY TO MM DD YY
19. RESERVED FOR LOCAL USE
20. OUTSIDE LAB? YES NO $ CHARGES
21. DIAGNOSIS OR NATURE OF ILLNESS OR INJURY. (RELATE ITEMS 1,2,3 OR 4 TO ITEM 24E BY LINE)
1. ___ . ___ 3. ___ . ___
2. ___ . ___ 4. ___ . ___
22. MEDICAID RESUBMISSION CODE ORIGINAL REF. NO.
23. PRIOR AUTHORIZATION NUMBER

| 24. A DATE(S) OF SERVICE From MM DD YY To MM DD YY | B Place of Service | C Type of Service | D PROCEDURES, SERVICES, OR SUPPLIES (Explain Unusual Circumstances) CPT/HCPCS MODIFIER | E DIAGNOSIS CODE | F $ CHARGES | G DAYS OR UNITS | H EPSDT Family Plan | I EMG | J COB | K RESERVED FOR LOCAL USE |
|---|---|---|---|---|---|---|---|---|---|---|
| 1 | | | | | | | | | | |
| 2 | | | | | | | | | | |
| 3 | | | | | | | | | | |
| 4 | | | | | | | | | | |
| 5 | | | | | | | | | | |
| 6 | | | | | | | | | | |

25. FEDERAL TAX I.D. NUMBER SSN EIN
26. PATIENT'S ACCOUNT NO.
27. ACCEPT ASSIGNMENT? (For govt. claims, see back) YES NO
28. TOTAL CHARGE $
29. AMOUNT PAID $
30. BALANCE DUE $
31. SIGNATURE OF PHYSICIAN OR SUPPLIER INCLUDING DEGREES OR CREDENTIALS (I certify that the statements on the reverse apply to this bill and are made a part thereof.)
SIGNED DATE
32. NAME AND ADDRESS OF FACILITY WHERE SERVICES WERE RENDERED (If other than home or office)
33. PHYSICIAN'S, SUPPLIER'S BILLING NAME, ADDRESS, ZIP CODE & PHONE #
PIN# GRP#

PHYSICIAN OR SUPPLIER INFORMATION

(APPROVED BY AMA COUNCIL ON MEDICAL SERVICE 8/88) ***PLEASE PRINT OR TYPE*** APPROVED OMB-0938-0008 FORM CMS-1500 (12/90), FORM RRB-1500, APPROVED OMB-1215-0055 FORM OWCP-1500, APPROVED OMB-0720-0001 (CHAMPUS)

**Figure 11.2** The CMS-1500 medical insurance form.

the procedure must be included with the claim form. An outline for a narrative report is given in *Box 11.4*. A sample narrative report is given in Chapter 22.

## INSURANCE CLAIM FOLLOW-UP UNTIL REIMBURSEMENT

Out-of-network providers charge according to their fee schedule and submit insurance claims as a service to the patient. The patient is responsible for all amounts not paid by

**BOX 11.4** *Outline for a Narrative Report*

Report date
Patient name and age
Date of treatment or services
Patient's chief complaint
Patient's medical and dental history
Other treatments for the disorder
Description of accident, incident, or illness, including cause
Objective clinical findings
Diagnosis
Treatment
Prognosis
Enclosures (e.g., insurance forms, radiographs, periodontal charting)

the insurance carrier. The patient must be informed of these additional costs as mandated by the Federal Truth in Lending Act when the cost of dental care exceeds $100. **Fee-for-service** dental practices require the patient to pay for treatment in advance, based on the fee schedule, in an attempt to expedite payment for services rendered. The patient then submits the insurance claim for direct reimbursement.

A thorough understanding of limitations, such as filing procedures for preauthorizations and coordination of benefits, avoids claim rejection, treatment denial, and incorrect payment. Before treatment is begun, the dental staff seeks **preauthorization** from the patient's insurance company, sending a detailed list of proposed procedure codes to the carrier for review. The carrier determines the patient's eligibility, covered services, payment amounts, co-payments, deductibles, and plan maximums. Preauthorization is usually not required for dental hygiene services.

**Coordination of benefits** occurs when a patient has dental insurance coverage from more than one insurance plan. Insurance guidelines generally do not allow dual coverage, which is stated in a nonduplication of benefits clause. When dental and medical insurance offer dual coverage, coordination of benefits or subrogation is decided between the insurance companies for primary and secondary coverage. Insurance claim forms contain spaces for this information to be documented. Dental and medical insurance codes do not correspond; therefore, the total case fee is bundled so that it is the same for both submissions. Most patients assume that dual coverage indicates no out-of-pocket expenses, so communication between the patient and business dental assistant is necessary for informed consent.

## Filing the Insurance Claim

Insurance claims are submitted by mail or fax or are filed online. Electronically filed claims are paperless and efficient, decrease processing time, and expedite claims payment, especially when payments can be directly deposited into the dental office's bank account. Electronically generated claims are submitted to a clearinghouse, which directs them to a specific carrier or a claim processing system via the Internet. Additional documentation, such as narratives, periodontal charts, photographs, and radiographs, are attached when applicable.

## Monitoring the Insurance Claim

Dental insurance claims are monitored to improve the chances for payment; unpaid insurance claims are unsettled accounts receivable that must be collected. Many state regulations mandate that claim payment or denial be made within 1 month. Phone calls to the carrier to resolve nonpayment issues must be made after 30 days past due. Reasons for nonpayment can include a lost, incomplete, or incorrect claim. Some dental offices make formal complaints to state insurance commissions to expedite the process. Dental insurance companies can refuse to pay unsettled claims 1 calendar year after treatment.

## Claim Reimbursement

Dental insurance payment checks are accompanied by an **explanation of benefits** (EOB) report that verifies procedure codes. This itemized statement details benefit payment information, reasons for a rejected claim (such as incomplete information, incorrect coding, or uncovered patient/procedure), and how payment was made according to the plan's benefit guidelines. All EOB statements should be checked for errors and payment information; if necessary, the claim should be corrected immediately for resubmission.

## Insurance Fraud

All practitioners who submit insurance claims are monitored by groups that search for fraudulent claims; federal and state agencies and political watchdog groups do this monitoring. **Insurance fraud** is the intentional attempt to falsify insurance claims (*Box 11.5*). When a higher fee is warranted because of unusual circumstances, a narrative report is needed to explain the higher fee. Insurance companies review claims for any discrepancies and report their findings to state insurance commissions, who investigate and prosecute fraud. Penalties handed down with fraud convictions include payment of fines and restitution, probation, confinement or incarceration, and loss of license. National groups that compile names to investigate insurance fraud are the U.S. Healthcare Fraud Task Force, National Fraud Information Center, Medicare Fraud and Abuse, National Insurance Crime Bureau, AISG Insurance Fraud Management Committee, and the National Health Care Anti-Fraud Association. Fraud is also investigated at the state level.

---

**BOX 11.5** *Examples of Insurance Fraud*

Adding unnecessary charges
Billing for more expensive services than performed
Billing for services not performed
Falsifying records
Filing incorrect charges or codes

Filing claims for full coverage to both medical *and* dental insurers
Not charging the patient the co-payment
Participating in kickbacks and rebates

## CONCEPT SUMMARY

- Many entities are involved in insurance claim processing: dental patients, the dental practice, insurance companies, clearinghouses, regulatory agencies, and fraud units.
- Comprehensive oral hygiene services are submitted for reimbursement to dental and medical insurance companies.
- Verification of coverage must be completed for each client.
- Two insurance forms are used to submit claims: the ADA attending dentist's statement dental insurance form and the CMS-1500 medical insurance form.
- Insurance claims are processed and monitored immediately after dental treatment.
- Dental and medical insurance companies may request a narrative report to support the need for treatment.

# REVIEW QUESTIONS

1. Define each of the following insurance terms.
   A. Cross-coding
   B. Co-payment
   C. Usual, customary, and reasonable (UCR)
   D. Schedule of benefits
   E. Subrogation
   F. ADA attending dentist's statement dental insurance form
   G. CMS-1500 medical insurance form
   H. Fee for service
   I. Preauthorization
   J. Bundling
   K. Narrative report
   L. Explanation of benefits
   M. Insurance fraud

## Assignment: Narrative Report

Use the narrative report outline given in *Box 11.4* to write a narrative report on a case study patient to submit to an insurance company.

# Production

## PRODUCTION

The globalization of manufactured products and services affects all of us. For example, if your computer starts to malfunction you will make a call to the manufacturer's technical support line. It is likely that you will speak to a service sector person who lives in India. Dental hygiene is a service sector occupation that requires marketing, performance of unique tasks, and distribution of products in return for money. Comprehensive oral healthcare services are delivered to clients in a specific geographical area, and it is likely that one day dental hygiene functions will be performed in the same manner whether the professional is in Australia, California, the United Kingdom, or New Zealand.

The efficient operation of the dental practice is achieved by implementing work processes that enable fiscal success. Office operations are based on the "Five Ms" of management: manpower, machines, methods, materials, and money. When applied to dental hygiene, manpower comes from the oral healthcare workers; machines are the equipment and technology used to deliver care; methods are procedures followed, products sold, and information learned and presented; materials are the goods used to deliver oral healthcare; and money is the financing, public relations, compensation, and paperwork.

## CONTROLLING AND MONITORING PRODUCTION

The principal reason for controlling and monitoring production is to determine why the dental practice spends money, where the money is spent, and how much is spent. The controlling and monitoring of production are ways to guarantee the financial success of the practice. Business owners secure the practice's financial stability by scheduling for production. **Production** is the number of primary, secondary, and tertiary oral health-care procedures performed by the appropriate oral healthcare provider. It is a flexible process implemented by oral healthcare providers who adapt to new information, equipment, procedures, regulations, and schedule changes.

The hygiene department can be compared to a car's engine: It runs the practice. Dental hygienists provide distinctive services, charge for them, and should be paid what they are worth. Without a strong hygiene department, the dental office will experience slow growth because the hygienist diagnoses treatment needs during assessment activities. One estimate is that 40% of returning patients have untreated diagnosed restorative needs. Once the oral healthcare services performed by the dental hygienist are identified, planning and controlling strategies are initiated.

Through **production blocking**, time is set aside each day for specific high-production-value procedures, called primary procedures. **Primary dental hygiene procedures** are periodontal therapies—specifically scaling and root planning—with high production value. Scaling and root planning should account for at least half of the daily hygiene production output. **Secondary dental hygiene procedures** have lower production value and represent all other comprehensive dental hygiene services. **Tertiary dental hygiene procedures** are performed at no cost and thus have no production value; however, they are necessary for patient care. Some dental practices do not charge a fee for oral hygiene instruction or office visits for a short reassessment to evaluate a condition. Primary dental hygiene procedures are not more important than low production value procedures. The patient's care and comfort needs must be met, regardless of any fees attached to the service.

## DENTAL HYGIENE PRODUCTION

Dental office production totals are calculated based on the office and procedure code numbers performed by each oral healthcare provider. The totals are measured in daily, weekly, monthly, quarterly, and yearly reports for each provider in the office and are generated by the dental practice management software program. Short-term production goals are based on daily or weekly planning, whereas long-term goals are estimated based on monthly or yearly planning. **Benchmarking** is the selection of a standard of practice that represents the best available system. One industry benchmark for production in the dental hygiene department is the generation of 33% of the practice's total production. Other accepted productivity levels for the hygiene department are given in *Box 12.1*. Dental hygiene production, like the practice's total production, can be assessed by the hour, week, month, quarter, and/or year, and is based on growth markers of forecasting, total quality management, service design and process, inventory, scheduling, and production analysis reports.

## Forecasting

**Forecasting** is the prediction of events using mathematical formulas or subjective assessments to estimate future demand for services. Formulas used to determine staffing needs are given in *Box 12.2*. The dental office practice management software system can calculate the number of active patients in the practice. That number is used by managers or owners to estimate the number of employees needed based on production totals (*Box 12.2*).

## Total Quality Management

First-class customer service mandates quality care and attention to patient comfort to satisfy patient needs. Quality affects the entire practice, from the office manager's leadership to employee commitment to the devoted patient base. Quality is also important to productivity, reputation, and legal liability. In manufacturing, companies strive to meet the criteria for quality set by the International Organization for Standardization (ISO). In the service sector, the **total quality management** (TQM) system is a commitment to excellence in service delivery and to meet the dental consumer's expectations. TQM turns patient desires into specific procedures and products they can benefit from. For example, if a patient notes on the dental history form that he or she is concerned about breath malodor, then emphasis should be placed on procedures and products that address this concern. To build long-term devoted patient relationships, give patients what they want and involve them in their care.

In addition to clinical excellence, quality care also involves the recommendation for urgent care and periodontal treatment, which can mean holding back on case presentation for major restorative work until the patient returns for routine recare. This low-key approach demonstrates business savvy to help rein in any big case aggressiveness. As noted earlier, patients often have thousands of dollars worth of need yet spend under $200 per year on their oral health. Aggressive selling of services will turn off some clients. Urgent and periodontal care recommendations help build trust.

What are the distinctive tasks of the dental hygienist that are crucial to success? One example is painless dental injections and other patient care and comfort extras provided

---

**BOX 12.1** *Dental Hygiene Productivity*

Accepted productivity levels for the dental hygiene department are 25%, 30%, 33%, and 35% of the practice's total production.

during the delivery of dental hygiene services. Patient care services include providing tooth-whitening systems, using lasers, treating breath malodor, designing a weight loss–control oral appliance, performing an orthodontic procedure, and offering spa-like extras that are lacking in other local practices. The use of any unique procedure should reflect the mission, vision, or philosophy statement of the practice; remember, each employee has ownership in these statements. These issues are addressed further in Chapter 24.

## Return on Investment

Unique or distinctive tasks may also include the use of new equipment or involve some other type of capital outlay. In some instances, the dental hygienist may have the responsibility of calculating and reporting the return on investment for an expenditure. **Return on investment** (ROI) is an accounting method used to determine when the amount paid for an item or service is recuperated. ROI is influenced by the lifespan of the product or service, the money invested, depreciation, and the length of time from the purchase to a positive cash inflow. For example, a practice purchases a light-activated tooth whitening system that requires 10 whitening sessions before ROI occurs. After the 11th patient is treated for tooth whitening with the new system, profitability begins, and the dental hygienist can then report the ROI to the dentist or staff.

## SERVICE DESIGN AND PROCESS

Current research and changes in technology require constant monitoring to remain competitive. Comprehensive oral hygiene services are designed for the patient's interaction with the healthcare provider. The patient participates in the delivery of oral healthcare by selecting the procedures to be performed, giving accurate information about his or her health status, paying for services rendered, keeping appointments, and following directions. Service design is the selection and delivery of quality customized procedures unique to the patient to improve health. Because this level of individualized care is labor intensive (one on one), the focus of the dental hygienist is on providing the patient with good customer service.

Changes in the economy, either up or down, affect the process of oral healthcare delivery. A patient retention rate of 80–85% is necessary for a healthy hygiene department. The typical retention rate is estimated to be in the 50–65% range.

## Increased Demand

Several options are available when the demand for dental hygiene services exceeds the ability to meet it. Once it has been determined that the demand is sustainable, the management may decide to increase fees, hire more staff, allow longer than 2-week waits for appointments, or examine work processes.

By examining work processes, it is possible to determine ways to decrease time per patient and increase the number of patients seen each day. Increasing the number of patients seen each day can be accomplished with the help of technology or a dental assistant for the dental hygiene department. It is recommended that 2 hours be set aside each week for nonpatient planning time to assist in implementation of new work processes.

## Dental Assistant for the Hygiene Department

Legal delegation of duties to properly credentialed staff greatly enhances production totals. In the private dental practice, a staff meeting helps in planning for the proper use of dental auxiliary and treatment rooms. In an established independent practice, the use of a dental assistant can increase the number of patients scheduled and build the practice's monthly income by $20,000–$40,000. Hygiene partnering with a credentialed dental assistant can be a real asset because legally allowable procedures can be delegated, reducing stress for the dental hygienist. As is true with all employees, the assistant must buy into the office philosophy of periodontal therapy and work well with the dental hygienist.

The production schedule can be double booked using a staggered schedule format when two dental operatories are available for use. An example of double booking is shown in *Box 12.3*; notice how the dental assistant and dental hygienist work together as the hygienist performs dental assisting skills. Compare the number of patients treated in the double-booking example (*Box 12.3*) with that in the single-booking example given in *Box 12.4*. Remember that the inventory supply and number of dental instruments must be doubled and that sterilization and communication requirements will also increase.

## Inventory Management

Spending less money on supplies improves the bottom line of operational costs. It may be a job requirement to count the number of products dispensed in an effort to monitor spending and estimate future costs. Once again, the dental office practice management software program can help when office procedure codes have been added to the database of insurance procedure codes. This helps in the calculation of specific products sold to patients because a general insurance procedure code number does not differentiate among products.

## Dental Product Sales

A variety of products can be made available from the dental practice and can be promoted and sold to patients to individualize and improve their care. Many products, drugs, medicaments, and therapies may be available only from the office. Good customer service focuses on the specific needs and wants of each patient. If the patient is sound periodontally yet is caries prone, the hygienist may dispense prescription rinses, take-home fluorides, toothpastes, automated toothbrushes, and saliva substitutes.

Should dental hygienists be uncomfortable recommending personal care products that enhance health and well-being? No. Just as people purchase hair care products from

**BOX 12.3** *Double Booking in the Hygiene Department (Half Day)*

**8:00—Woody Trail**
*Seated; MDHX update;[a] 4 bitewing x-rays*
8:10 Oral cancer examination; periodontal charting with assistant
8:20 Adult prophylaxis; scaling
8:30

8:40 *Coronal polishing; adult fluoride; periodic examination with dentist; dispense breath malodor kit; dispense sonic toothbrush; patient education*
8:50 *Dismiss patient; clean room*
9:00
9:10

9:20

**9:30 Lucy Little**
*Seated; MDHX update; full-mouth x-rays*
9:40 Oral cancer examination, periodontal charting with assistant
9:50 Periodontal maintenance; scaling
10:00 Dispense take-home fluoride

10:10 *Coronal polishing; adult fluoride; periodic examination with dentist; patient education*
10:20 *Dismiss patient; clean room*

**10:30 Bill Fold**
*Seated; MDHX update*
10:40 Office visit for evaluation; periodontal débridement
10:50 Site-specific antibiotic injection; *dismiss patient; clean room*

**11:00 Jade B. Green**
*Seated; MDHX update; 4 bitewing x-rays*
11:10 Child prophylaxis; scaling
11:20 *Coronal polishing; child fluoride; periodic examination with dentist; patient education*
11:30 *Dismiss patient; clean room*

11:40

11:50

**12:00 Robin Bird**
*Seated; MDHX update*
12:10 Full-mouth débridement

12:20 Patient education; dispense chlorhexidine
12:30 *Dismiss patient; clean room*

---

8:00

8:10

8:20

**8:30 Luke Warm**
*Seated; MDHX update*
8:40 Upper and lower right periodontal scaling; root planing 4 or more teeth; local anesthesia

8:50
9:00
9:10 Dispense chlorhexidine; 8 site-specific antibiotic injections
9:20 *Patient education; postoperative check; dismiss patient; clean room*

9:30

9:40

9:50

**10:00 Bill Board**
*Seated; MDHX update*
10:10 *Full-mouth x-rays*

10:20 Oral cancer examination; periodontal charting with assistant
10:30 Periodontal maintenance; scaling

10:40 Dispense take-home fluoride

10:50 *Coronal polishing; adult fluoride; periodic examination with dentist; patient education*
11:00 *Dismiss patient; clean room*

11:10
11:20

**11:30 Holly Berry**
*Seated; MDHX update*
11:40 Oral cancer examination; periodontal charting with assistant
11:50 Periodontal maintenance; scaling
12:00 Dispense take-home fluoride

12:10 *Coronal polishing; adult fluoride; periodic examination with dentist; patient education*
12:20 *Dismiss patient; clean room*

12:30

[a]Italics denotes functions of the dental assistant. *MDHX*, medical and dental history.

**BOX 12.4** *Single Booking in the Hygiene Department (Half Day)*

**8:00—Woody Trail**
    4 bitewing x-rays
    Adult prophylaxis
    Periodic examination
    Adult fluoride

    Dispense breath malodor kit
    Dispense sonic toothbrush
    Patient education

**9:00—Luke Warm**
    Upper and lower right periodontal scaling
       and root planing on 4 or more teeth

    Dispense chlorhexidine
    8 site-specific antibiotic injections

**10:00—Lucy Little**
    Full-mouth x-rays
    Periodontal maintenance
    Dispense take-home fluoride

    Adult fluoride
    Patient education

**11:00—Bill Board**
    Full-mouth x-rays
    Periodontal maintenance
    Dispense take-home fluoride

    Adult fluoride
    Patient education

**12:00—Bill Fold**
    Office visit for evaluation
    Periodontal débridement per tooth
      (unspecified periodontal treatment
      by report)

    1 site-specific antibiotic injection

a stylist or foods from specialty shops, patients purchase oral care products from the hygienist. Such products may include prescription fluoride rinses and gels, prescription systematic antibiotics, desensitizing agents, viral infection medications, oral sore healing rinses, salivary substitutes, and breath malodor, lip care, and oral hygiene products.

## SCHEDULING FOR PRODUCTION

Daily production goals are based on the anticipated yearly gross, which is first divided into monthly production goals and then divided by the number of workdays patients will be scheduled that month. For example, if the monthly goal for the hygiene department is $32,000 and the office will be open 20 days that month, the dental hygiene department must earn $1,600 per day. Being aware of the necessary total daily production goal helps staff efficiently schedule appointments and personnel.

Careful time management keeps the department at the maximum productivity level, avoids the need to rush, and helps prevent staff from falling behind schedule. The daily schedule should be mixed, with a variety of primary, secondary, and tertiary procedures. Most practices preblock for high-value, primary procedures, fitting secondary procedures with lower fees and tertiary (no-fee) procedures around that time.

If the production goal is $2,000 per day, 4 days per week, 4 weeks per month, 12 months per year, the dental hygiene department should expect to earn $384,000 a year. Primary procedures should bring in approximately half of the daily production. For example, assume the practice preblocks 2 hours each day for four quadrants of periodontal scaling, carefully scheduling these difficult procedures for the dental hygienist's preferred time slot. If the fee per quadrant is $200, then the hygiene department is guaranteed $800 (for four quadrants) per day, which is near the $1,000 needed for primary procedures (half of daily production). Secondary and tertiary procedures are then scheduled around the primary procedure appointments in the amount needed to meet the daily goal.

## Increasing Hygiene Production

Dental hygiene oral healthcare services and product sales are tracked via office or procedure code numbers to determine expenses, costs, and estimated production. For example, suppose the office generates a list of the number of child prophylaxis procedures performed in August and then generates the same list for February (the 6-month recare interval); the staff can then check that the numbers coincide. From this comparison, the office can identify clients who need appointments so recare activities can be directed specifically toward them.

It may be difficult some months to meet the monthly production goal because of time out of the office, no shows, or cancellations. Monitoring and compensating for these situations improves production totals and keeps the schedule full, preventing any open unscheduled time. One action plan to compensate for an anticipated decrease in income is to add a couple of extra days of work in the month preceding or following the shortfall. Another method for increasing daily production is to schedule more patients for several days that month until the production goal is met. Maintaining an effective recare system helps keep the schedule booked. Many consultants agree it is vitally important to the health of the practice to continually monitor daily production totals.

## Another Approach

A few dental practices do not follow the production system with a daily production goal because they do not want to meet specific numbers. What they do instead is determine how much they must charge per hour to meet costs and then adjust their fees accordingly. This approach is found in dental practices that do not participate in any insurance programs and are not fee-for-service practices.

## MANAGING FEE INCREASES

Fees are increased each year or when the demand for dental hygiene services increases. The cost of living increases yearly by 3–4%; therefore, fees should increase yearly by at least this amount. Increasing fees by 10% compensates for a one-third attrition rate, meaning the professional could lose one-third of his or her patients and still remain at the same level of profit. Increasing fees by 20% compensates for the loss of half the patients while remaining at the same profit level. There should be no guilt or any other negative emotion associated with fee increases because dental hygienists render valuable services.

## PRODUCTION ANALYSIS

A variety of formulas can be used to gauge the financial health of the dental practice. One method of measuring the economic health of a business is net margin. **Net margin** is the proportion of gross billings remaining after all costs have been paid. It is com-

**BOX 12.5** *Calculating Net Margin*

$$(\text{Gross billings} - \text{Expenses}) \div \text{Gross billings} = \text{Net margin}$$

Gross billings = \$384,000        Expenses = \$222,720

$$(\$384,000 - \$222,720) = \$161,280 \div \$384,000 = 0.42$$

The net margin for the dental hygiene department is 0.42 or 42%.

puted by subtracting expenses from revenues and dividing the result by gross billings (*Box 12.5*). Although the average net margin is 40%, it can be as high as 50% and as low as 31%. Net margin does not measure financial success, but it does allow the office to monitor production relative to costs. The net margin is only as accurate and current as the information used in the calculation. The most logical methods for improving the net margin are to ensure adequate production, charge cost-effective fees, schedule all available appointment times, and deliver oral healthcare efficiently.

## CONCEPT SUMMARY

- Dental hygiene services are crucial to the financial health and growth of the dental practice.
- Dental hygiene production ranges from 25% to 35% of the total production in a general dentistry practice.
- Production blocking is a technique used to set aside time in the schedule for primary procedures.
- Forecasting growth attributes is needed to determine practice expansion.
- Total quality management, service design and process, inventory, and scheduling are methods to improve production and customer service.
- Product sales increase dental hygiene production totals.
- A net margin analysis is one method for assessing the financial health of the practice.

# REVIEW QUESTIONS

1. How does practice production affect the success of the practice?
2. How important is the dental hygiene department to the financial health of the dental practice?
3. What is the difference between primary, secondary, and tertiary dental hygiene procedures?
4. What is production blocking?
5. What is the benchmark for dental hygiene department production?
6. What growth markers are needed for practice expansion?
7. What is total quality management and how does it affect customer service?
8. Why is service design and process necessary for a service sector businesses?
9. What effect can a dental assistant have on production in the hygiene department?
10. How can managing and controlling inventory affect the dental practice?
11. How does product sales promotion improve production totals?
12. What is practice net margin?

## Assignment: Determining Production

1. Determine the production total for the single-booked hygiene schedule given in *Box 12.4*. Use the fee schedule provided in *Box 12.6*.
2. Determine the production total for the double-booked hygiene schedule given in *Box 12.3*. Use the fee schedule provided in *Box 12.6*. By how much did production increase as a result of the double-booked schedule?
3. Determine the total production loss assuming that the following appointments were canceled. Then calculate the average lost hourly income.
   Single-booked day: cancellation of Luke Warm.
   Double-booked day: cancellation of Luke Warm and Robin Bird.
4. Determine the production totals for the double-booked day per hour, per 8-hour day, per 4-day week, per 4-week month, per 3-month quarter, and per 12-month year.
5. Use the monthly production total calculated in Problem 4 to determine the number of employees needed for an independent practice.
6. Use the daily production total calculated for the double-booked day in Problem 3 (with two cancellations) to determine the hourly, daily, weekly, monthly, quarterly, and yearly total income lost.

---

**BOX 12.6**  *Sample Fee Schedule*

| | |
|---|---|
| Periodic examination | ($40) |
| 2 bitewings radiographs | $41 |
| 4 bitewings radiographs | $61 |
| Adult prophylaxis | $84 |
| Child prophylaxis | $60 |
| Child/adult fluoride | $35 |
| Full-mouth débridement | $145 |
| Full-mouth x-rays | $120 |
| Local anesthesia | no charge |
| Localized delivery of chemotherapeutic agents | $35 |
| Office visit for observation | $35 |
| Oral hygiene instruction | no charge |
| Periodontal maintenance | $120 |
| Scaling and root planing, 1–3 teeth per quadrant | $150 |
| Scaling and root planing, 4 or more teeth per quadrant | $200 |
| Unspecified periodontal procedure by report | $20 |
| | |
| Dispensing medicaments | |
| Breath malodor kit | $25 |
| Chlorhexidine | $15 |
| Sonic toothbrush | $125 |
| Take home fluoride gel | $10 |

# Credit and Collections

## LEARNING OUTCOMES

Upon mastery of the content of this chapter, the student should be able to:
- Recognize the importance of a 30-day accounts receivable.
- Characterize the payment options used by dental practitioners.
- Identify federal regulations related to credit and collections.
- Recognize potential credit risk patients.
- Determine when a collection agency or small claims court is needed for collection activity.

## KEY TERMS

collections

credit

creditor

fee for service

incidental credit

pro bono

## CREDIT AND COLLECTIONS

After the discussion with the patient regarding his or her diagnosis and possible treatment options, an arrangement is made for the payment of services to be rendered; the patient must be fully informed before any services are performed. Patients must be made aware of not only their dental needs but of the value of the services rendered; furthermore, patients must give informed consent and must understand the office's policies on matters of credit and collections.

**Credit** is the extension of payment for goods and/or services based on the good manner in which a patient conducts his or her personal finances. A **creditor** grants to customers the right to defer payment for purchased goods or services. Creditors report their customers' business transactions and payment deferrals to financial institutions, called credit bureaus, which rate the financial behaviors on a credit report. Major credit-reporting agencies include Experian, TransUnion, and Equifax. Some dental offices obtain a copy of the patient's credit report from one of these credit bureaus when first accepting the patient into the practice. The reports help the staff determine whether the patient presents a risk for nonpayment. Because some clients do not fulfill their financial obligations, it becomes necessary for dental practices to use collection techniques. **Collections**

are a series of activities undertaken to obtain payment of monies owed to the dental practice.

# CREDIT

A common business philosophy held by many healthcare practitioners is to not extend credit to patients. Many aspects of credit law may be better handled by banks, lending institutions, and credit companies, who deal with these issues more frequently than does the dental office. Lending institutions, stores, and other businesses do not extend credit to all customers, and the dental office should not give credit to every patient. In such instances, clients who want to use credit as a means to finance oral healthcare are directed to seek the assistance of a lending source.

If the dental practice does extend credit, several procedures must be followed. According to the U.S. Federal Deposit Insurance Corporation (FDIC) Truth-in-Lending Act, healthcare providers become creditors when procedures are performed at a cost that exceeds $100, which is not paid within 90 days. The U.S. Internal Revenue Service (IRS) assumes that any account carried over 90 days accrues interest regardless of whether an interest charge is stated. Patients are asked to sign a federal truth-in-lending disclosure statement when the oral healthcare provider is going to carry a balance; the statement informs them of the interest charges that accrue after 90 days.

**Incidental credit** is a type of credit extended for personal, family, or household purposes, which is granted for 90 days. The debt is not subject to any finance charge or interest during that time. It is commonly called "90 days same as cash." Incidental credit is given when a multiple payment plan will not last longer than 90 days. After 90 days, such credit is no longer called incidental credit because finance charges can be applied.

## Equal Credit Opportunity Act

The U.S. Equal Credit Opportunity Act bars discrimination in all areas of credit to ensure that credit is available fairly and impartially. It prohibits discrimination because of race, color, religion, national origin, sex, marital status, or age, or because the customer receives income from any public assistance program. This act allows creditors to grant credit to defer payment for goods and services. Because of the complexity of this issue, the practice is advised to have a third-party lender extend credit to dental patients to avoid any misinterpretation of the law or claims of discrimination. To be sure fair practices are in use, standardized forms collect the same information from each and every client.

## Financial Arrangements

Once the patient's dental needs have been explained and value is created, financial arrangements are made. Clients are directed to a payment option that takes into account the needed treatment, number of appointments, costs, and preferences. Financial arrangements are negotiations that have the ultimate goal of clearing the account balance as quickly as possible, usually within 60 days, although 30 days is optimum. To keep in line with U.S. credit law, outstanding balances beyond 90 days change the terms of the agreement and allow finance charge accrual.

Preferably, financial arrangements are done in person, but they can be conducted by telephone. Negotiation of terms is likely to be most successful when all possible problems are identified and remedied, resulting in a mutual agreement and consent. The finalized agreement is formalized in writing, and the written record of negotiations is placed into the patient's record. Any future discussions or agreement modifications are also documented and stored in the record.

## Payment Options

Payment options allow patients to pay for their care within 60 days to keep accounts receivable totals low. Any payment plan made available by the practitioner should be agreeable to the patient. An unhappy patient is more likely to file a lawsuit against the practice than is a satisfied one. A preestablished office policy should be based on the financial philosophy of the practice, socioeconomic status of the patient, and the operational costs of the office (*Box 13.1*).

Multiple payment plans have two basic scenarios: one-third payment or one-half payment. The one-third multiple payment plan requires that the first third of the balance be paid at the appointment time, the next third within 30 days, and the final third within 60 days. The one-third payment option clears the account balance within 60 days. The one-half multiple payment plan requires that the first half of the balance be paid at the appointment time, and the final half within 30 days. The one-half payment plan clears the account within 30 days.

Another form of multiple payment plan is the issuance of postdated checks submitted by the patient at the start of treatment. The checks can then be deposited by the dental practice according to the prearranged dates of the payment plan.

Third-party payment plans are programs sponsored by lending sources such as credit cards, banks, healthcare financing programs, local dental professional societies, or insurance programs. With third-party payment plans, the entire account balance is paid in full before treatment begins, and there is no remaining balance over 30 days. Using a credit card for account payments zeros out the balance on the account at each visit. Bank loans enable the patient to pay for his or her entire treatment before it begins and thus to receive possible incentives such as a 5% fee reduction. Healthcare financing programs such as Care Credit and the Dental Fee Plan also pay for the entire costs before treatment is rendered. Local professional dental societies may have financing programs available for the patients of member dentists.

---

### BOX 13.1 *Payment Options*

Cash, check, or credit card payment at each appointment
Cash or check for entire amount before treatment begins receives a courtesy fee reduction of 5%
Loan from a bank, credit card, or finance company
Multiple payment plan to be completed within 90 days
Pro bono oral healthcare services
Senior citizen discount of 10%
Statement billing

Dental insurance as the third-party lender can be used in two ways: with reimbursement to the dentist or to the patient. When the reimbursement is sent to the dentist, the insurance claim is filed with the carrier, and the patient pays his or her anticipated percentage. When the reimbursement is sent to the patient, he or she pays for treatment directly to the dental practice and then receives a check from the insurance company.

**Pro bono** oral healthcare services are procedures performed for the patient at no charge. Some oral healthcare providers offer pro bono care to people in need. The no-fee or "pay when you can" philosophy of a dental practice may be broadcast throughout the community via word of mouth. Thus, oral healthcare providers should know what their limits of free care are and exercise caution once they adopt this policy owing to the potential for attracting high-credit-risk clients who are seeking free or reduced-fee care.

## Credit Risks

Unfortunately, some people have no intention of paying for their oral healthcare; their goal is to receive free services. It is important to try to identify such individuals. The poor-credit-risk patient may have one or more of the following characteristics:

- Moves from dental practice to dental practice.
- States he or she has dental insurance, but after verification procedures is found to not be covered.
- Has insurance that is expiring and asks for care to be done in a short period of time.
- Overreacts when asked to pay.
- Complains or finds fault with the care received.
- Changes jobs in a short period of time.
- Has moved often.
- Has family problems—separation, divorce, large number of children.
- Has dental needs caused by an accidental injury.

Several methods can improve the likelihood of being paid in these scenarios. Make a copy of the patient's driver's license and obtain the number of a valid credit card so any remaining balances can be charged. Generate a credit report from a credit bureau to help determine whether to extend credit based on past credit history. Discover whether homeowners' or automobile insurance will cover the costs of an accidental injury and try to establish who is responsible for payment. If possible, do not schedule further appointments until the outstanding balances are paid in full.

## Fee for Service

It is widely known that the longer the time lapse, the less likely the patient will pay for his or her care. The financially successful practice has a 30-day or less accounts receivable collection rate. This financial principle makes it mandatory that payment be made at the time the services are rendered. A **fee-for-service** office policy demands payment at the appointment time in the form of cash, check, credit card, or payment from another lending source. Many dental consultants recommend that dental offices establish a policy of no financing and no lending.

The business office that follows the fee-for-service model does not submit dental insurance claims as a courtesy to the patient; the patient pays the costs up front. The patient must communicate with his or her insurance company by submitting an itemized receipt stapled to a blank insurance form requesting reimbursement be sent directly to him or her. The oral healthcare provider does not become a creditor for these clients, and no billing statements need to be sent each month. Many offices are moving to this system of accounts receivable owing to denials of and delays in payment from insurance companies and patients.

## Account Aging

Account aging is a business procedure that determines outstanding account balances to provide basic information for collection of delinquent payments. Account age analysis reports are generated by computer to identify patients who have not paid for services, to determine how much is owed, and to discover the length of time without payment. Patient accounts are reviewed weekly to prevent an accounts receivable beyond 90 days. The patient with an outstanding unpaid balance has a reason for not paying, and the best way to obtain payment is to determine those reasons via telephone and to avoid jeopardizing future relations.

## COLLECTIONS

Collection procedures are usually outlined in the office policy and procedures manual. Having an awareness of accounts receivables plus a proactive collection system in place helps in these matters. The most successful method of collection is to inform the patient via the treatment plan of the cost for each procedure performed and the amount he or she must pay at the end of each appointment. Collection activities are listed in *Box 13.2.* Collection protocols differ from office to office; one example is given in *Box 13.3.*

After statements are sent, telephone contact has been made, and a series of three collection letters have been mailed, a decision is made whether to pursue the matter in small claims court or to send the account to a collection agency. All contact with the person responsible for the account should be documented in the patient's record. Scripts are followed when making collection telephone calls. Sample collection letters are found in dental office software programs and are written in a business format in 40 words or less to increase readership. Motivating phrases that appeal to basic human needs with catch phrases such as "we provided good service," are found in collection letters. A sample final collection letter is given in Chapter 22.

## Fair Debt Collection Practices Act

Federal law states that collection calls to demand payment cannot be made to a person at his or her workplace. According to the federal Fair Debt Collection Practices Act,

---

**BOX 13.2** *Collection Activities*

Informed consent forms that include pricing
Monthly statements
Assorted sticker messages placed on statements
A series of collection letters

Telephone calls
A collection agency
Small claims court

## BOX 13.3  *Collection Protocol*

| | |
|---|---|
| 30 days | Send statement with a sticker message |
| 45 days | Send first collection form letter |
| 60 days | Telephone call and second collection form letter |
| 75 days | Send final collection form letter with a warning of collection |
| 90 days | Send account to a collection agency or small claims court |

however, telephone contact can be made with the workplace to determine if the patient is employed there. It is also lawful to call the patient at work to arrange a convenient time to call him or her at home to discuss the account.

### Collection Agencies

When choosing a collection agency, make sure that it deals with dental accounts, follows federal laws, and attempts to collect on any dollar amount. Patient accounts are handed over to collection agencies when office systems have been unable to collect outstanding balances. The office policy and procedure manual should have guidelines as to when accounts are turned over to collection agencies. Collection agencies use the following information, which may be in the patient's dental record, to make contact with the patient: a copy of the driver's license, the Social Security number, the credit report, the patient registration information, and the financial records. Accounts are handed over to the agency at 90 days to improve the chance for account settlement. Collection agencies attempt to collect outstanding accounts for a fee (usually half of what is collected).

All payments or contacts received by the dental practice are reported to the agency at once to prevent legal liability. Debtors commonly assert that they will pay when they receive a check from the insurance company or when the dental office corrects an error in the bill. When the debtor claims that the insurance company will pay, be sure to provide the collection agency with copies of any rejection letters from the insurance company. Be sure to clearly explain and outline all bills so the patient is less likely to have a basis for questioning the validity of the outstanding balance.

### Small Claims Court

Some dental offices pursue delinquent accounts in the legal system instead of using collection agencies because of the diminishing return on amounts paid. Small claims court allows the dentist to present delinquent accounts to a judge in an attempt to collect outstanding debt. The business dental assistant may act as an agent for the dentist to appear in court at the scheduled time. The same patient records that are provided to a collection agency may be used as evidence in court. When the judge rules in favor of the dental office, several events may occur. If the patient shows up in court, he or she will have to pay the court clerk after the hearing. If the patient does not show up in court, the court can place a lien at the patient's place of employment to garnish his or her wages until the debt is repaid. If the patient is not employed, the court can seize property to be sold at public auction until the debt is paid.

## CONCEPT SUMMARY

- The financial success of a dental practice can be measured by a 30-day accounts receivable.
- Payment options used by dental practitioners help clients finance their dental care.
- Federal regulations in credit and collections provide for equality and nondiscriminatory actions in financial matters.
- Some dental clients are potential credit risks and have no intention of paying for dental care.
- A collection agency and small claims court are final options when attempts to collect outstanding balances have failed.

## REVIEW QUESTIONS

1. When is the oral healthcare provider not a creditor?
2. Why is it not a good policy to extend credit to patients?
3. What is incidental credit and how is it applicable in dentistry?
4. Is it necessary to make financial arrangements with patients who have dental insurance? If yes, when is this done?
5. List the payment options used in dental practices.
6. What should be considered when payment options are selected?
7. What is the difference among the federal acts regulating credit and collections?
8. Why is federal legislation necessary for matters of credit and collection?
9. Who is potentially a credit risk?
10. What is a fee-for-service practice?
11. Why are account aging reports generated?
12. What is of the utmost importance for preventing collection problems?
13. List the collection activities commonly found in dental offices.
14. How do collection agencies operate?
15. When a favorable small claims court judgment has been made, how is the debt collected?

## CRITICAL THINKING GROUP ACTIVITY

1. Why should the dental practice collect fees within 30 days?
2. Is it a good policy to extend credit to patients?
3. Why don't some people pay their dental financial obligations?
4. Could you recognize a credit risk?
5. What demands are placed on a person's finances that could make him or her unable to pay the dental account balance? Does this make the individual a "deadbeat"? Does the dental practice need to be paid?
6. Should oral healthcare providers provide pro bono dental services?
7. Would you provide the number of a valid credit card to be charged for any remaining balances?
8. If you were in independent practice in a small community, would you send your accounts to a collection agency or pursue the debt in small claims court?

# 14

# Records Management

Upon mastery of the content of this chapter, the student should be able to:

- Appreciate the complexity, specialization, and importance of records management.
- Differentiate between clinical and financial patient records.
- Characterize the three basic records management systems used in medical and dental practice.
- Describe how technology has enhanced records management.
- Recognize the scope and intent of the Health Insurance Portability and Accountability Act (HIPAA) privacy laws.

## KEY TERMS

active files

alphabetical filing

bar code systems

chart audit

filing

inactive files

indexing

numeric filing

records management

terminal digit filing

## RECORDS MANAGEMENT

In the healthcare industry, records management has become an important and necessary function for handling private medical information. Dental office systems are modeled after medical records management systems, and business dental assistants implement and maintain the dental office records. Although medical records specialists have more focused and specialized education, business dental assistants are also qualified to work with the clinical and financial data of patients. Dental hygienists may be asked to perform records management activities during the course of the business day.

Data collection, documentation, information storage and retrieval, and records maintenance must be organized for quality assurance and risk management. **Records management** is the organization, maintenance, and protection of client information either electronically or on paper. The patients' clinical and financial records are kept separately in dental practices. Fully computerized offices keep financial data in electronic databases, which are backed up daily; the clinical records are stored adjacent to the reception area.

In noncomputerized dental practices, financial ledger cards used in accounting board systems are stored in a different file box from that of the clinical records. **Filing** is the storage of sorted data.

There are three primary types of filing systems: alphabetical, numeric, and terminal digit. In **alphabetical filing** systems, stored data are arranged according to the letters of the alphabet. In **numeric filing** systems, stored data are arranged according to numbers, such as account, policy, license, or case numbers. In **terminal digit filing** systems, stored data are arranged according to three sets of numbers corresponding to terminals, sections, and file folders. Other filing system variations include geographical filing and subject and chronological filing.

## FILING SYSTEMS

### Alphabetical Filing

Alphabetical filing systems are recommended for practices with up to 10,000 patient files. The average number of active files for an independent practice hygienist is about 2,000. The basic idea of alphabetical filing is to sort the files starting with the patients whose last names begin with the letter *A* and ending with the patients' whose last names begin with the letter *Z*. Alphabetical filing may be based on names, geographic location or ZIP code, or chronology and subject area.

#### NAME INDEXING

The most common form of alphabetical filing is the indexing of client names. **Indexing** is the division of a patient's name in a rank order for information storage (*Box 14.1*). All patient information is first sorted by last, first, and middle name. *Box 14.2* provides an example of how a name is indexed.

The common universal rule to remember when filing is that "nothing comes before something." If, for example, one patient is named Bill Slate and another is named Bill S. Slate, the rule indicates that the name Bill Slate is filed before the name Bill S. Slate. Surnames with prefixes—such as De, De La, Del, La, Mac, Mc, O', St, Ste, and Van—are indexed as if the prefix is part of the surname. Names with abbreviated prefixes are indexed as if the prefix were spelled out. For example, Renee Ste. Jacques is sorted as Sainte Jacques, Renee. Hyphenated surnames are considered as one word and are indexed on the first word in the name. For example, Mary Makie-Farrar is stored under M for Makie-Farrar,

---

**BOX 14.1** *Order of Indexing Names*

Last name (family name, surname)
    First name
        Middle name, initial, or maiden name
            Seniority (Senior/Junior), rank (Captain, Lieutenant), title (Lord, Lady)
                Courtesy title (Mr., Mrs., Ms)

Mary. Titles, college degrees, and courtesy titles (Mr., Mrs., Ms) are informational and used only to differentiate between two individuals who share the same name, such as Robert Johnson and Robert Johnson, PhD. Finally, names with abbreviations that indicate seniority, such as Jr. and Sr., are indexed alphabetically as if the abbreviations were spelled out (junior and senior); similarly, names with Roman numerals that indicate seniority, such as II and III, are sorted as if the numerals were spelled out (second and third).

### GEOGRAPHICAL FILING AND ZIP CODE FILING

Geographical filing, a variation of alphabetical filing, is used to sort information based on states and cities. The name of the state and city where a person or business is located are the first items indexed. For example, the file for Sue H. Smith from Mobile, Alabama, is sorted first on Alabama, then on Mobile, then on Smith, then on Sue, and finally on H. In dental practices, sorting charts by city is more common than sorting by state.

ZIP code filing sorts patients' files according to their post office ZIP codes. The ZIP code is indexed first, and then files are sorted by the alphabetical indexing of patients' names within each ZIP code. Businesses that use bundle bulk mail use ZIP code filing to take advantage of reduced postal rates. Furthermore, ZIP codes are frequently bar coded; and in **bar code systems**, files are marked with a label containing the bar code identifier. Information for file and label creation is downloaded from the computer software program used for bar coding.

### SUBJECT AND CHRONOLOGICAL FILING

Subject filing is used to sort information by subject area, such as orthodontic and periodontal patients. The patient records are filed alphabetically within the subject area. Chronological filing is used to sort information by date of visit and is used most effectively with recare card files of preaddressed appointment-reminder postcards.

## Numeric Filing

Numeric filing sorts information by numbers instead of names and is recommended for practices that manage more than 10,000 patient files. In this filing system, the first file is labeled 00000, and the remaining files are given consecutive numbers through 50000. Dental offices, insurance companies, legal firms, and government agencies use numeric filing to maintain paperwork by account, policy, license, or case number. This system is best used by large companies that must take care of large numbers of records.

Note that in a numeric filing system, the records of a single family are not stored together; therefore, each patient must be located by file number before his or her record can be found. This is a little more time-consuming, because staff members must first search for the account number in the computer or in an accession book. An accession book is a cross-referencing tool used to register the numbers assigned to patients. It prevents two patients from having the same number by showing the next available number. An accession book is also used to find missing numeric files by providing the name that has been assigned to that number.

## Terminal Digit Filing

A terminal digit filing system is indicated for high-volume practices with 50,000 or more patients; it is a simple method of filing. The numbering system consists of three pairs of digits, which are assigned to each patient from a master control list. It is built around three simple principles: the filing area is divided into 100 terminals, each terminal is divided into 100 sections and each section is divided into 100 file folders. A file with the number 152003 is located at terminal 15, section 20, file 03. This filing system eliminates problems with identical names; furthermore, locating a file is easy and the system will not reach full capacity. Using color coding (see below) further helps eliminate misfiled records.

## CHART AUDITING

The oral healthcare provider performs a **chart audit** before placing a patient record into the filing system. The audit involves checking the contents for completeness and making sure the folder contains no improperly placed materials. It is beneficial to assign a business staff member to double-check each file before it is returned to the storage area as part of a quality assurance program. Insurance company representatives may ask the practice administrator to review the files of their clients. After their review, the representatives send a report to document the visit and their findings. Such auditors are reviewing files for the following types of information: medical history updates that are signed and dated at each visit, documentation of oral cancer screening results, proper flagging of medical conditions, accurate recording of services rendered, and radiographs.

## RECORD STORAGE

Shelf files are the most efficient and cost-effective paper document filing system. Open shelf filing systems allow visual recognition of records; are fast; are convenient; and can handle records in a variety of media from paper documents to optical disks, magnetic media, and microfilm. Archived paper records should be stored in tightly packed fireproof metal filing cabinets. Some legal authorities recommend that archived records be retained for 10 years; others recommend that such records be kept forever, even after the death of the patient and/or healthcare provider.

## Active versus Inactive Files

There are two principal types of files: active and inactive. **Active files** are the current records of patients who have been seen within the previous 3 years. **Inactive files** are the records of patients who have stopped treatment or who have not been seen for 3 years. Transfer of records from active to inactive should be performed periodically throughout the year. Date tabs or stickers are attached to patients' files for aging purposes; they indicate the year in which the patients were last seen in the office. Inactive files are purged; placed into labeled boxes, shelves, or cabinets; and stored either in or out of the office. In some instances, data may be duplicated onto microfiche for electronic information storage and the paper records then shredded and recycled.

## Color Coding

Color coding is used to enhance record management. At a distance, the human eye sees colors and patterns faster than it recognizes letters and numbers. Color-coded systems work well when more than one person has regular access to the records; it also allows immediate recognition of filing errors. The color-coding system uses colored folders, tabs, and/or stickers and is available in all three filing systems, but it proves most beneficial when used with terminal digit filing.

## Bar Coding

Bar code filing is used in the oral healthcare setting to streamline office systems; these identification and data collection systems rely on high-tech scanner and labeling equipment. Owing to increasing office operational costs and stricter privacy laws, healthcare providers have turned to cost-effective technological solutions to secure patient information and documents. Bar coding allows offices to control items that need to be tracked, such as patient files, x-rays, other images, and diagnostic test results. A computer software program generates the bar codes, which can then be printed onto labels. Handheld scanners read the bar codes to track the movement of patient information. This enhances security, reduces loss, locates documents, tracks files, and keeps a record of the chain of custody. Computer-generated reports monitor and manage chart location and the media within.

## Electronic Imaged Documents

State-of-the-art document processing uses document imaging and optically stored programs to convert business documents into electronic data. These processes save time, expense, and paper, and are legally admissible forms of records that can be used in court. Digital computer information, document imaging, and bar coding help the dental practice meet growing business and regulatory demands.

Electronic imaging is a cost-effective way to handle documents and share information with employees and business associates. Document management systems convert paper documents into a format that is electronically accessible via the Internet using a standard Web browser. A computerized management system scans documents, indexes and stores documents, creates cross-references and links among the electronic files, and allows file sharing and document retrieval.

By using electronically generated files, the dental office reduces its reliance on paper, photographic and/or x-ray film, and storage equipment; a single CD-ROM can store as much information as a 15-drawer file cabinet. Electronic storage is important for any disaster recovery strategy because it allows the secure storage of documents both on and off site. A file storage service allows offices to transfer copies of their electronic files to a central data center using data encryption; the service then indexes, compresses, and stores the documents until needed for viewing, printing, faxing, or emailing. Document retrieval is performed using a search engine that is available 24/7 via an Internet connection.

## Missing Files

In most cases, missing files have been misplaced, not lost. Missing charts or items from charts may be in the custody of another staff member, may have been placed in a location that disguises its presence, or may have been misfiled. The situation is taken seriously if a search does not reveal the file's location, and a temporary chart is then started. If the patient is aware of the missing information, he or she must be assured that it will be located. A quick check of the patient's financial record can provide information on what procedures were completed and when. This will also help the clinician determine what needs to be done in the event the patient's treatment plan is unavailable.

## HEALTH INSURANCE PORTABILITY AND ACCOUNTABILITY ACT

To help American citizens keep medical insurance coverage after termination of employment and to keep personal health information private, Congress enacted (and then revised) the Health Insurance Portability and Accountability Act (HIPAA). HIPAA is administered by the Centers for Medicare and Medicaid Services (CMS) within the U.S. Department of Health and Human Services. One component of the law allows ex-employees to maintain their medical benefits for up to 18 months after losing their job; it is frequently referred to as COBRA for the Consolidated Omnibus Budget Reconciliation Act. The COBRA benefit is time limited, however, and patient insurance coverage should be verified at the time of oral healthcare delivery.

HIPAA also defines patient privacy practices and the rights of patients to access their clinical records. After reading a statement explaining the privacy practices, clients sign a notice acknowledging that they have been informed of the practices. HIPAA's changes came about after complaints were made to Congress regarding the sale of patients' personal information by healthcare providers to companies for use in direct marketing of supplies and services to particular patients.

## Privacy Practices

Under HIPAA, the dental office is required to keep health information private, to notify patients regarding privacy practices, and to inform patients of their legal rights. Staff members must be trained in HIPAA practices and undergo periodic updates. Patients sign a HIPAA form titled "Notice of Privacy Practices" after being apprised of the office policy and implementation of the privacy act. If a patient refuses to sign or is unable to sign, the office documents the barriers or situations that prevented the patient from signing the acknowledgment. The patient is entitled to a copy of the Notice of Privacy

**BOX 14.3** *Health Information Disclosure*

| | |
|---|---|
| Credentialing activities | Provider performance reviews |
| Criminal justice system | Quality assessment and improvement activities |
| Messages for appointment reminders | Social services |
| Military authority | Training programs |
| Physicians/other healthcare providers | |

Practices and a copy is placed in the patient's file. Health information is disclosed to many entities (*Box 14.3*), and financial information is disclosed to outside sources to obtain payment for services (such as dental insurance companies, collection agencies, and the legal system).

## Access to Records

Patients have a legal right to look at or request a copy of their records and make any additions or corrections to their file. Requests must be placed in writing using an appropriate HIPAA form. In the instance of a copy request, a reasonable fee may be charged for duplication of the records and radiographs and for staff time and postage. The dental practice has 30 days to comply with a patient's request. If a patient believes any violation of his or her privacy rights has occurred, a complaint may be filed with the CMS.

## Business Associate Contracts

Business associate agreements are made with any person or entity that has access to or uses protected health information within the dental practice. The business associate may be the person performing legal, actuarial, accounting, consulting, data aggregation, management, administration, accreditation, or financial services that concern protected health information. A written agreement with each separate business associate protects the patients' private health information yet allows for the use and disclosure of private health information so the associates can complete their fiduciary duties. The agreement may be terminated if there is any breach of contract by giving written notice, and the business associate must return all client records or data compiled from the records.

## CONCEPT SUMMARY

- Records management is used for clinical and financial patient records.
- The three basic records management systems used in medical and dental practices are alphabetical, numeric, and terminal digit filing.
- Technology has enhanced records management by the use of bar coding, scanning, and electronic duplication and storage of data.
- The HIPAA privacy laws have affected dental practices by mandating records management systems that ensure information privacy.

# REVIEW QUESTIONS

1. What is records management and why do some people specialize in it?
2. What is the difference between active and inactive files?
3. What is the system capacity for each of the three methods of filing medical and dental records?
   A. Alphabetical
   B. Numeric
   C. Terminal digit
4. How does the office computer system affect records management?
5. How would a barcode system work in private practice?
6. Why is electronic imaging a viable office process?
7. Why did HIPAA privacy legislation come to pass?
8. What are the basic elements of HIPAA?
9. Is it mandatory to give the patient a copy of his or her records when requested?
10. How are business associate contracts implemented?
11. Place the following names in the correct indexing order.
    Kay O'Pectate     Roger Overendoute
    Bill Overdeaux    Keri Onward
    Al Oye            Patty O'Cover
12. Place the following names in the correct indexing order.
    John Johnson        Johnny Johnson Sr.
    John St. John       John Robert Johnson III
    J. R. Johnson       John Thomas Johnson II
    J. T. Johnson Jr.

# Appointment Scheduling Systems

## LEARNING OUTCOMES

Upon mastery of the content of this chapter, the student should be able to:
- Recognize times when the oral healthcare provider is unavailable to see patients.
- Distinguish among the characteristics of appointment scheduling for production.
- Follow appointment scheduling suggestions.
- List patient priority for appointment scheduling.
- Identify the principles of appointment confirmation and for handling broken appointments, late arrivals, and cancellations.
- Use daily treatment schedules.
- Initiate referrals.

## KEY TERMS

Broken appointments
Double booking
Flex time

Scheduling coordinator
Time management

## APPOINTMENT SCHEDULING SYSTEMS

Appointment scheduling is an office system that uses time management. **Time management** is the efficient scheduling of work so that a maximum productivity level can be achieved without causing the dental professional to rush through oral healthcare services or fall behind in the schedule. Dental practice profits improve when the appointment schedule is varied and stress free and without no-shows, cancellations, and gaps. Knowing when to schedule is the basis for handling appointments. Appointments are scheduled around blocked-out time (which cannot be used) and for available open time. The blocked-out areas are reserved for times when the oral healthcare providers are not available to treat patients or for times when only selected types of procedures are performed.

## SCHEDULING

A patient's appointment is made in a manner similar to almost any reservation. An appointment is a reserved time set aside specifically for a single patient. Patients are informed of their next appointment time, and the staff emphasizes that the time is reserved just for them. This is done to prevent rescheduling, cancellations, and no-shows. Stress-free days consist of patients arriving on time and leaving on time, indicating that the office schedule was adequately planned and managed.

Sometimes the oral healthcare provider is in the dental office yet unavailable to treat patients. Such periods are blocked out to prevent staff from scheduling patient appointments. *Box 15.1* lists typical daily and yearly blocked-out periods in a dental office. When possible, professionals plan their time out of the office at least 6 months in advance, and at a minimum, 30 days in advance, to avoid inconveniencing patients.

Just one person should perform appointment scheduling because errors occur when many people make appointment reservations. When one person manages the appointment schedule, he or she has control over planning work and makes fewer errors. Some dental practice consultants believe the person who takes on these duties should be the dental hygienist; other consultants recommend that an office staff member handle appointment scheduling because the best use of the dental hygienist's time is rendering comprehensive oral healthcare services. Be advised that appointment scheduling varies from dental practice to dental practice, making this a subject to be discussed during employment negotiations.

Scheduled appointments are entered into the office computer system or an appointment book. The pages or computer screens are dated and viewed one day or one week at a time. Each operatory and/or oral healthcare provider has a column set aside for appointment scheduling (*Fig. 15.1*). A predetermined time limit for each oral healthcare service is established and blocked by 10- or 15-minute increments. The time required for dental procedures varies according to patient needs, provider ability, and available assistance.

## Production Blocking

Efficiently scheduling appointments is one of the most important aspects of a well-managed dental practice because this system is tantamount to the practice's productivity and financial security. Based on a daily production goal, production blocking for primary procedures ensures the necessary open time for high-production-value appointments. Preblocked time should be filled at least 72 hours in advance; if the time is not filled with primary dental hygiene procedures by then, secondary and tertiary procedures should be scheduled instead.

---

**BOX 15.1** *Blocked-Out Office Time*

Time is blocked out of the dental office schedule so staff members have time for the following activities.

| | |
|---|---|
| Continuing education courses | Recare scheduling |
| Conventions or meetings | Staff meetings |
| Days out of the office | Staff performance review |
| Flex time | Treatment planning |
| Lunchtime or dinnertime | Vacations and holidays |

*D. Floss*                    **Daily Schedule**           *T. Brushe*

M   T   W   Th   F   Sa                    Date _____

| | | |
|---|---|---|
| | 8:00 | |
| | 8:10 | |
| | 8:20 | |
| | 8:30 | |
| | 8:40 | |
| | 8:50 | |
| | 9:00 | |
| | 9:10 | |
| | 9:20 | |
| | 9:30 | |
| | 9:40 | |
| | 9:50 | |
| | 10:00 | |
| | 10:10 | |
| | 10:20 | |
| | 10:30 | |
| | 10:40 | |
| | 10:50 | |
| | 11:00 | |
| | 11:10 | |

**Figure 15.1** An example of a two-column daily schedule.

## Scheduling Suggestions

Appointment scheduling is more than placing names into available time slots. The dental hygiene treatment plan provides appointment details, such as amount of time needed for each appointment, oral healthcare services to be rendered by insurance code, and time interval needed between each appointment. Difficult cases are best scheduled during the peak effectiveness time of the provider. For example, a morning person performs better earlier in the day. An afternoon or evening person performs better later in the day. For more on peak times and physiologic clocks, see Chapter 29.

It is generally recommended that the same time and day of the week be reserved for each patient based on his or her availability. If a patient favors Monday afternoon appointments, schedule a series of them. The patient will be less likely to forget the appointment times because he or she will associate a specific time and day with the dentist's office.

Plan flexible time around the lunch hour to reduce stress. This allows for the performance of other job tasks and helps maintain the time schedule if the office is running late. Flexibility allows time for complications, late arrivals, and other job-related responsibilities. **Flex time** is unscheduled appointment time that can be used for planning; making calls to pharmacies or patients for recare or wellness checks; writing letters or narratives; and performing other tasks. Flex time provides space in the schedule for such tasks and helps maintain the daily schedule so staff can compensate if anyone begins to fall behind.

The **scheduling coordinator** is a business dental assistant with responsibility for managing and maintaining the appointment calendar. The amount of time needed for specific procedures and the gap between appointments are predetermined and listed on the treatment plan or in the office manual protocols.

The scheduling coordinator must also take into consideration the time needed to clean and set up the operatory between patients, the number of available instruments, and the capability of the sterilization area to process those instruments for the next appointment. The daily schedule must account for the time needed for such repeated procedures. Sterilization time is a minimum of 30 minutes, depending on the equipment in use. When possible, the office should have an adequate inventory of instruments and supplies to reduce the stress caused by waiting for sterilization to finish, to improve production, and to avoid making patients wait or sending them away without providing treatment.

The scheduling coordinator is expected to build variety into each day. Whenever possible, the coordinator avoids scheduling two consecutive appointments for the same type of treatment to prevent staff boredom and stress. Variety makes the day more pleasurable and improves efficiency while decreasing monotony, errors, and stress. A stress-free day can be achieved by reducing scheduling errors. The oral healthcare provider becomes stressed when two patients arrive at the same time for an appointment, when the office begins to run behind schedule, when patients arrive late or cancel, and when there is unscheduled production time.

## Dental Patient Priority

Patients are scheduled according to priority. The top-priority dental hygiene patient is the patient of record who is in an active course of periodontal therapy. This patient has been informed of services to be rendered, and needs periodontal scaling or root planing, periodontal maintenance, periodontal evaluation, periodontal reevaluation, or other periodontal-related procedure. The second-priority dental hygiene patient has had an examination and requires a consultation appointment to obtain informed consent for needed treatment. If too much time elapses before this patient is seen, he or she may lose the motivation to return to the office, resulting in wasted staff time.

The third-priority patient is the new patient. Production time should be blocked each day for the scheduling of new patients for prophylaxis because new patients help the practice grow. Without new patients and practice growth, production income stands still or drops. The fourth-priority patient is the patient of record who needs a periodic examination and prophylaxis. These appointments are frequently scheduled in advance. The fifth-priority patient is the patient requesting a single service. He or she wants only prophylaxis; dental practices usually do not perform a single service for a patient who is not a patient of record, but exceptions are made based on individual office policy.

## Appointment Confirmation

Appointment cards are written in ink and given to the patient to serve as an exact documentation of the patient's next visit. This card may be professionally designed and includes the dental practice and provider's name, location, and telephone number. Space is provided for the staff to write in the patient's name and appointment date and time. Some appointment cards serve as informed consent, noting procedures and estimated fee quotes and requiring a patient signature. This type of card serves as a written confirmation about the appointment reservation and can be used to document the patient's approval of the conditions established for the appointment. Giving the patient a written reminder and telling him or her of the importance of the reserved time slot reinforce the message that the patient is expected to show up for the appointment.

Telephone appointment confirmation is made by a staff person or an automated service. Confirmation of appointments 24–72 hours in advance is a courtesy performed for the patient and reduces last-minute cancellations and no-shows. Not all healthcare providers call to confirm appointments. Patients who do not come to their appointments are called no-shows or **broken appointments.** Last-minute open time is difficult to fill and represents a loss of production, creating a compensation challenge. For these reasons, patients who are 5 minutes late are called using all available telephone numbers to determine whether or not they are coming. The dental hygienist coordinates with the business office regarding who will make these calls. A message is left at each number regarding the appointment time, asking if everything is okay, and requesting a return call when the patient receives the message. This is done to make the patient accountable for missed appointment time. Each phone call is documented and made a part of the patient's permanent record so that future missed-appointment fees can be charged and a case can be made to dismiss the patient from the practice owing to absenteeism, if necessary.

## NO-SHOWS AND CANCELLATIONS

### Handling Broken Appointments

Patients report a variety of reasons for missing appointments. Illness, death, unforeseen business obligations, and slow traffic are typical excuses. Some or all of these may be considered legitimate in dental practices. Unspoken or nonlegitimate reasons for missing an appointment are lack of money, fear, absentmindedness, and lack of value attached to healthcare issues. In many dental offices, cancellations without due notice and broken appointments incur a penalty. Staff should be reminded not to contribute to patients' ability to cancel appointments by suggesting or recommending that if an appointment is inconvenient they may "just give us a call"; instead, patients should be informed that violating their duty to show for dental appointments can result in fees and dismissal. Broken-appointment fees increase with each infraction and eventually lead to termination of the patient–dentist relationship as a result of this breach of duty by the patient.

Late arrivals are handled according to office policy. Some offices charge a broken appointment fee; others reschedule the appointment. Some may schedule an appointment but tell the patient the time is 15–30 minutes earlier than it really is.

### Cancellations

Dental offices handle cancellations in a variety of ways (*Box 15.2*). Many dental practices institute a fee when inadequate time is given to cancel or change the appointment time or when the patient fails to show. The amount of time needed to fill open appointments is generally between 24 and 72 hours. Cancellation fees can range from $25 to more than $100, depending on the oral healthcare provider or the number of times the patient has canceled.

**BOX 15.2** *Preventing Cancellations*

When scheduling, orally reinforce the need to keep the next appointment.
Charge a fee that increases with each patient breach of duty.
Confirm appointments.
Do not schedule again for that time slot.
Double book the patient.
Make the patient accountable by requiring that he or she contact the office when running at least 5 minutes late.
Schedule appointments at more convenient times.
Schedule during last-minute openings.

A cancellation list contains the names of patients who are waiting for an appointment or who can come in on short notice before their already scheduled appointment. Cancellation lists contain the patient's name, phone number, length of time needed for the treatment, and procedures to be performed. **Double booking** is the scheduling of two patients for the same time. It is done when the staff doubts that one of the two patients will show for the reserved time. This can present a problem and increase the stress level of patients and employees if both patients do arrive for the same appointment. Another method for handling difficult-to-schedule patients is to ask them to call on a day when they are available for a last-minute opening. They may or may not be able to be seen at their request, but this technique can help fill unforeseen and difficult-to-fill last-minute cancellations.

## DAILY TREATMENT SCHEDULES

Easy access to the schedule helps keep the staff informed of the patients who are expected to arrive. Daily treatment schedules list the patient names, appointment times, services to be rendered, and phone numbers to call in the event of a delayed arrival. These schedules are placed everywhere the staff may be located—in every operatory and in the laboratory, lounge, front desk, and even the darkroom. Patient information is protected by Health Insurance Portability and Accountability Act (HIPAA) regulations and daily treatment schedules must be kept from view of the patients.

## INITIATE REFERRALS

When the oral healthcare provider encounters a patient who has needs beyond his or her expertise, it is necessary to use the services of another healthcare provider or specialist. Referrals may be made to medical doctors, dental specialists, or healthcare providers with expertise in a discipline. The patient is referred via a phone call, a written referral letter, or a preprinted referral form kept on file in the dental office. A series of letters are sent as follow-up to any telephone calls between the two dental offices concerning the patient's treatment and outcomes. Once the specialist accepts the patient, the following items may be mailed to him or her: referral letter or form, clinical record/health history, radiographs, diagnosis/prognosis, and treatment received. A sample referral letter written to a patient from a general dentist can be found in Chapter 22.

# REVIEW QUESTIONS

1. Why is one person given the responsibility of making dental appointments?
2. Why is production blocking performed?
3. How are the oral healthcare provider's personal characteristics considered?
4. Which patient has priority on the healthcare provider's time?
5. How is the patient made accountable for appointment scheduling?
6. What legitimate reasons might patients have for breaking appointments?
7. What nonlegitimate reasons might patients have for breaking appointments?
8. What information is found on the cancellation list?
9. How are daily treatment schedules used?
10. When is the patient referred to another healthcare provider?

# CRITICAL THINKING ACTIVITY

1. Set up a form similar to the one provided in *Figure 15.1*. Schedule appointments on it using the following general information and patient information, creating names and phone numbers for each patient.

   General information

   Daily office hours: 9:00 A.M. to 6:00 P.M. Monday, Tuesday, Thursday, and Friday; 8:00 A.M. to 2:00 P.M. Saturday

   Lunch break: 12:00 P.M. to 1:00 P.M.

   One unit of time: 10 minutes

   Standing appointment: Mr. Mason Jarr, dental salesman, 9:00 A.M. every Tuesday

   Patient information

   4 child prophylaxis appointments, including periodic examination, fluoride, and 2 bitewing radiographs at 3 units each

   4 adult prophylaxis appointments, including periodic examination and 4 bitewing radiographs at 5 units each

6 periodontal maintenance appointments with periodontal evaluation at
    6 units each

10 two-quadrant scaling and root planing appointments at 6 units each

5 limited oral examination appointments, including three tooth débridements
    and locally applied antibiotic at 3 units each

2 full-mouth radiograph series appointments, including comprehensive oral
    examination at 3 units each

1 alginate impressions appointment for tooth-whitening procedures at 2 units

1 full-mouth débridement appointment, including a panoramic radiograph at
    4 units

1 suture removal office visit at 1 unit

8 office visits for reevaluation at 3 units each

1 desensitization appointment at 2 units

2 sealant of first molar appointments at 3 units each

2. Create and discuss the "perfect" hygiene schedule, complete with primary, secondary, and tertiary procedures.

## Assignment: Writing Referral Letters

Write a referral letter that will be sent to a physician for a patient with moderate chronic adult periodontitis.

# Chapter

# 16

# Recare Systems

## LEARNING OUTCOMES

Upon mastery of the content of this chapter, the student should be able to:
- Discuss the benefits and shortcomings of the three common recare systems.
- Apply principles of recare maintenance.
- Calculate recare intervals.
- Use a recare tracking system.
- Recognize recare system failure.

## KEY TERMS

advance appointment recare system
continuing care
mailed notice recare system

recall
recare systems
telephone recare system

## RECARE SYSTEMS

**Recare systems** are a component of the appointment scheduling system meant to inform the patient that it is time to schedule a dental hygiene visit. Sometimes called **recall** or **continuing care**, this office system helps maintain patient oral health and appearance, prevent pain and disease, protect previous treatment, and reduce the need for extensive/expensive dental treatment. Adding new patients increases the dental practice, whereas treating recare patients generates a steady source of income. The financial success and viability of a dental practice depends on this recurring client care. In addition, regular oral healthcare maintenance prevents disease and provides for early diagnosis. Patients must understand that dental hygiene treatment is important; educated patients value oral healthcare, as well as general physical health, and realize that dental costs can be minimized through regular office visits.

After the initial oral healthcare visit, the patient's oral health status is evaluated to determine treatment regimens. The patient's preventative or periodontal needs should be assessed and monitored at each visit, and the recare interval adjusted if the patient's oral health conditions change.

Who is responsible for the recare system in the dental office is the subject of some debate. In many practices, the business dental assistant manages and maintains the appointment system, of which recare is a component. An appointment coordinator may have the general responsibility to schedule appointments and keep the schedule fully booked. Using this assumption, the best use of the dental hygienist's time is providing oral healthcare services. In some dental practices, the dental hygienist maintains the recare system chairside, during down time or during time that is designated for recall.

## TYPES OF RECARE SYSTEMS

There are three types of recare systems: advanced appointment, mailed notice, and telephone call. Dental practices employ a combination of all three systems to keep patients returning to the office.

### Advance Appointment Recare System

The **advance appointment recare system** is the scheduling of the next appointment at the end of the current appointment. This is recognized as the most efficient method of recare because it saves time by preappointing the dental hygienist. In addition, the patient schedules the appointment and makes the commitment to return. The hygienist may fill out a postcard with the next appointment information and ask the patient to address it; the card is then mailed 2 weeks before the prescheduled appointment. A courtesy telephone confirmation call regarding the reserved time is made 48–72 hours before the scheduled appointment.

Because the appointments are prescheduled, the hygiene schedule is booked in advance, making it necessary to keep a list of patients to call when openings occur. Although some patients may be unable to predict their future schedule, patients are more likely to reschedule an appointment than to schedule one from a mailed or telephone reminder.

### Mailed Notice Recare System

The **mailed notice recare system** is the mailing of a preprinted decorative postcard to inform the patient it is time to call to schedule his or her hygiene appointment. The least-effective recare system, mailed notices are personalized, stamped, and labeled to be sent a month in advance of the expected appointment time. The office identifies patients needing recall notices via a computer-generated list, printed labels, or previously completed postcards. At the beginning of each month, the cards are stamped, labeled, and mailed. A variety of professionally designed cards are available, and messages can be selected especially for each type of patient. For example, the staff member may send a child patient a cartoon card and an adult a seasonal card. The card serves as a tangible reminder for the patient to call for an appointment. Disadvantages to mailed recare systems include the cost of postage for large mailings and the lack of patient response, making it necessary to make follow-up telephone calls.

### Telephone Recare Systems

Using the **telephone recare system,** the dental office calls patients to schedule recare appointments. Immediate personal contact with the patient is good when contact can be made; however, because of caller ID, voicemail, answering machines, cellular phones, and multiple phone lines, personal patient contact can be difficult to achieve and office personnel may need to leave a voice message. This method is cost effective for smaller offices whose patients are in a local calling area, but when office staff must spend a lot of time calling many patients who have multiple telephone numbers that require long distance fees, the costs begin to accumulate.

In this system, patients are contacted by telephone 1 month before their targeted treatment dates to schedule recare visits. An alphabetical list containing patient names—along with their telephone numbers, date of last appointment, and suggested recall date—is generated monthly by the computer. Dental office software not only can produce patient lists but also can be used to produce mail merge letters, printed envelopes or postcards, and labels. All attempts to contact patients by telephone and mail are documented in the patients' records.

## Email Notification

An emerging technique for recare is email notification. Email notification entails sending an electronic message to inform the client that he or she should call to schedule an appointment.

## MANAGING RECARE SCHEDULING

### Calculating Recare Intervals

Each patient returns to the dental office at different times based on his or her oral health-care needs. Typically, 6-month recare appointments are suggested for adult and child prophylaxis, whereas periodontal therapy may require a 1-, 2-, 3-, or 4-month interval. To compute recall intervals in the first half of the year, add 6 months. To compute recall intervals in the last half of the year, subtract 6 months.

### Recare Tracking Systems

A recare tracking system should be in place to monitor patient contacts and determine whether appropriate attempts to schedule have been made; this avoids any possibility of abandonment. Any and all attempts to contact the patient are documented, including conversations, voice messages, and email messages. Recorded data for recare include scheduled, broken, canceled, and rescheduled appointments. Recare tracking can be done on an index card, recall card, log, or other form, or in the patient record. The date, type of contact, and results of contact are entered in the recare tracking form. Based on the individualized recare interval, patient contact is usually attempted at 30 days past due, 90 days past due, 12 months past due, and 18 months past due. Phone calls can be made at any time. *Figure 16.1* provides an example of a 90-day past due letter.

### Recare System Failure

If the final attempt to schedule an appointment fails, some practices will make the patient account inactive. No further attempts are made to contact the patient, and the

*Forever Smiles Dental Offices*
*123 Main Street, Anytown, Anystate 12345 Phone: 888-555-1515*

February 13, 2006

Mrs. Robin Bird
111 Any Avenue
Anyvillage, Anystate 12345-6789

Dear Mrs. Bird:

You are now more than 90 days past due for your oral healthcare visit. We are concerned about your continued health because dental problems rarely have symptoms until they reach the point at which extensive treatment is needed. For this reason, we are sending you this letter. We know from experience that conditions in the mouth change over time. While there may be no problems at all, it is a risk to postpone necessary dental visits. If you do have a developing problem, we can find it early, when it is easy to remedy.

The oral health services our patients have come to expect include oral cancer screening, periodontal assessment, dental cleaning and periodontal treatment, examination, and home care instructions. We know that with an individualized program of home care and professional visits, you can maintain your oral and physical health.

We understand that many people need to watch their expenses, but the investment in prevention is usually less expensive than treatment costs. If you have not returned because you are not happy with how you were treated, we apologize and hope that you will let us know so we can improve our services, learn from our mistakes, and welcome you back into the office.

Your oral health can be maintained with minor expense and minimally invasive procedures. Don't let pain bring you back for care. Please call our office to avoid unnecessary dental pain.

Sincerely,


Dr. Tooth Drawer

**Figure 16.1** Example of a recare tracking letter.

patient record is purged from the active records. A viable recare system is not a guarantee that patients will return for continued care if they are unhappy with their experience. Reduced recare appointments may be the result of a transient community, a slow economy, or a new and developing practice without a large client base; on the other hand, some patients may be unhappy with the office.

If the office notes repeated failed attempts to bring back patients, staff must evaluate the practice for in-office problems. The most effective method for determining why a patient is not returning is a telephone conversation. Begin by asking the patient if he or she was offended in some way or if there was a problem with the treatment. Exit surveys and/or patient questionnaires displayed in a prominent place in the reception area can help the office learn why patients are not returning. The survey should guarantee patients' anonymity. Feedback from patients will help assess if there is an office, personnel, or treatment problem.

**CONCEPT SUMMARY**

- The common recare systems are advanced appointment, mailed notice, and telephone call.
- Each client returns at a customized recare interval.
- A recare tracking system is used to monitor contacts to determine whether appropriate attempts to schedule have been made.
- After a series of attempts to inform the client of his or her need for an appointment have failed, the patient is given inactive status.

# REVIEW QUESTIONS

1. Define the following terminology:
   A. Advance appointment recare system
   B. Continuing care
   C. Mailed notice recare system
   D. Recall
   E. Recare systems
   F. Telephone call recare system
2. Why are recare procedures performed?
3. What is the difference between advance appointment, mailed notice, and telephone recare?
4. Which is the most effective recare system? Why?
5. Which is the least effective recare system? Why?
6. Why is recare activity tracked?
7. How does the dental office software program assist in recare activity?

8. Calculate recare intervals for the following individuals:
   A. In February, Justin Tyme is placed on a 6-month recall. When is his next scheduled visit to the dental office?
   B. In July, Fay Slift, is placed on a 3-month recall. When is her next scheduled visit to the dental office?
   C. Polly Ester is placed on a 6-month recall in November. When is her next scheduled visit to the dental office?
   D. Frank Furter is placed on a 3-month recall in September. When is his next scheduled visit to the dental office?
   E. B. Stalling is placed on a 4-month recall in May. When is her next scheduled visit to the dental office?

# Payroll and Taxation

Upon mastery of the content of this chapter, the student should be able to:
- Differentiate between gross and net pay, wages, and salary.
- Describe payroll earnings and deduction calculations.
- Recognize an accounts payable employee ledger card.
- Describe payroll tax reporting and calendar year-end procedures.
- Briefly discuss an IRS tax audit.
- Use common formulas for calculating dental hygiene salaries.

| | |
|---|---|
| gross pay | regular hours |
| net pay | salaries |
| overtime hours | taxation |
| payroll | wages |

## PAYROLL AND TAXATION

Payroll encompasses the accurate computation of earned wages or salary and taxes withheld and other deductions. Whether you are employed in a private or group practice, partnership, or corporation, or are in independent practice, you will be verifying the accuracy of your paycheck and possibly calculating the paychecks of other employees. **Payroll** is an office system used to calculate and record employee earnings. There are two main items to determine for payroll: earnings and deductions. Payroll is calculated by entering data into a payroll software program or by reading tax tables and performing mathematical functions to determine gross and net pay; some dental offices employ a business accountant to handle these functions. The total wages earned during a pay period before deductions comprise **gross pay**; the total wages earned during a pay period after deductions comprise **net pay**. Simply stated, gross pay minus deductions equals net pay.

Payroll **taxation** calculations are used to compute the tax responsibility of employers and employees; the tax is reported and paid to government entities. Taxation calculated at the end of the year is based on the exchange of goods and services by the dental office (small business); the calculation is usually completed by an accountant or accounting service. The U.S. Department of the Treasury Internal Revenue Service (IRS) is the branch of the U.S. government to which federal taxes are paid. State and local taxes are paid to the respective government departments. Calculations of payroll taxes to be withheld and payment of those taxes are accomplished using forms obtained from the IRS and appropriate state and local government offices.

## PAYROLL

The U.S. Department of Labor administers the Fair Labor Standards Act (FLSA), which sets forth working conditions. A regular workweek is considered to be 40 hours, which are called **regular hours**; when an employee works more than 40 hours in a week, the extra time is called **overtime hours**, which must be paid at time and a half for nonexempt employees. Other provisions of FLSA are given in Chapter 28.

Personal income and earnings are confidential issues that should not be discussed in social situations with anyone in the workplace. Unnecessary office gossip and resentment can stem from sharing this type of information with coworkers. It is advisable not to reveal your earnings to others; when coworkers ask about your pay, it is appropriate to change the subject. Another tack is to turn the situation around by asking why they want to know or by stating firmly it is none of their business.

Office gossip may occur during performance review time or when collection or production bonuses are distributed. Resentment may occur among coworkers if production bonuses are given to the dental hygienist, even though such bonuses are based on comprehensive oral hygiene services and are usually negotiated employment terms. It is important to remember that dental hygienists perform billable procedures. Furthermore, dental hygiene practice requires advanced study in anatomy, physiology, microbiology, chemistry, pharmacology, periodontology, and patient care. Professionals merit extra pay and bonuses based on this level of education and on their production performance.

Total earnings paid at an hourly rate for a specific period are known as **wages**. The pay period, which is set by the dental practice, is based on the calendar dates worked. Total earnings at a fixed rate during a pay period, regardless of the number of hours worked, are called **salaries**. Wages and salaries can be calculated daily, weekly, every two weeks, twice a month, monthly, or yearly. Dental hygiene contractors earn daily wages and may be paid accordingly. Dental hygiene providers in private practice earn daily wages and may be paid weekly, every two weeks, or twice a month. Dental hygiene educators earn daily income based on a yearly salary and may be paid every two weeks, twice a month, or monthly. Dental hygienists in independent practice are paid according to the business rule of law determined by the business model—that is, proprietorship or partnership.

### Payroll Withholdings

On the first day of employment and every time there is a change, employees complete or modify an Employee's Withholding Allowance Certificate, also known as IRS Form W-4, to determine their tax exemptions (*Fig. 17.1*). This form indicates how many people (usually his or her dependent children) legally need the employee's care. An employee's taxes are calculated based on the number of exemptions; each exemption increases the net (take-home) pay. The number of exemptions determines the amount of federal, state,

# Form W-4 (2006)

**Purpose.** Complete Form W-4 so that your employer can withhold the correct federal income tax from your pay. Because your tax situation may change, you may want to refigure your withholding each year.

**Exemption from withholding.** If you are exempt, complete only lines 1, 2, 3, 4, and 7 and sign the form to validate it. Your exemption for 2006 expires February 16, 2007. See Pub. 505, Tax Withholding and Estimated Tax.

**Note.** You cannot claim exemption from withholding if (a) your income exceeds $850 and includes more than $300 of unearned income (for example, interest and dividends) and (b) another person can claim you as a dependent on their tax return.

**Basic instructions.** If you are not exempt, complete the **Personal Allowances Worksheet** below. The worksheets on page 2 adjust your withholding allowances based on itemized deductions, certain credits, adjustments to income, or two-earner/two-job situations. Complete all worksheets that apply. However, you may claim fewer (or zero) allowances.

**Head of household.** Generally, you may claim head of household filing status on your tax return only if you are unmarried and pay more than 50% of the costs of keeping up a home for yourself and your dependent(s) or other qualifying individuals. See line E below.

**Tax credits.** You can take projected tax credits into account in figuring your allowable number of withholding allowances. Credits for child or dependent care expenses and the child tax credit may be claimed using the **Personal Allowances Worksheet** below. See Pub. 919, How Do I Adjust My Tax Withholding, for information on converting your other credits into withholding allowances.

**Nonwage income.** If you have a large amount of nonwage income, such as interest or dividends, consider making estimated tax payments using Form 1040-ES, Estimated Tax for Individuals. Otherwise, you may owe additional tax.

**Two earners/two jobs.** If you have a working spouse or more than one job, figure the total number of allowances you are entitled to claim on all jobs using worksheets from only one Form W-4. Your withholding usually will be most accurate when all allowances are claimed on the Form W-4 for the highest paying job and zero allowances are claimed on the others.

**Nonresident alien.** If you are a nonresident alien, see the Instructions for Form 8233 before completing this Form W-4.

**Check your withholding.** After your Form W-4 takes effect, use Pub. 919 to see how the dollar amount you are having withheld compares to your projected total tax for 2006. See Pub. 919, especially if your earnings exceed $130,000 (Single) or $180,000 (Married).

**Recent name change?** If your name on line 1 differs from that shown on your social security card, call 1-800-772-1213 to initiate a name change and obtain a social security card showing your correct name.

---

**Personal Allowances Worksheet** (Keep for your records.)

**A** Enter "1" for **yourself** if no one else can claim you as a dependent . . . . . . . . . . . **A** _____

**B** Enter "1" if:
- You are single and have only one job; or
- You are married, have only one job, and your spouse does not work; or
- Your wages from a second job or your spouse's wages (or the total of both) are $1,000 or less.

**B** _____

**C** Enter "1" for your **spouse.** But, you may choose to enter "-0-" if you are married and have either a working spouse or more than one job. (Entering "-0-" may help you avoid having too little tax withheld.) . . . . . . . . . . **C** _____

**D** Enter number of **dependents** (other than your spouse or yourself) you will claim on your tax return . . . . **D** _____

**E** Enter "1" if you will file as **head of household** on your tax return (see conditions under **Head of household** above) . **E** _____

**F** Enter "1" if you have at least $1,500 of **child or dependent care expenses** for which you plan to claim a credit . . **F** _____

(**Note.** Do **not** include child support payments. See **Pub. 503,** Child and Dependent Care Expenses, for details.)

**G** **Child Tax Credit** (including additional child tax credit):
- If your total income will be less than $55,000 ($82,000 if married), enter "2" for each eligible child.
- If your total income will be between $55,000 and $84,000 ($82,000 and $119,000 if married), enter "1" for each eligible child plus "1" **additional** if you have four or more eligible children.

**G** _____

**H** Add lines A through G and enter total here. (**Note.** This may be different from the number of exemptions you claim on your tax return.) ▶ **H** _____

For accuracy, complete all worksheets that apply.
- If you plan to **itemize or claim adjustments to income** and want to reduce your withholding, see the **Deductions and Adjustments Worksheet** on page 2.
- If you have **more than one job** or are **married and you and your spouse both work** and the combined earnings from all jobs exceed $35,000 ($25,000 if married) see the **Two-Earner/Two-Job Worksheet** on page 2 to avoid having too little tax withheld.
- If **neither** of the above situations applies, **stop here** and enter the number from line H on line 5 of Form W-4 below.

---

- - - - - - - - - - - - - - - - - - - - **Cut here and give Form W-4 to your employer. Keep the top part for your records.** - - - - - - - - - - - - - - - - - - -

Form **W-4**

Department of the Treasury
Internal Revenue Service

## Employee's Withholding Allowance Certificate

▶ Whether you are entitled to claim a certain number of allowances or exemption from withholding is subject to review by the IRS. Your employer may be required to send a copy of this form to the IRS.

OMB No. 1545-0074

2006

| 1 Type or print your first name and middle initial. | Last name | | 2 Your social security number |
|---|---|---|---|

| Home address (number and street or rural route) | 3 ☐ Single ☐ Married ☐ Married, but withhold at higher Single rate. |
|---|---|
| | **Note.** If married, but legally separated, or spouse is a nonresident alien, check the "Single" box. |
| City or town, state, and ZIP code | 4 If your last name differs from that shown on your social security card, check here. You must call 1-800-772-1213 for a new card. ▶ ☐ |

| 5 | Total number of allowances you are claiming (from line **H** above **or** from the applicable worksheet on page 2) | **5** | |
|---|---|---|---|
| 6 | Additional amount, if any, you want withheld from each paycheck . . . . . . . . . . . . . | **6** | $ |
| 7 | I claim exemption from withholding for 2006, and I certify that I meet **both** of the following conditions for exemption. | | |

- Last year I had a right to a refund of **all** federal income tax withheld because I had **no** tax liability **and**
- This year I expect a refund of **all** federal income tax withheld because I expect to have **no** tax liability.

If you meet both conditions, write "Exempt" here . . . . . . . . . . . . . . ▶ | **7** |

Under penalties of perjury, I declare that I have examined this certificate and to the best of my knowledge and belief, it is true, correct, and complete.

**Employee's signature**
(Form is not valid unless you sign it.) ▶ _____ Date ▶ _____

| 8 Employer's name and address (Employer: Complete lines 8 and 10 only if sending to the IRS.) | 9 Office code (optional) | 10 Employer identification number (EIN) |
|---|---|---|

**For Privacy Act and Paperwork Reduction Act Notice, see page 2.**　　Cat. No. 10220Q　　Form **W-4** (2006)

**Figure 17.1** IRS Form W-4, Employee's Withholding Allowance Certificate.

and local income tax that is withheld, or subtracted from the pay and sent directly to the IRS, state, and/or local government. Federal, state, and local withholding income taxes are the first dollar amounts deducted from an employee's gross pay for each pay period. The income tax burden for U.S. taxpayers of all combined taxes (federal, state, and local) ranges from 32.3% to 23.6%, depending on the state and local district of residency. The income tax burden for combined state and local taxes ranges from 12.9% to 6.3%, depending on residency [e.g., New York ranks first (highest), and Alaska ranks 50th (lowest)].

The U.S. Federal Insurance Contribution Act sets forth the withholding of Social Security taxes placed into an individual Federal Insurance Contribution Account (FICA). FICA (or Social Security) taxes are deducted from an employee's gross pay for each pay period. Social Security is a federal entitlement program for individuals over age 65 years, for families of deceased persons, and for disabled persons. Employees and employers pay Social Security taxes to the federal government to provide a minimal monthly income to qualified individuals. FICA taxes are calculated at a rate of 0.124 of the employee's gross pay. The employer matches the amount paid by the employee.

Medicare is a federal healthcare insurance program that is available to elderly citizens. It is an entitlement program that provides minimal medical benefits to senior citizens. Medicare taxes are calculated at a rate of 0.029 of the employee's gross pay. Combined, FICA and Medicare result in a deduction of 0.153 (15.3%) from the employee's gross pay for each pay period. Additional deductions that may be taken from an employee's gross pay include health insurance payments, disability insurance, repayment of an office loan, or parking fees.

By the end of each January, employers must provide employees with IRS Form W-2 Wage and Tax Statement (*Fig. 17.2*). The W-2 records the dollar amounts for the employee's previous calendar year's earnings and the taxes withheld by the employer.

## Completing Accounts Payable

Recall from Chapter 10 that the accounts payable office system may record earnings, taxes, and deductions for each employee for each pay period on a ledger card, which is completed in the accounts payable disbursement journal as gross earnings minus deductions. The accounts payable disbursement journal has columns for listing specific withholdings. As shown in *Figure 17.3*, the earning record includes the employee's name, Social Security number, number of exemptions, date of payroll computation, hours worked, rate of pay, and gross pay, along with columns for withheld federal, state, and local income tax; net pay; and a summary by month/year. A payroll software program installed on the office computer or a spreadsheet program in an integrated software package may be used to compute payroll. Some dental practices hire an outside company or accountant to calculate payroll.

## TAXATION REPORTING

The payment of payroll taxes is made each pay period according to the selected pay period model used by the practice. These taxes are deposited into federal reserve depository accounts for businesses and corporations for the transfer of federal, state, and local

| a Control number | | | | |
|---|---|---|---|---|
| | | OMB No. 1545-0008 | Safe, accurate, FAST! Use  IRS e-file | Visit the IRS website at www.irs.gov/efile. |

| b Employer identification number (EIN) | 1 Wages, tips, other compensation | 2 Federal income tax withheld |
|---|---|---|
| c Employer's name, address, and ZIP code | 3 Social security wages | 4 Social security tax withheld |
| | 5 Medicare wages and tips | 6 Medicare tax withheld |
| | 7 Social security tips | 8 Allocated tips |
| d Employee's social security number | 9 Advance EIC payment | 10 Dependent care benefits |
| e Employee's first name and initial     Last name | 11 Nonqualified plans | 12a See instructions for box 12 |
| | 13 Statutory employee ☐  Retirement plan ☐  Third-party sick pay ☐ | 12b |
| | 14 Other | 12c |
| | | 12d |
| f Employee's address and ZIP code | | |

| 15 State   Employer's state ID number | 16 State wages, tips, etc. | 17 State income tax | 18 Local wages, tips, etc. | 19 Local income tax | 20 Locality name |
|---|---|---|---|---|---|
| | | | | | |

Form **W-2**  **Wage and Tax Statement**     **2005**     Department of the Treasury—Internal Revenue Service

**Copy B—To Be Filed With Employee's FEDERAL Tax Return.**
This information is being furnished to the Internal Revenue Service.

**Figure 17.2** IRS Form W-2, Wage and Tax Statement.

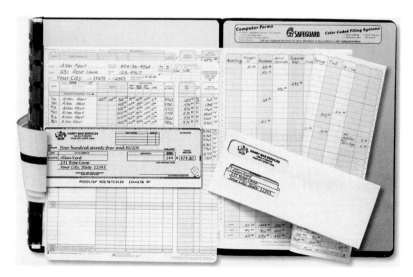

**Figure 17.3** Employees earning record ledger card. Courtesy of Safeguard Business Systems.

government taxes. Each month, the federal government sends a federal depository receipt form to the dental office. Private practices, group practices, partnerships, corporations, and independent practices must calculate and verify the accuracy of the payroll taxes on a quarterly tax report.

In some instances, the business dental assistant or person in charge of payroll submits the quarterly tax forms. Federal tax, FICA, and Medicare are reported on IRS Form 941 Employer's Quarterly Federal Tax Return. The completed form is sent to the IRS, and one copy is maintained for the office records. A check from the federal depository account is written to the IRS to pay the withheld quarterly taxes. Discovery of any error after the form has been forwarded is amended using IRS Form 941C, which must be completed and mailed to document and correct the error. In some instances, a monthly withdrawal of taxes is made to the federal government from the dental practice's federal depository account. In return, the federal government sends the federal depository receipt form.

## Calendar Year End

At the end of the year, several federal government forms must be completed. They include the W-2 Wage and Tax Statement forms for taxes withheld for each employee, the W-3 Transmittal of Income and Tax Statements form, and the W-4 Employee's Withholding Allowance Certificate for exemptions. Besides these three forms, the IRS provides the dental practice with federal depository receipts, the 941 Employer's Quarterly Federal Tax Return form, the Federal Unemployment Tax form (FUTA), and Circular E (employer tax guide tables). Generally, the state government will provide forms for quarterly tax return reports, state unemployment tax forms, employer tax guide tables, and worker's compensation forms.

Worker's compensation is a state fee paid by employers for employees. Revenues from this tax go into a fund for injured workers, who can access the money if they are injured on the job and the injury prevents them from working.

## Tax Audit

A **tax audit** is an IRS review of accounting business records, including payroll records, to search for discrepancies, fraud, and unreported income. When the oral healthcare provider is audited, a lawyer, accountant, and bookkeeper are also involved. When being audited, the business owner may receive a notice via the U.S. Postal Service or a federal agent of the IRS may arrive at the office to inform the receptionist that he or she is there to audit the books. The auditor will have a federal subpoena to enter the office. Usually the dentist or independent practitioner will ask that legal counsel and an accountant or bookkeeper be present for any proceedings. Chances are the office will be closed to cooperate fully with the tax authority.

## SALARY

As an employer, the dentist is in a position to periodically review job performance and give merit raises. Staff need a vested benefit in the practice to remain motivated to per-

**BOX 17.1** *Earnings Formulas*

Wages
- Hourly rate of pay multiplied by number of hours worked in a pay period

Commission salary
- one quarter of production
- one third of production
- another percentage between 25% and 35% of production

form at a peak level. Owing to ever-increasing overhead costs and variable economic conditions, dental practices use a variety of salary formulas to determine the pay of their dental hygienists. (Production is discussed in Chapter 12.)

An understanding of how dental hygiene earnings can be determined is straightforward once an earnings formula has been selected. Staff salaries generally equal 20–25% of overhead; although some are even higher. Most dental hygienists work for an hourly wage, based on local averages. The average hourly rate for dental hygiene professionals is between $12.50 and $33.50, depending on the state of residence. Hourly wage earners are paid for the time on the job; the amount of hygiene production is not factored in. This model works well in an established practice with a steady flow of patient visits, because it guarantees a constant wage based on a 40-hour week. However, an hourly wage earner can be scheduled for fewer hours when business is slower and unscheduled time occurs. The addition of a bonus plan can make hourly pay an attractive choice for dental hygienists.

Some dental hygienists are paid a salary based on a wage times a 40-hour workweek— for example $30 per hour × 40 hours = $1200 gross pay per week or $2400 every two weeks. Note that salaried employees who meet the FLSA definition of "exempt" are not further compensated for working more than 40 hours per week; when extra hours are required, the professional should cheerfully complete his or her work. Examples of earnings formulas are given in *Box 17.1.*

## CONCEPT SUMMARY

- Payroll is calculated based on gross earnings and deductions to arrive at net pay.
- Payroll is computed by a staff member manually or via computer software, or through an outside service.
- Payroll tax payments are made each pay period and are filed with the government quarterly and at the end of the year. Several federal government forms must be completed as part of this process.
- An IRS tax audit is a review of the accounting business records to search for discrepancies, fraud, and unreported income.
- Dental hygienists are paid an hourly wage or a salary and may earn commissions or be given bonuses.

# REVIEW QUESTIONS

1. What is the difference between gross and net pay, wages, and salary?
2. What are the two components of payroll?
3. What federally required form is completed by new employees?
4. List the federal taxes withheld from every employee's earnings.
5. List the other deductions that may be made from an employee's earnings.
6. What taxes are paid by the employer yearly?
7. Which tax forms are mailed by the federal government to the dental office?
8. Which tax forms are mailed by state and local entities to the dental office?
9. To whom is a check written to pay withheld taxes?
10. What is a federal depository receipt form?
11. What two forms are filed annually for employees?
12. What procedures are involved in an audit?

## CRITICAL THINKING GROUP ACTIVITY

Let's dream large. You want to earn $100,000 in salary in addition to receiving bonuses. Make a plan that outlines the level of performance required to earn that salary and bonuses. How many hours per week and per year do you want to work to earn $100,000? What would your hourly earnings need to be and at what production level would you need to perform? *Hint:* Most people want at least 2 weeks of vacation a year.

## CRITICAL THINKING ACTIVITY

- Assume an employee has an hourly wage of $30 and works 40 hours a week to earn $1200 per week. Compute the employee's net pay for the year (52 weeks) with an overall tax burden of 30%.
- Assume a dental practice grosses $600,000 per year. Determine the dental hygienist's earnings based on one quarter of gross production. Determine the dental hygienist's earnings based on one third of gross production.

# Inventory Maintenance

Upon mastery of the content of this chapter, the student should be able to:
- Describe inventory maintenance systems.
- Determine purchasing methods and sources for employment settings.
- Explain how costs and time are considerations when purchasing merchandise.
- Handle incoming supply deliveries and store merchandise.
- Comply with "right to know" regulations related to dental merchandise.

**KEY TERMS**

back orders
business office items
capital items
expendable supplies
material safety data sheets
nonexpendable supplies

Occupational Safety and Health
  Administration
professional items
purchase orders
right to know

## INVENTORY MAINTENANCE

The purchase and use of equipment and supplies are necessary to provide oral health-care services to patients. Inventory maintenance systems are used to monitor purchasing, maintaining the level of supplies and equipment to enable a steady flow of production. Without an adequate inventory, dental procedures cannot be performed. Purchasing methods and sources are selected based on costs and time constraints. The storage of incoming delivered supplies and merchandise purchased from stores must comply with federal regulations. Special storage conditions are required for many dental products, and the improper storage of supplies can be hazardous and costly.

## LOCATING AND ORDERING SUPPLIES

Dental assistants monitor and place orders for 90% of dental practices. Dental hygienists select, use, and recommend dental products for purchasing and reordering. These products may be used once or many times before being discarded or recycled. Dental hygienists also use different types of equipment that must be maintained according to manufacturer's directions. Selection and ordering of supplies are frequently based on minimizing costs and speeding delivery. When replacing equipment and supplies, the hygienist must consider cost, ease of use, and suitability for the practice. After selecting the best purchase rate and quantity, the professional takes into account the total cost of the order and capital available so a cost-effective decision can be made.

**Expendable supplies** generally cost less than $50 and have a useful life of less than 3 years. Items that are expendable include gauze sponges, cotton rolls, and anesthetics. **Nonexpendable supplies** cost more than $50 and last longer, such as hand instruments, ultrasonic inserts, and syringes for locally applied antibiotics.

## Types of Supplies

Supplies can be divided into three main categories: capital items, professional items, and business office items. **Capital items** generally cost more than $1,000 and include the operatory equipment and office furniture—dental chairs, chairside computers, nitrous oxide–oxygen delivery system, curing light, and autoclave. Master lists of capital inventory are alphabetized and maintained room by room. These lists contain the item name, date of purchase, purchase cost, manufacturer, warranty information, and place of purchase.

**Professional items** are expendable and nonexpendable items used in the operatory and laboratory, such as prophylaxis handpieces and sealant kits. Alphabetized master inventory lists of all supplies are established and maintained in a manner similar to that used for the capital items. Product information is listed by name, date of purchase, amount of purchase, manufacturer name, supplier name, unit cost, and total cost. **Business office items** include personalized paper and plastic products such as letterhead stationery, recall cards, and printed bags for dispensing toothbrushes. Any item that requires personalized printing takes a longer time to produce; therefore, advanced ordering is necessary for these items.

## Purchasing Sources

There are many sources for and methods of purchasing supplies (*Box 18.1*). In some offices, a dental sales person from a dental supply house visits the practice to write up personal orders, allowing for "high-touch" customer service. Dental product information is also available from catalogs and websites. Dental offices make purchases via mail order, telephone calls, faxing, and the Internet. Payment on merchandise accounts can be made by cash, credit card, or office check. Educational, institutional, and government employment settings use purchase orders to pay for merchandise. **Purchase orders** are forms that authorize the purchase of items and use an identification number for a departmental budget reimbursement; these are submitted to supply companies.

Oral healthcare practitioners often have preferred dental supply houses, companies, and sales representatives (also called detail people). Dental supply houses such as Benco, Patterson Dental, Henry Schein, and Darby have many internal departments (e.g., business office supplies; drugs and medications; equipment sales, installation, service, and repair; gold; merchandise and miscellaneous supplies; sales representatives; and tooth). Some dental supply companies may specialize in a particular type of supply or have a department dedicated to personalized recall cards, greeting cards, seasonal cards, sta-

**BOX 18.1**  *Sources of Dental Supplies: Where to Go for What*

**Business supply company**
  Office items
**Dental manufacturer**
  Dental materials
  Equipment
**Dental supply house**
  Dental materials
  Equipment
**Grocery, discount, or department store**
  Coffee
  Cleaning supplies
**Medical supply company**
  Masks
  Gloves
  Gauze

**Occupational safety supply company**
  Safety items
  OSHA products
**Pharmacy**
  Prescription drugs
  First aid supplies
**Professional association**
  Patient education materials
**Toy manufacturing company, discount store**
  Gifts for pediatric patients
**Uniform manufacturer**
  Clothing

tionery, accounting forms, and other items. Prescription drugs and medications, such as home-use fluoride, must be ordered using a dentist's drug/narcotic license number. Once an account is established, the supplier maintains the numbers on file for future purchases. Equipment is often purchased from dental supply houses because installation, service, and repair agreements are provided and implemented by expert technicians employed by the supply house.

Certified pure gold, gold alloy, and other precious metal alloys are purchased by dental laboratories from dental supply houses for the manufacturing of dental appliances. The cost of precious metal alloys is variable, changing with the daily stock market trading value.

Plastic teeth used for the fabrication of dental appliances are purchased by dental laboratory technicians from the tooth departments of dental supply houses. Miscellaneous supplies purchased from dental supply houses can include toys for children, uniforms for staff, and personal grooming items such as hand lotions. Sales departments have offices and support services for their sales force representatives. Merchandise is the area of focus for most dental supply house catalogs and websites.

Grocery, discount, department, local pharmacy stores, and business/office supply stores provide items necessary for use in dental offices, such as cleaning supplies, beverages, personal hygiene items, and general business supplies.

## Merchandise Purchasing

Purchasing is spread throughout the year based on a supply budget. Dental practice supply budgets are usually limited to 6% of the office fee collection (*Box 18.2*). For example, if the monthly collection is $50,000, then $3,000 (6% of $50,000) is available for monthly supplies. A variety of merchandise purchasing systems can be used to monitor and maintain inventory by dental office personnel. Whatever system is used, information is documented for each purchase (*Box 18.3*). To adequately maintain inventory, the staff determines the maximum and minimum levels of needed inventory based on rate of use, shelf life, cost, delivery time, and available storage space. *Box 18.4* lists monitoring systems used to maintain inventory levels. The hygienist must determine when to reorder and how much to buy to maintain supplies between the maximum and the minimum inventories in an attempt to avoid both overstocking and running out of a supply item. Costs increase when items expire before they can be used (over supply), are stored incorrectly (e.g., in terms of temperature or light exposure), or are purchased on short notice without adequate planning.

Seasonal issues also affect the timing of purchases. For example, developer and fixer chemicals are adversely affected by the freezing temperatures of winter so are best ordered in warmer weather. Time of year also affects sales, especially around annual convention time when dental hygiene instruments are available at reduced costs to stimulate convention sales. The cost of some items is based on the stock market; for example, the price of dental x-ray film increases when the value of silver goes up.

The staff must monitor the availability of supplies because some items may be discontinued by manufacturers or may be offered for only a limited time. Again, items that require personalized printing, such as toothbrushes, must be ordered well before the office inventory has been depleted.

## Supply Delivery

Deliveries arrive at the dental office daily from a variety of sources—the postal service, United Parcel Service, Federal Express, DHL, and other freight and delivery companies; dental laboratory pick up and delivery service; and sales and manufacturer representatives. One person is assigned responsibility for unpacking and inspecting shipments. Usually this is a task performed by a dental assistant; however, the dental hygienist may be responsible for the items used in the hygiene department.

The opening of packages may be confined to a particular area of the dental office, such as the storage room, owing to the possibility of contamination. Assuming that

**BOX 18.4** *Monitoring Systems*

Bar code technology
Colored tape/stickers or red flag tags placed on merchandise
Index card file of all inventory items
Master supply lists or computer database of all inventory items
Notebook, clipboard, or eraser board of running lists of wanted and needed items

packages are safe to open, a box-cutter razor blade is used to slice through strapping or packing tape. Once the package is opened, the packing list and/or shipping invoice is located. A packing list is an itemized statement of the package contents. A shipping invoice is a billing statement demanding payment. The packing list or invoice is dated on arrival, and the package contents are checked against the invoice to verify that all itemized merchandise was received. The original purchase request is compared to the packing list or invoice to verify that all ordered merchandise was received. Any items or substitutions that are unacceptable are returned to the company, and further monitoring is needed until a credit slip or voucher has been sent from the supplier.

Any items that were not shipped because of a temporary lack of availability are called **back orders.** Further monitoring is needed until all backordered items have arrived at the dental office. Usually a staff member calls the company to determine the estimated shipment date if it is not noted on the packing list or invoice. When items do not arrive as a result of oversight or back order, purchases can be canceled and other sources can be contacted.

## SUPPLY STORAGE

After the purchase is verified for completeness and accuracy, the staff must store the items. The amount of storage space required and type of space required are taken into consideration, as are the need to rotate stock, stock expiration dates, and special storage requirements. Incoming merchandise is placed behind currently stocked supplies. Expiration dates are checked to determine an item's shelf life. Special storage conditions include lead-lined boxes; cool, dark, and/or dry areas; refrigeration; and special considerations for chemical, combustible, and flammable items.

### Managing Inventory

To adequately maintain inventory, the practice must establish reorder times and monitor supplies. Managing inventory can be achieved by using running lists; index cards; master supply lists; colored tape, stickers, or tags; and bar code technology. Bar code systems, which use scanners, mobile computers, and software, allow inventory control of consumable supplies and check in/check out of inventory items. Check in/check out items, such as dental radiographs, instruments, and equipment, are shared or reused and need to be tracked for longer periods of times. Frequently, the bar code system is used in large practices, hospital/clinic settings, and educational institutions.

## OCCUPATIONAL SAFETY AND HEALTH

The **Occupational Safety and Health Administration** (OSHA) (www.osha.gov), administered by the U.S. Department of Labor, has targeted the healthcare industry as one of the top 100 most hazardous workplaces in the United States. In 1970, the Occupational Safety and Health Act was adopted to establish national guidelines for worker health and safety, including workplace safety, building safety, fire safety, and "right to know." In the dental office, right to know laws apply to merchandise found in use and in storage. Part of the right to know laws are hazard communication standards that require employers to inform workers about handling potentially harmful chemicals and products (*Box 18.5*). Practice owners are responsible for implementing and maintaining a hazard communication training manual for their workplace to inform and train employees about hazards found in the office.

### Chemical Hazard Communication Programs

There are several basic elements of an OSHA hazard communication program. A hazard communication program for the use of chemical products consists of a training manual, posters, wall charts, material safety data sheets (MSDSs), labeling, and a training program. A training manual, available to all employees, should contain the following:

- Communication of hazards that identifies and lists hazardous chemicals, via the manual, posters, and wall charts.
- MSDSs.

---

**BOX 18.5**  *Right to Know Employer Requirements*

Implement and maintain a chemical hazard communication program for employees that:
    identifies and lists hazardous chemicals,
    provides MSDSs and labels for each hazardous chemical, and
    trains staff in chemical safety.
Post notices to keep employees informed of their rights and responsibilities under the law.
Provide occupational health and safety training:
    to newly assigned employees,
    to all employees annually, and
    whenever a new hazard is introduced to the workplace.
Identify, control, or eliminate possible causes of accidental injury.
Provide personal protective equipment at no cost to employees.
Provide sanitary conditions in passageways, storerooms, and service rooms.
Provide properly grounded electrical equipment.
Provide emergency exits.
Provide properly functioning fire extinguishers.
Provide emergency protocols to ensure safety during emergencies.
Maintain a record-keeping system of accident reports and employee medical records.
Regularly review safety and health responsibilities.

- Labeling information for each hazardous chemical.
- Training about hazardous materials.

Dental practices with more than one office must have a hazard communication program for each location. Right to know posters should be located in a prominent location, such as lounge areas, making it easy for employees to read and keeping employees informed of their rights and responsibilities under the law.

## Material Safety Data Sheets (MSDS)

**Material safety data sheets** are forms provided by chemical product manufacturers that describe product contents and potential health hazards from exposure. Safe handling and the use of chemical products are the responsibility of the employer, employee, and chemical manufacturer. Chemical manufacturers provide MSDSs and product labels for each hazardous chemical, and employers keep the MSDSs in a single location in the dental office. Of particular interest on an MSDS to the allied dental professional is "Section VIII: Control Measures." This section provides recommendations regarding types of control measures and protective devices that are necessary for worker safety (*Fig. 18.1*).

Employee rights under the right to know laws with respect to MSDSs are as follows:

- Accessibility to MSDSs.
- Nondiscrimination for employees who exercise their rights.
- Notification of and directions for locating any new or revised MSDSs that arrive in shipments.

| | | |
|---|---|---|
| Respiratory protection (specify type) ________ | | |
| Ventilation: | Local exhaust ________ | Special ________ |
| | Mechanical (general) ________ | Other ________ |
| Protective gloves ________ | Eye protection ________ | |
| Other protective clothing or equipment ________ | | |
| Work/hygienic practices ________ | | |

**Figure 18.1** MSDS Section VIII: Control Measures.

- Access to a conveniently located poster announcing the location of the MSDSs and another poster listing all the newly arrived or revised MSDSs.

## Merchandise Labeling

The dental employee should recognize, understand, and use the information on product labels written in English. Labels must contain the product name, physical hazards (such as flammable or combustible), and health hazards (such as eye irritant). Cabinets used for storage may also be labeled to identify the products inside. Color-coded labels are used for very small containers or bottles to alert the employee to the hazard. Larger labels have the required target organs and routes of entry information plus color-coded National Fire Protection Association (NFPA) identification symbols (*Table 18.1*).

Radiation caution labels are required on radiographic equipment (*Fig. 18.2A*). Biohazard warning labels are fluorescent orange or orange-red and include the biohazard symbol (*Fig 18.2B*). They are required on trash receptacles in each operatory; on refrigerators and freezers containing blood or other potentially infectious material; and on containers used for storage, transport, shipment, or disposal of infectious materials. Wall chart labeling systems allow healthcare workers to quickly reference protective equipment needs. Rating codes and pictorials help workers prepare chemical products.

## Exposure Control Plans

The second area of OSHA authority relating to dentistry is infection control. Each employer in a workplace where occupational exposure to blood and other potentially infectious materials may result must establish a written exposure control plan, provide employee training and personal protective equipment, and meet housekeeping and record-keeping requirements.

## OSHA Inspection

When OSHA inspectors visit a dental office, there are five standards they investigate for compliance with the law:

- General-duty clause—discovery of any unsafe violations not specified in the standards.
- Personal protective equipment—staff follow the guidelines while treating any patient.
- Labeling—all products and containers are labeled appropriately.

| TABLE 18.1 NFPA Identification Symbols | | | |
|---|---|---|---|
| **Class** | **Fire Hazard (Red)** | **Health Hazard (Blue)** | **Reactivity (Yellow)** |
| 0 | Will not burn | No hazard | Stable |
| 1 | Above 200°F | Slightly hazardous | Unstable if heated |
| 2 | Below 200°F | Hazardous | Violent chemical |
| 3 | Below 100°F | Extreme hazardous | Shock/heat may detonate |
| 4 | Below 73°F | Deadly | May detonate |

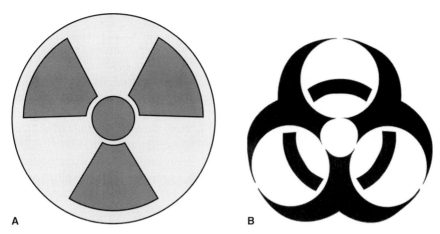

A                                          B

Figure 18.2 **A.** The symbol for radiation. Reprinted with permission from LifeART.
© 2006 Lippincott Williams & Wilkins. All rights reserved. **B.** The symbol for biohazard.

- Housekeeping—written plans exist for appropriate cleaning of hazardous spills.
- Hazardous waste disposal—written plans exist for appropriate disposal of waste.

## CITATIONS AND PENALTIES

Inspectors may discuss their tentative findings with the practice owner and file a report to the OSHA area director. The area director determines what citations and penalties will be imposed for any infraction. A citation is a legal warning for violations of the law that is mailed to the practice owner and that may list how and when the owner must correct the problem(s). Financial fines may be attached to a citation. Citations must be posted in a prominent location for employees to read. Fines and penalties may be contested within 15 working days from the date the citation is received.

## CONCEPT SUMMARY

- A variety of office systems are designed for monitoring and maintaining adequate supply inventory.
- Expendable supplies cost less than $50 and have a useful life of less than 3 years; nonexpendable supplies cost more than $50 and last longer.
- Capital items, professional items, and business office items are the three categories of dental supplies.
- Dental supplies are purchased from a variety of sources.
- Supply shipment and delivery are verified via a packing slip or invoice.
- Storage is unique for each dental product.
- The Occupational Safety and Health Act was adopted to establish national guidelines for worker health and safety, including workplace safety, building safety, fire safety, and "right to know." Potentially hazardous dental supplies must be handled in accordance with OSHA's guidelines.

# R E V I E W   Q U E S T I O N S

1. What is the purpose of inventory control?
2. What is the difference between expendable and nonexpendable supplies?
3. What are capital items?
4. What are professional supplies?
5. Why should office supplies be purchased in advance?
6. List four types of purchasing systems.
7. How and why are reorder and purchase quantities established?
8. What information is needed to maintain inventory?
9. What are the divisions of a dental supply house?
10. Besides a dental supply house, where else can items be purchased?
11. How is an incoming shipment handled?
12. Why must you verify the invoice with the merchandise received?
13. When items are returned, what is received from that company?
14. How does the shelf life of an item affect the quantity purchased?
15. How are incoming shipments stored?
16. List four items that require special storage.
17. What are some safety requirements for storage?
18. What are the right-to-know laws?
19. What is an MSDS and how is it used?
20. What are the three employee rights relating to an MSDS?

## Assignment: Inventory

- Develop an inventory file for dental hygiene supplies. Use a spreadsheet computer program to collect information on five different merchandise items and addresses the following pieces of information:
  Product category
  Product brand name
  Manufacturer (address, city, state, ZIP)
  Purchase quantity
  Purchase price per unit
  Dental supplier (address, city, state, ZIP)
  Location of MSDSs
- Visit the website of a dental supply company to practice placing an online purchase of five different dental hygiene merchandise items.

# Office Management

*Dental Hygiene Domain Competencies*[1]

## PROFESSIONALISM AND ETHICS

### Professional Behavior

- Assume responsibility for dental hygiene services.
- Provide accurate documentation when serving in professional roles.
- Communicate effectively using verbal, nonverbal, written, and electronic skills.

### Ethical Behavior

- Integrate the American Dental Hygienists' Association (ADHA) code of ethics in all professional endeavors.
- Adhere to federal, state, and local laws.
- Apply principles of risk management to prevent legal liability.

### Professional Commitment

- Advance the values of the profession by affiliation with professional and public organizations.
- Assume the role of clinician, educator, researcher, change agent, consumer advocate, and administrator as defined by the ADHA.
- Assume responsibility for lifelong learning.
- Evaluate scientific literature to make evidence-based decisions that advance the dental hygiene profession.

## ORAL HEALTH PROMOTION AND COMMUNITY HEALTH

- Identify the goals, values, beliefs, and preference of the patient concerning oral health and general wellness for promotion, prevention, and maintenance.
- Communicate effectively with individuals and groups from diverse populations both orally and in writing.
- Participate in service activities and community affiliations using the human needs model of patient care to advance oral healthcare.
- Screen, educate, and refer services that allow patients access to the resources of the healthcare system.

---

[1]Adapted from American Dental Education Association. Competencies for Entry into the Profession of Dental Hygiene (as approved by the 2003 House of Delegates). Reprinted by permission of *Journal of Dental Education*, Volume 68, Issue 7 (July 2004). Copyright 2004 by the American Dental Education Association.

- Facilitate patient access to oral healthcare services through a variety of healthcare settings as a member of a multidisciplinary team.

## DENTAL HYGIENE PROCESS OF CARE

### Patient Assessment

- Assess client concerns, goals, values, and preferences when guiding client care.
- Obtain, review, update, and interpret the patient's medical and dental history, radiographs, and vital signs.

### Patient Diagnosis

- Analyze and interpret data to formulate a dental hygiene diagnosis.
- Obtain consultations as appropriate.
- Refer clients to other healthcare providers as needed.

### Implementation

- Educate clients to prevent or control risk factors that contribute to oral disease.

### Evaluation and Maintenance

- Determine the outcomes of dental hygiene services using indices, instruments, examination techniques, and client self-reports.
- Compare actual outcomes to expected outcomes and reevaluate goals, diagnosis, and services when expected outcomes are not achieved.
- Develop and maintain a periodontal maintenance program.
- Determine client satisfaction with care received and oral health status achieved.

### REFERENCES & RESOURCES

**Organizations**
ADA Council on Dental Benefit Programs (www.ada.org/prof/resources/topics)
Agency for Healthcare Policy and Research (www.ahcpr.gov/clinic/index.html)
American Association of Oral and Maxillofacial Surgeons (www.aaoms.org)
American Dental Association (www.ada.org)
American Dental Hygienists' Association: government affairs updates (www.adha.org/governmental_affairs/stateline. htm)
Centers for Medicaid and Medicare Services (www.cms.hcfa.gov)
Cochrane Group (www.cochrane-oral.man.ac.uk)
Insurance Commissioners (members.tripod.com/proagency/insurance3.html)

National Conference of State Legislatures (www.ncsl.org/programs/health/dentalhy.htm)
National Fire Protection Association (www.nfpa.org)
National Guideline Clearinghouse (www.guideline.gov)
Occupational Safety and Health Administration (www.osha.gov)
State Children's Health Insurance Program (new.cms.hhs.gov/home/schip.asp)
U.S. Department of Labor (www.dol.gov)
U.S. Internal Revenue Service (www.irs.gov)
WorldView, Ltd. (www.worldviewltd.com/asp)

**Online Resources**
Accounting (www.health-infosys-dir.com)
AMA and the CPT (www.ama-assn.org/ama/pub/category/3113.html)

Automated telephone confirmation services (www.televox.com)

Bar coding (www.barcoding.com)

Bartering (www.bbu.com; www.barteradvantage.com)

Business dental assisting (www.dentalassisting.org)

Business plans (www.masterplanz.com; www.businessplans.org)

CMS for the ICD-9-CM 1991 (www.cms.hhs.gov/home/medicare.asp)

Collection agencies (www.collectionagencyservices.net/resources/Insurance-Health.html)

Dental hygiene production (www.dentalbootkamp.com; www.hygienistonline.com)

Dental office design (www.pattersondental.com; www.burkhartdental.com; www.dentalrep.com; www.smilefinder.com; www.ada.org/prof/resources/pubs/epubs/brief/brief_0310.pdf; www.unthank.com; www.designergonomics.com)

Dental program software (www.kodak.com/global/en/health/dental/productsForDentists/practiceworksOffice/index.jhtml; www.kodak.com/global/en/health/dental/productsForDentists/softDent/index.jhtml; www.dentrix.com; www.genesissoftware.com; www.mogo.com; http://patterson.eaglesoft.net/index.htm)

Dental spas (www.oraspa-RDH.com)

Embezzlement (www.criminal-law.freeadvice.com)

Encyclopaedia Britannica, 1994–2002 (www.britannica.com)

Equal Credit Opportunity Act (www.ftc.gov/bcp/conline/pubs/credit/ecoa.htm)

Fair Debt Collections Practices Act (www.fdic.gov/regulations/laws/rules/6500-1300.html#6500titleviiidcp)

HIPAA (www.cms.hhs.gov/hipaageninfo)

Insurance Solutions Newsletter (www.dental-ins-solutions.com)

PubMed (www.ncbi.nlm.nih.gov)

Republic Data Information System, The Guide: Medical—Dental Cross-Coding (www.rdsguide.com/Guide2.html)

Small claims court (www.am-lrc.org)

Supervision and ADHP information (www.adha.gov)

Tax Foundation, Income Tax Burden 2004 (www.taxfoundation.org/research/topic/9.htm)

Telephone techniques (www.businesstrainingworks.com; www.etiquetteexpert.com; www.speaking.com/articles_html/JoliAndre_1083.html)

Truth-in-Lending Act (part of the Consumer Credit Protection Act) (www.fdic.gov/regulations/laws/rules/6500-200.html)

### Pamphlets, Dissertations, Papers, and Software

American Academy of Periodontology. Periodontal procedures: Coding for submission to medical plans, 28.

American Dental Hygienists' Association. Advanced dental hygiene practitioner fact sheet. Available at: www.adha.org/media/facts/adhp.htm. Accessed November 2004.

Crowson B. Business letter module. Oakland Technical Center, 1980.

Dental Practice Management [Software]. Waco, TX: Complete Systems, Inc. (www.completesys.com).

Drahos G. Medical history. Power Point lecture presented at the University of Illinois at Chicago, College of Dentistry, September 2002.

Genrke K. Diagnosis and treatment planning. Power Point lecture presented at the University of Illinois at Chicago, College of Dentistry, November 2002.

Govoni M. HIPAA What it means for dental practices. Seminar presented at the Michigan Dental Assistants Association, Mt. Pleasant, December 2002.

Gurenlian JR. Client assessment and diagnostic testing. Paper presented at the Old Dominion University Dental Hygiene/Dental Assisting Symposium, September 1995.

Haisch MA. Oral risk assessment—Early intervention system. Lecture presented by Procter & Gamble at the Minnesota State University at Mankato, October 2000.

Insurance Solutions. Fraudulent medical claims. February 2002.

McKenzie S. Small change: Feel awkward selling products? Get over it! Automated plaque-removal products supplement.

Safeguard Business Systems. Private practice—Are you ready? [Form 801113].

Spellicy D. Dental office management. OTC-NW, Clarkston, MI, 1986.

Turner VC. Personal communication. May 2002.

Virtual Vision RX. Breakthrough patient management system. Redmond, WA, 1994.

Vargo, R. Internal controls for physicians.

Zarb JP. EBD. Power Point lecture presented at the University of Illinois at Chicago, College of Dentistry, March 2003.

Zarb JP. Evidence-based clinical practice. Power Point lecture presented at the University of Illinois at Chicago, College of Dentistry, October 2002.

### Articles

American Dental Assistants Association. Tipsheet. Dent Assist 2.

American Dental Assistants Association. Tipsheet: Dental computers: Programming effective office management. 1984.

American Dental Hygienists' Association. ADHA responds to ADA dental hygiene practice study. Access 2005:11–14.

American Dental Hygienists' Association. Independent practice. 2003.

American Medical Association. Current procedural terminology. 2001.

Andrews EK. Continuing education: complementary and alternative therapy. J Contemp Dent Prac 2001;2:73.

Andrews EK. Continuing education: Insurance cross coding: submitting medical insurance. J Contemp Dent Prac 2002;4:73.

Berger EK, Gutkowski S. Diagnostic tools for dental hygiene practice. Contemp Oral Hyg 2004:10–14.

Bernardi AE, Bernardi RA. Is the hygiene operatory a . . . profit center . . . or just a convenience for the patients? RDH 2004:44, 46, 48, 105.

Bernhardt C. Scheduling for production. Dent Teamwork 1989:138–140.

Bernie KM. Politics of independence—ADHP-A future reality for dental hygiene. Contemp Oral Hyg 2005:32.

Bernie KM. Politics of independence—"Faux-gienist" proposal still alive in Missouri. Contemp Oral Hyg 2004: 22–23.

Bernie KM. Politics of independence—Responses to reader queries about ADHP. Contemp Oral Hyg 2005:20–21.

Brown K. The puzzle of the appointment book. Dent Assist.

Bryan S. Computer integration: a challenge for dental assisting education. ADAA J 1991:4–6.

Chandler-Cousins L. Self-regulation is not unique, not radical, not impractical—it's what professions do. RDH 1996:22, 23, 55.

Cohen BE. Use of aromatherapy and music therapy to reduce anxiety and pain perception in dental hygiene. Access 2001:34–41.

Computers in dentistry—A panel of experts answer common computer questions. Dent Econ 1991:100–103.

DaCosta V. Computer reports mean money! RDH 2004:50.

Danner V. Defining quality care. ADHA 2002:26–34.

D'Autremont P. The dental history considerations for optimal client care and compliance. Dent Hyg News 8:19.

De St. Georges J. Don't lose patients in the chair or the charts. Dent Today 2004:142, 144, 146.

DePalma AC. Habits of effective offices. RDH 2004:38, 40, 42.

Dietz E. Office manager: one-write bookkeeping. Dent Assist 21–24, 36.

DiGangi P. Solving the mysteries of patient records. Contemp Oral Hyg 2004:32–34.

Drayer K. Q & A: Making your practice more productive. Dent Assist 2004:16, 25.

Ehrlich A. The computers are coming! Dent Assist 1983:29.

Ehrlich A. Filing systems: the ABC's of spring cleaning. Rules for alphabetical filing [Tipsheet]. Dent Asst 1987.

Ehrlich A. Managing computerized dental bookkeeping. Dent Assist 1984:30–41.

Farran H. Patient financial arrangements: Make them profitable. J Am Dent Assoc 1993:111–114.

Fletcher BB. The HIPAA quiz: questions you should ask your vendors about compliance. Dent Assist 2004:10.

Forgionne G. Structuring prepaid dental plans to accommodate consumer tastes and preferences. Dent Assist 1985:11–18.

Forrest JL. Quality assurance: integrating it into private practice. Dent Hyg News 9:12, 13, 16.

Forrest JL, Miller SA. White paper: evidence-based decision making in dental hygiene education, practice, and research. J Dent Hyg 2001:50–63.

Frohn MA. Recall visits—Finding the right formula. Dent Assist 1991:7, 25.

Gervasi R. PPOs: scoring points in the busyness game. Dent Assist 1985:9–13.

Guignon AN. Sinking into a soothing . . . COCOON. RDH 2004:30–35.

Gutkowski S. Connectivity that's not therapy. Contemp Oral Hyg 2005:18.

Gutkowski S. Empowerment tools for dental hygiene profession. Contemp Oral Hyg 2004:18.

Gutkowski S. The Washington advantage. RDH 2004:18, 20, 22, 24.

Hainsfurther B. Claims processing simplified. Dent Teamwork 1988:96–98.

Hainsfurther B. For the office. Dent Teamwork 1988: 112–113.

Hall J. A computer enhanced our practice efficiency. Dent Econ 1990:45–48.

Harmon B. Tips on avoiding collection problems. Dent Teamwork 1991.

Hein C. Perio pathways advancing dental hygiene education to affect earlier diagnosis, better treatment, and appropriate referrals for specialist care of periodontal disease—Part 2. Contemp Oral Hyg 2004:28–30.

Hein C. Perio pathways etiology fast forwarded: the host-bacterial interaction theory and the risk continuum. Contemp Oral Hyg 2004:16–20.

Hutchinson L. Enhancing dental hygiene productivity. Dent Hyg News 6:21-22.

Jahn C. Evidence-based health care. RDH 2004:92–97.

Jameson C. Curbing patient cancellations, no shows. J Am Dent Assoc 1996:876–877.

Jameson C. The dental computer, a powerful marketing tool. Dent Assist 1993:9–12.

Jameson C. Scheduling for productivity, profitability and stress control. J Am Dent Assoc 1996:1777–1782.

Jamison L. Managing your insurance claims. Dent Teamwork 1993:35–37.

Jay A. Using computers . . . and actually liking it. Dent Mgmt 1990:30–31, 34, 36, 41.

Jones G, Woods M. The radiographic needs and policies of insurance carriers: hints for the dental office. Dent Assist 1993:6–9.

Kaiser K. Spice up hygiene services. RDH 2005:48, 50, 103.

Limoli T. Insurance reimbursement matters. Compend Contin Educ Dent 14:124–129.

Miles L. Effective hygiene recall. Access 1999:29–31.

Miles L. The eight phases of a dental visit. Dent Asst 1985.

Miles L. The new roles of today's dental team. Dent Asst 2005:12–13.

Miles L. Reign in your A/R–For good. Dent Prac Rept 2004.

Miles L. Staff compensation. Dent Asst 2004.

Miller K. Comprehensive care. RDH 2004:44, 46, 91.

Miller L. Presenting your case. RDH 1997:26, 28, 30, 58.

Morgans JP. Infection control for computer viruses. Dent Assist 1989:30–31.

Nash KD. What's your MOD net margin? J Am Dent Assoc 1992;123:92, 94, 96.

Nathe C. The oral exam, Part 1 of 3: historical outlook. Contemp Oral Hyg 2004:38–39.

Nathe C. The oral exam: the term diagnosis. Contemp Oral Hyg 2004:40.

Nimmons K. Putting together the puzzle pieces. RDH 2004: 52–54.

Nunn PJ. Medical history: why do we need to know all that personal stuff? Access 1993:33–36.

Nunn PJ. SOAP for whiter, brighter notes! Access 1994: 26–32.

Parks N. A dental insurance primer. Dent Assist 1983: 26–30.

Parks N. Efficient systems for handling dental insurance. Dent Assist 1982:25–26.

Perich P. Practice marketing: Whose job is it? Dent Teamwork 1990.

Pollack R. Helping the practice take flight. Dental Teamwork 1988.

Pollack R. Keeping the appointment book full. Dent Teamwork 1993:28–30.

Pollack RD. Inventory control: a system that works. Dent Teamwork 1990.

Pollack-Simon R. Hygiene partnering: optimizing the use of a hygiene assistant. J Pract Hyg 2001.

Pride J. Creating your practice philosophy: it's your chance to set goals. J Am Dent Assoc 1992:123.

Richards C. Electronic claim filing—Is it right for your office? Dent Assist 1990:30–31.

Ring T. The advanced dental hygiene practitioner. Access 2004:14–20.

Ring T. Trends in dental hygiene supervision. Access 2004:20–27.

Romano RV, Warner K. During economic uncertainty, patient comfort is king. Dent Asst 2004:30–31.

Sadler G. The benefits of dental electronic claims processing to the dental office. Dental Assist 1994:9.

Semple LG, Andrews EK. Continuing education: submitting dental insurance claims. J Contemp Dent Prac 2002;3:51.

Shinnawie R, Dmoch K. Creating a spa in Omaha. Dent Equip Mater 2004:61–66.

Stephenson B. Does your appointment book belong on your computer? Dent Today 1981.

Stephenson B. Simpler is better. Dent Econ 1990.

Stoeppler C. Computers in dentistry: avoid common mistakes with good preparation. Dent Econ 1991:67–70.

Sudimack L. Successful conversion to computerization. Dent Econ 1990:43–44.

Thomas RD. On their own. RDH 1994:14–26.

Von Buol P. Dental hygienists' business savvy boosts practice success. Access 1999:26–29.

Woodal I. Commentary support the hygienists who dare to be different. RDH 1985.

Zahrebelny O. Insurance solutions. Are dentists diagnosing medical problems? 2001.

Zuelke P. Take aim at solving insurance problems. Dent Econ 1986:49–58.

**Books**

American Dental Association. Advanced Dental Practice Management. Chicago: American Dental Association, 1970.

American Dental Association. Current Dental Terminology (4th ed.). Chicago: American Dental Association, 2003.

Ball VA, Halvorson EW. Managing the Dental Practice. San Francisco: Rinehart, 1974.

Darby ML, Walsh M. Dental Hygiene Theory and Practice (2nd ed.). St. Louis, MO: Saunders, 2003.

Dietz E. Dental Office Management. Albany, NY: Delmar Thomson Learning, 2000.

Douglas MA. Secretarial Dental Assistant. Delmar, 1976.

Earl E. Dental Assisting Manual: Professionalism, Legal Considerations and Office Management. Chapel Hill, NC: University of North Carolina Press, 1980.

Ehrlich A. Business Administration for the Dental Assistant (4th ed.). Champaign, IL: Colwell Systems, 1991.

Financial Management of a Dental Practice. Safeguard Business Systems, 1980.

Finkbeiner B. Practice Management for the Dental Team (3rd ed.). St. Louis: Mosby Year Book, 1991.

Finkbeiner B, Finkbeiner C. Practice Management for the Dental Team (5th ed.). St Louis: Mosby, 2001.

Harroch RD. Small Business Kit for Dummies. New York: Hungry Minds, 1998.

Malamed SF. Handbook of Local Anesthesia (5th ed.). St. Louis: Mosby, 2004.

McKeever M. How to Write a Business Plan. Berkeley, CA: Nolo, 1992.

Render B, Heizer J. Principles of Operations Management with Tutorials (2nd ed.). Upper Saddle River, NJ: Prentice Hall, 1997.

Schwartzrock, Jensen. Effective Dental Assisting. Brown Publications, 1991.

Slagon G. Dental Receptionist Procedure Manual. Devonshire Publishing Co., 1972.

St. Anthony's Publishing. Code Book for Outpatient Services. Vols. 1 and 2. 2002.

Stevens N. The ABC's of Filing: Basic Manual of Procedures. Lane Community College, 1983.

The Guide: Medical/Dental Cross-Coding, Republic Data Information Systems.

Torres H, Ehrlich A. Modern Dental Assisting (6th rev. ed.). Philadelphia, PA: Saunders, 2002.

Trump DJ, McIver M. How to Get Rich. New York: Random House, 2004.

U.S. Department of Health and Human Services, Public Health Service, Health Care Financing Administration. The World Health Organization International Classification of Diseases (9th rev.). Clinical Modification Codes. Washington DC: U.S. Government Printing Office.

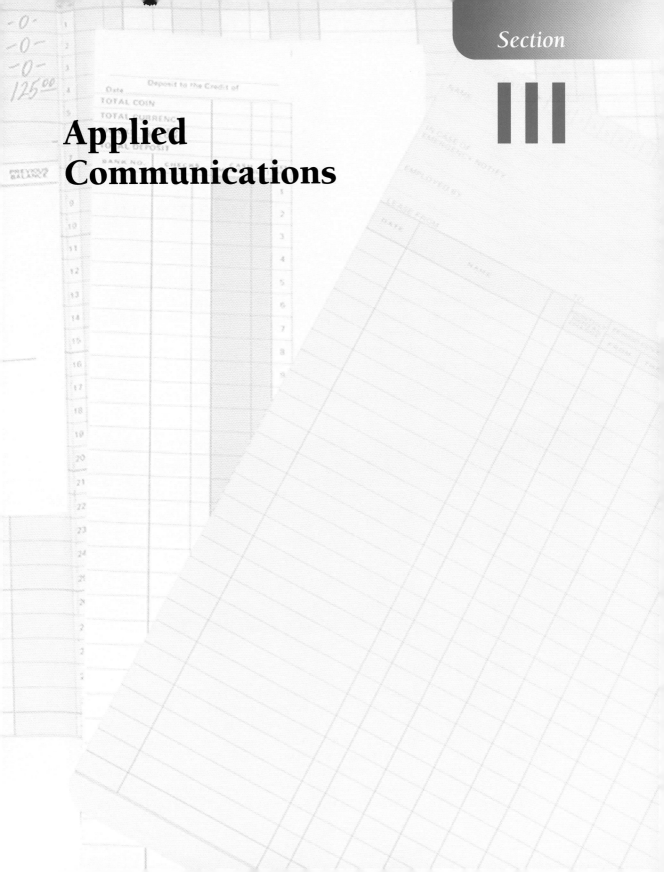

# Applied Communications

# Chapter

# 19

# Public Speaking Fundamentals

## LEARNING OUTCOMES

Upon mastery of the content of this chapter, the student should be able to:
- Communicate person to person with clients of differing needs.
- Communicate to an audience by presenting a case study, research paper, table clinic, or poster session.
- Create a case study to present to an audience.
- Research a topic by reviewing the literature and writing a paper to present to an audience.
- Create a table clinic and/or poster session and present it to an audience.

## KEY TERMS

abstract
affective learning
American Psychological Association
case study
clustering
cognitive learning
conductive deafness
International Committee of Medical
    Journal Editors
learning disabilities

personal space
poster sessions
psychomotor learning
research manuscripts
research papers
research poster
scripts
sensorineural deafness
sensory impairments
table clinics

## PUBLIC SPEAKING FUNDAMENTALS

Public speaking is the communication of thoughts and ideas from one person to an audience or group of people. Person-to-person communication is the one-on-one discourse between just two people. In the dental office, the latter type of communication often takes place between the dental professional and a person with different knowledge (most patients), different abilities (a pediatric patient), and different needs (an elderly patient). It is especially evident when the dental hygienist must instruct the patient or present a case. Dental professionals engage in some level of public communication when discussing a case study, writing a research paper, or presenting a table clinic or poster session.

# COMMUNICATION

Communication is simply the transfer of an idea from one person to another. Each day, the dental hygienist communicates with patients as well as coworkers and other business associates. It is important to realize that any method of communication may result in misunderstanding as a result of using vague language, inadvertently injuring feelings, invading the other's personal space, having poor listening skills, or displaying confusing body language.

# PERSON-TO-PERSON COMMUNICATIONS

Oral communication is the use of the spoken word to send a clear message using precise words or scripts. Because many English words contain more than one meaning, words must be well chosen so they are clearly understood by others. Some words may inadvertently hurt the feelings of others. When speaking, the professional should avoid using meaningless words and phrases such as "you know," "so," and "like." The use of these words cloud the message and detract from the dental hygienist's professional image and credibility; furthermore, the use of too many technical words may sound impressive, but the patient will not have understood their meaning.

The manner of speech is just as important as the words that are used. Consistent communication and doing what is said builds trust and enables people to have an open dialogue. When there is trust, the patient expects the oral healthcare provider to keep him or her from harm; when there is distrust, the patient may behave in a negative, defensive way. To build credibility, speak in a manner that is consistent with your professional beliefs, because people trust actions that support words.

In Chapter 8, the voice was mentioned as an important part of oral communication. The rate of speech and the tone and volume of the voice are involved in proper message transfer. Speaking too quickly, slowly, or softly may cause the listener to miss or ignore parts of the message. The message intended for the patient may be from a script or individualized, depending on the circumstances.

## Scripts

**Scripts** are written documents that outline what to say pertaining to a certain topic. Scripts are used for answering the telephone, giving patient instructions, making financial arrangements, and other often-repeated discussions. Although the dental professionals will not read the script directly, all staff members should memorize the same scripts and state information in a similar way to be sure accurate information is shared consistently.

## Legal Discussions

People may respond negatively if they perceive that they are being talked down to or are not valued. Treating others kindly using words that are neutral and not blaming helps make message transfers more accurate. It is the legal duty of the dental hygienist to inform the patient of his or her condition and to provide instructions on home care. Patient education (e.g., reiterating the need for daily flossing) combined with a statement noting your legal duty to inform patients, may help lend credence to the informational message.

## Communication Distance

The distance between people while they are interacting is another important aspect of message transfer, and it can be affected by cultural background or the use of power. **Personal space** is the area around an individual that is needed to feel safe and secure. The area is greater when communicating with a stranger and smaller when talking to a friend. The distance most Americans are comfortable with is arm's length (18–24 inches). Studies have shown that touching behaviors are frequently related to the use of power—that is, children are often touched; women are touched more than men; and employees more than supervisors.

## COMMUNICATING WITH PATIENTS

Some consultants recommend that patient conversations be centered on dental wants and needs, and that less than 25% of the conversation should be social in nature. There is a lot of information to impart to clients that needs to be consistent, accurate, and educational. The most frequent communications with patients are education or instructions and case presentation. As the speaker, the dental hygienist must be knowledgeable, be energetic, use an appropriate voice, and choose words wisely. The professional should limit distractions and interference from others to give the patient undivided attention while delivering the message.

### Presenting a Treatment Plan

As the expert on dental hygiene care, the dental hygienist may be asked to present the case facts on caries or periodontal disease to a patient. Patient education is reinforced by good communication skills, especially when discussing a treatment plan with a new patient, talking to a patient of record who has not been into the office for years, informing the patient of record about his or her onset of periodontal disease, or telling the periodontal maintenance patient there is recurrent infection. After reviewing assessment procedures to identify the needs, the dental hygienist makes a diagnosis and develops a treatment plan that states the expected outcomes and how they will be accomplished. The sequence of dental hygiene appointments intended to control, eliminate, prevent, stabilize, and reevaluate disease management is organized and planned and then presented to the patient.

The patient better understands the value for oral health treatment and maintenance when informed that periodontal health has a link to systemic well-being. Point the patient to websites and other sources that contain information about the relationship between oral health and heart disease, respiratory conditions, diabetes, and preterm or low birthweight babies. Recommend urgent care, such as palliative treatment of periapical abscesses, after the necessary nonsurgical periodontal therapy and regimens have been completed. Emphasize that periodontal maintenance is needed to reduce the progression of disease to prevent further loss of bone.

Dental hygiene therapy is performed according to a schedule of bundled procedures based on multiple sequenced appointments; patients are charged a single total case fee. The patient will be interested in what the out-of-pocket expenses will be, and the office manager or business dental assistant negotiates the financial payment plan. The dental hygienist keeps the treatment plan negotiations focused on patient education, planning his or her appointments, and answering any questions regarding dental care. The human needs deficits, care and comfort needs, pretreatment instructions, postoperative instructions, and other concerns are explained in detail at this time.

## Listening to the Patient

Patients express their emotions, and they should be encouraged to do so. One of the most difficult emotions to express is fear, and the healthcare professional who is uncomfortable with a patient's self-revelation may be tempted to discourage him or her from expressing that fear. If a patient has an infectious disease, he or she may fear rejection and fail to make a complete health history disclosure. Patients should be allowed to talk, and the professional should keep his or her reactions on a level that will help assure patients that they are worthwhile.

## Communicating with Children

Many adults adopt an artificial attitude when communicating with children by speaking in a higher pitched voice and more slowly or loudly, as if the child were hearing impaired. Children respond better when people talk to them in the same tone of voice used for adults. Communication is different with children because they live in the present and do not visualize the future. They understand the literal word and facts but do not fully understand all concepts. Speak truthfully and do not make any promises or guarantees to children or any patients. For example, suppose the dental hygienist tells the child that he or she is only going to take a look in the mouth. If a dental problem that needs immediate treatment is found, the provider will appear untrustworthy, and the child will lose confidence.

## Communicating with Adolescents

Adolescence—the teenage years—is the time of life during and after puberty. The adolescent may be moody and sensitive, making communication a challenge. Characteristics of this age group include resistance to advice from authority figures and to rules and regulations from parents or teachers. Teenagers are often more communicative to the dental professional when they are not in the presence of their parents or peers. Adolescents respond well if spoken to in the same tone used for adults. The dental professional should not judge a teenager based on his or her attitude or appearance; being nonjudgmental leads to the development of trust and open communication. Teenagers may wish to speak to the dental hygienist regarding a personal issue, and the adult should listen to them, allowing any disclosure.

## Communicating with the Elderly

Individuals over the age of 65 years (the basic retirement age as defined by Social Security), are referred to as the elderly, senior citizens, the aged, and older adults. Because this is such a diverse group of individuals, the best description is simply "people aged 65 or older." Today's senior citizens are not the stereotyped pill-popping grandparents portrayed in the media but are healthy, well-educated, politically aware, and financially secure adults actively engaged in life. Age discrimination based on different health needs, stereotypes, lower income, and other prejudices is frequently a challenge for the elderly. Most older adults maintain active lifestyles with expectations for extended lifespans and overall good health.

Traditionally in the United States, the elderly population had the lowest median income of any group. In recent years, there has been a dramatic decrease in the percentage of elderly living below the poverty level. More and more senior citizens have insurance coverage and continue to increase their use of insurance benefits. A major concern of the elderly is that their healthcare benefits will be not be enough to cover the cost of healthcare as they grow older. Also, they must cope with an increasing number of physical and psychological health concerns. An older person, like anyone else, wants the opportunity to finish speaking his or her thoughts; therefore, the dental professional must listen carefully and attempt to eliminate any barriers to oral healthcare.

Biomedical research and improved living environments are two reasons for the increase in the elderly population. These changes affect the way people live, and the attitudes toward older adults are changing to reflect the lifestyles of older Americans. Extended lifespans place the focus on the quality of the years remaining, not on withholding treatment because the patient has only a few years left to live. The demand for dental services by the elderly has increased more than for any other group. Because the elderly represent a growing number of patients seeking dental treatment, they have increased expectations and demands for health services.

The dental professional may need to modify his or her communication techniques if the older adult patient has cognitive deficiencies, sensory disturbances, physical impairments, or other age-related problems. After age 65, most individuals begin to notice some gradual changes in these arenas. An example of a cognitive deficiency is forgetfulness, and it can be frustrating for an older person. Another cognitive change in older individuals is an altered perception of time and movement. Alzheimer disease causes a decrease in intellectual functioning and is characterized by confusion and memory failure.

## EMOTIONAL NEEDS

One emotional characteristic of the aged is depression or frustration related to limited physical power and lack of physical control. Depression in the elderly, as well as in the general population, may be associated with loneliness, loss of family or friends, and changes in physical appearance. Some senior citizens are insecure owing to a reduced economic status and/or the inability to work. All people, and especially the elderly, have a strong desire to feel needed and derive a sense of personal importance when their needs and opinions are respected. Many older adults need to feel accepted and find the use of touch reassuring.

# Communicating through Language Barriers

English is the predominant language in the United States and in most parts of the Western world. Although English is the predominant language in the United States, not everyone speaks English as a primary language, resulting in a language barrier between the oral healthcare provider and the patient. The inability to communicate orally in English may make it difficult to gain the proper consent for dental treatment, which is required by most jurisdictions. Because educating the patient in proper oral healthcare is a vital function of the dental professional, special modifications are necessary to communicate with a person whose first language is not English.

If the office anticipates a language challenge, finding an interpreter who can help with communication during treatment may be the best choice. Communicating with the patient through the interpreter allows the staff to explain dental treatment, to gain consent, and to give instructions. Some practices may invest in commercially available language boards or chairside translator cards to help with communication; such items can be found at dental association websites. Sometimes a dental team member is able to speak the language of the patient and can facilitate patient communication with the non-English-speaking person.

## COMMUNICATING WITH CHALLENGED PATIENTS

All patients have unique and different human needs, goals, and experiences. Communication-challenged individuals include those who have a learning disability or hearing impairment. **Sensory impairments** are handicaps that affect the senses, such as learning disabilities and visual and hearing impairments. The oral healthcare provider must remain flexible when dealing with all patients but especially handicap-challenged individuals because each of these patients has unique needs. Many people who have a disability have had a great deal of contact with the healthcare establishment and are often involved in discussions concerning their abilities. Sensitivity and empathy are necessary when discussions may be emotionally hurtful.

Communicating with challenged patients requires the use of appropriate terminology as defined in the Americans with Disabilities Act. By using proper communication techniques with handicapped patients, the oral healthcare provider earns their trust and improves rapport.

### Patients with Learning Impairments

The term **learning disabilities** encompasses a multitude of conditions by which individuals have difficulty assimilating new information. Patient education for clients with a learning disability depends on each patient's specific needs and involves a variety of teaching techniques. There are three basic learning styles: cognitive, psychomotor, and affective. **Cognitive learning** is the process of perceiving knowledge using sight, sound, and thinking; the dental healthcare professional teaches such patients via pamphlets, models, and instructional videos. **Psychomotor learning** is the process of perceiving knowledge from demonstration or physical practice; the dental hygienist can, for example, demonstrate the act of tooth brushing in the patient's mouth. **Affective learning** is the process of perceiving knowledge by feeling emotions or reflecting attitudes; when the professional teaches such a patient, he or she should use praise to address the client's well-being. Some people with a learning disability may respond to all three types of learning. Remember that part of the natural aging process involves slower thinking and learning; therefore, allow older adults more time to learn and respond.

## Patients with Sensory Impairments

The visually impaired depend on eyeglasses, so be sure to return them to the patient before giving any instructions. Give the patient printed pamphlets and postoperative instructions to help with home care compliance.

There are two types of hearing impairment: conductive and sensorineural deafness. **Conductive deafness** is a condition in which the organs of the ear cannot conduct sound waves owing to interference caused by injury or disease. This type of deafness can be treated with hearing aids. Patients with hearing aids should be advised to turn them off during sonic or ultrasonic therapy. **Sensorineural deafness** is an incurable condition frequently associated with aging in which the organs that perceive sound, such as the inner ear, auditory nerve, and auditory center of the brain, malfunction; individuals with sensorineural deafness my experience dizziness. Measles, complications of upper respiratory infections, allergies, sinusitis, tonsillitis, and adenoid disease have been associated with sensorineural deafness.

Hearing loss is frequently found in people of advanced years and can be recognized if the patient asks the professional to repeat sentences, places a hand to the ear, turns one ear toward the speaker, speaks loudly, or responds inappropriately to requests. The hearing impaired have problems with background noises, multiple talkers, telephones, and other people's perceptions. Basic communication techniques used with such patients may include lip reading, sign language, writing messages on paper, or the use of an interpreter. When communicating orally, the oral healthcare provider should give these patients undivided attention, eliminate background noise, and speak at a slow rate while facing the patient (to aid in lip reading). Dental hygienists use gestures and visual aids to assist in discussions with patients, such as pointing to a poster or brochure. The hearing impaired may use sign language or finger spelling to communicate and may respond better to cognitive learning techniques.

## DEVELOPMENT AND PRESENTATION OF CASE STUDIES

Case study presentations are a form of person-to-person communication performed by the dental hygienist. A **case study** is a comprehensive patient profile that reviews existing conditions, contains a client-centered dental hygiene intervention care plan, and reports the results of treatment. Presentations relating to patient conditions, treatment plan, and evaluation of progress occur during an office visit or consultation appointment.

To learn how to make presentations to patients, dental hygiene students are given a clinic patient profile and are asked to prepare and present a case study to an audience of peers. Case study presentations are problem-based learning assignments that apply critical thinking skills in assessment, planning, and evaluation of a patient scenario in a clinical course. Case studies based on actual patients allow students to apply and synthesize theory, science, and clinical practice to evidence-based, patient-centered care.

The ability to plan and implement treatment takes experience, and case study assignments help increase confidence for future planning and evaluation decisions. The development and presentation of a case study help students learn about treatment successes and failures, prepare computer-generated reports for writing-intensive course requirements, and improve audience presentation skills. The ability to communicate and use critical thinking reflects educational success; these skills are reinforced when students write reports. Written communication is also important to employers because the abil-

**BOX 19.1** *Evaluation Criteria for Case Studies*

Preparation

| | |
|---|---|
| Rationale of presentation | 5% |
| Patient information | 5% |
| Dental, medical, social history | 10% |
| Clinical assessment data | 15% |
| Human needs deficits | 10% |
| Treatment plan | 15% |
| Treatment evaluation | 10% |
| Discussion of case | 10% |
| Spelling, grammar, diction, punctuation | 5% |
| Use of pertinent records to support findings | 10% |
| Three board-style questions | 5% |

Presentation

| | |
|---|---|
| Eye-contact, mannerisms | 10% |
| Rate of speech | 10% |
| Tone and volume of voice | 10% |
| Well rehearsed | 15% |
| Enthusiasm for subject | 10% |
| Visual aids | 15% |
| Phrase variety | 15% |
| Answered questions | 15% |

ity to communicate is one of the top skills for job success. *Box 19.1* provides the criteria instructors and faculty typically use for evaluation of case study presentations.

Published or previously presented case studies can be used as a guide for developing a new case study. Case studies are readily available through websites of colleges, universities, and dental companies; professional journals; and textbooks, and can be used to assist in this learning process.

## Selecting Patients

To be of value as learning and teaching tools, case studies should have the following elements. Generally, they should be based on actual clients, situations, assessment data, and physical, pathologic, ethical, legal, psychosocial, or epidemiologic problems or disorders that affect clients' health. *Box 19.2* lists the types of information needed to prepare a case study.

## PERSON-TO-AUDIENCE COMMUNICATION

Most people consider communicating person to person to be more comfortable than speaking to an audience. One of the most difficult and feared of all experiences is talking in front of a group of people. Applied communications skill assignments require that the student present a written product to a group of peers. *Box 19.3* lists general themes for professional presentations.

**BOX 19.2** *Data Needed for Case Studies*

| | |
|---|---|
| Rationale for patient selection | Human needs deficits |
| Patient information | Care and comfort needs |
| Chief complaint | Treatment plan |
| Dental history | Results of treatment |
| Medical history | Radiographs |
| Social history | Intraoral and extraoral photographs |
| Oral risk assessment | Dental, plaque, and periodontal charting |
| Clinical findings | Study models |

## Professional Presentations

Research papers, table clinics, and poster sessions are typical projects that dental hygiene students prepare during a course of study. For each type of assignment, students practice writing skills to develop higher cognitive critical thinking skills by actively participating in the learning process. The presentation of these assignments gives students public speaking practice and experience. Every project requires the learner to review the literature on an approved topic, prepare a written report, and present the findings to peers; each assignment has a higher level of difficulty. The great thing about such projects is the opportunity for personal growth and advancement. To keep the task enjoyable, the student should select a topic of interest or one in which he or she has had previous experience.

## Research Papers

Most of the **research papers** students write are thesis-type essays that review the scientific literature and are presented to a group of peers. Assigned at the beginning of the semester, research papers are presented at midterm or at the end of the term. These reports are assigned by college and university professors to prepare students for more

**BOX 19.3** *Topics for Professional Research Papers, Table Clinics, and Poster Sessions*

| | |
|---|---|
| Clinical research findings | New procedures |
| Dental disciplines | New products |
| Dental diseases | New techniques |
| Disease prevention | Prescription drugs |
| Ethics, jurisprudence, risk management | Special needs |
| General dentistry | Specialty dentistry |
| Government regulations | Systemic diseases |
| International dental care | Technology |
| Medical emergencies | |

difficult projects and to promote learning and scholarly activity. The benchmark for a typical research paper is three double-spaced typed pages, presented in 5 minutes with a discussion at the end. There are three principal phases of this type of assignment: preparation, presentation, and evaluation.

**Research manuscripts** are unpublished reports of clinical biomedical studies in which research methods and findings are described. They are submitted to peer-reviewed professional journals for publication, thus becoming part of the scientific literature and meeting national standards. Research findings are presented at the national meetings of professional associations, as poster sessions, or in speeches.

The American Psychological Association (APA) publishes a style guide titled *Publication Manual of the APA,* which assists both students and professionals in preparing scholarly papers. The APA is the most common writing style used by college and university students. The **International Committee of Medical Journal Editors** (ICMJE) created a style guide for research manuscripts submitted to biomedical journals to help authors, researchers, and editors create clear reports. The ICMJE style, sometimes called the Vancouver style, uses the American National Standards Institute (ANSI) reference style adopted by the National Library of Medicine (NLM) for its databases.

## PREPARATION

All writing assignments begin with an original idea. The topic can be found through the process of clustering and then thinking about (or reflecting on) those clusters. **Clustering** is a way of discovering several topics that are related to a central idea through stream-of-consciousness writing. A general topic is written in the center of a piece of paper; all ideas that stem from the initial topic are written on the paper as they come to mind and lines or arrows join similar topics. The process takes 3–5 minutes. When finished, the student reflects on the resulting clusters to discover a specific topic for the paper. In most cases, the faculty must approve the subject matter before the student begins working on the report.

The next step is to investigate information sources and keep track of any reference materials. Once the information on the topic has been gathered and read, the student begins to prepare a "zero draft." Many instructors want to see the zero draft activities to verify originality, timely work progress, and appropriateness of materials. The zero draft may be written as an outline, on index cards, as clustering or free writing, or in lists. At this stage of development, faculty provides input and feedback to help the student stay on track.

The first, or rough, draft of the paper should contain a title page, introduction, body, conclusion, and list of references cited and should be printed out from the computer. While writing the rough draft, the student should be aware of the possible evaluation criteria (*Box 19.4*). The rough draft may undergo a peer review.

In the next stage, the student works the rough draft into the final paper. The cover page should contain the title of the paper, the student's name, the date, the course title, and the name of the teacher or professor. The body of the paper should be three pages, with footnotes, and is followed by the reference list. Many colleges and universities accept only original work and require students to pledge by signature that the work is theirs and original to them. Students should refer to their school's policy concerning plagiarism and original work.

**BOX 19.4**  *Typical Criteria for Evaluating Research Papers*

Context
    Purpose (clearly stated central idea)    10%
    Tone, style    10%
    Audience (other dental professionals)    10%
    Mode (description, comparison)    10%
    Point of view (authority)    10%
Mechanics
    Organization (APA or ICMJE style)    5%
    Paragraph structure    5%
    Phrase variety    5%
    Sentence structure    5%
    Diction (word choice)    5%
    Coherence (clarity of thought)    5%
    Preparation (title page, word processed, 12-point font, name,    4%
        course name, date, topic)
    Spelling    4%
    Punctuation (commas, apostrophes, colons, semicolons)    4%
    Margins and spacing (double-spaced with 1-inch margins)    4%
    Footnotes (APA or ANSI style; cite three footnotes) and    4%
        bibliography (at least four forms of current reference materials;
        3 references must be from current periodicals; other
        references from textbooks, Internet, pamphlets, interviews)

## PRESENTATION

Before presenting any paper or talk, it is important to rehearse the material to become comfortable saying it out loud. Some people practice in front of a mirror; others in front of other people. Whichever practice technique is preferred, be sure to practice and to keep the presentation within the allotted time frame. Evaluators pay attention to communication skills, knowledge of the subject, polish of the presentation, grammar, professional demeanor, style of delivery, and ability to answer questions (*Box 19.5*).

## EVALUATION

The process of writing a research paper helps students develop cognitive and professional skills. Generally, students are evaluated throughout the assignment, including the zero draft, peer review, written research paper, and oral presentation.

# Table Clinics

**Table clinics** offer a chance to exchange instructions, information, and ideas using a tabletop display and handout materials. They are presented by individuals or a collaborative group to peers. Assigned at the beginning of a semester, the table clinics are offered during professional association meetings to promote professional interaction at the

**BOX 19.5** *Typical Criteria for Evaluating Research Paper Presentations*

| | |
|---|---|
| Stated purpose | 10% |
| Organization | 10% |
| Eye-contact, mannerisms | 10% |
| Rate of speech | 10% |
| Tone and volume of voice | 10% |
| Well rehearsed | 10% |
| Enthusiasm for subject | 10% |
| Visual aids | 10% |
| Phrase variety | 10% |
| Answered questions | 10% |

local, state, or national level. This assignment is a little more difficult than the research paper because the audience includes experienced oral healthcare providers who are accustomed to attending table clinics to promote continued learning and scholarly activity. Table clinics are competitive; and faculty assign first-, second-, and third-place awards. The benchmark for a table clinic is a 5-minute presentation of original content that can be easily repeated. There are three principal phases for this type of assignment: preparation, presentation, and evaluation.

## PREPARATION

As with any college-level writing assignment, the student must present a unique idea and original work and use an approved writing style (APA or ICMJE). The specific topic can be found through the processes of clustering and reflection, whether the table clinic is an individual or group project. After faculty approval of the selected subject, the next phase is to research and obtain information. Instead of writing a research paper, the student develops a script that is delivered during table clinic demonstrations. The script should be based on a review of scientific literature and should contain many of the components found in a research paper: title, introduction, body, and conclusion. Sometimes the student will be required to write an abstract.

### The Abstract

An **abstract** is a condensed summary of a scientific article, literary piece, or address that is submitted to a review board for consideration for publication, presentation, or a table clinic or poster session. For most competitions open to the dental hygiene student, the abstract must adhere to specific guidelines, such as the following. The abstract should begin with a title of 10 words or less and should appear on the top line. The author's name is placed two lines below the title. When there are multiple authors, the names may be alphabetized or ordered by amount of contribution; sometimes the presenting author is listed first. The next line contains the authors' affiliation, such as school, workplace, or company. (Note that for some competitions, the affiliation must *not* appear.) Two lines below the affiliation (or authors' names) is the abstract. Frequently, the abstract is limited to 50–250 words. Most word-processing software includes a tool for counting the number of words. The abstract must meet the requirements for font size and style as well as page set up; these are defined by the table clinic rules or by following APA or ICMJE style.

### Visual Aids

Many times the table clinic presenters construct a trifold board that contains print material and visual aids, which rests on the table. Sometimes the competition allows an easel stand for the visual aids. Other presenters display materials directly on the tabletop. The table is usually 30 inches by 30 inches by 72 inches; sometimes the facility provides a cover for the table or presenters may bring a tablecloth and drape. Visual aids, whether words or pictures, should support the presentation and be neat, concise, and creative. Pamphlets, products, props, models, and/or electrical devices are placed on the table in front of the trifold board. Note that electronics, such as view boxes, electronic media, and projectors (if allowed), need electrical outlets and extension cords and may require special requests or reservations. Table clinic rules usually disallow advertising and promotion of specific products. Thus, commercial products, professional materials, and drugs must not be identified by trade names or acronyms in the written material and should not be recognizable in displays. For example, it may be necessary to cover any manufacturer's name or model number that appears on instruments and equipment.

### Handouts

Brochures or pamphlets are created, assembled, and given to the audience at each talk. This material is prepared in a manner similar to the abstract. Each handout should include the title of the table clinic, the date, the objective, a brief abstract or outline, and a list of references. Brochures may be created from a bifolded or trifolded piece of paper that contains a front cover (title, authors, date, and perhaps a graphic), a page with the outline or abstract, and a page with the list of references. It is always appropriate to acknowledge in writing those who assisted in the preparation of the table clinic.

### Rehearsal

Practice allows the presenter to become comfortable reciting the script out loud. As noted earlier, some people practice in front of a mirror and others in front of other people. Be sure to keep the presentation within the allotted time. As for research papers, evaluators pay attention to communication skills, knowledge of the subject, polish of the presentation, grammar, professional demeanor, style of delivery, and ability to answer questions.

### PRESENTATION

Remember that the script is not read; the student may have small note cards with cues, but a well-rehearsed presentation is noteworthy. Table clinics require a specific dress code. Students may be asked to wear uniforms, scrubs, or business attire that is neat, clean, and ironed. The shoes should be clean. Personal appearance includes no heavy fragrance, hair in neat and clean condition, and no jewelry or nail polish.

## EVALUATION

Communication skills, organization, delivery, grammar, professionalism, poise, and the appearance of the clinic materials are all evaluated. Judging criteria are given in *Box 19.6*. Evaluators will not necessarily make themselves known to the presenter during the demonstration. When table clinics are presented at professional meetings, the participants usually receive a certificate of recognition that can be placed in their portfolios. Practicing oral healthcare providers who attend table clinic presentations receive a one-credit continuing education certificate that can be used toward their yearly requirements.

The table clinic winners are awarded a free membership renewal, a cash prize, and/or the opportunity to present their table clinic at the next level of competition (at the state or national association's annual session). Some associations award financial support to help the table clinic winners pay for travel expenses to the next competition.

## Poster Sessions

**Poster sessions** are an oral exchange of instructions, information, and ideas, or a demonstration of a procedure or technique using a poster display. For the dental hygiene student, poster sessions are competitive presentations performed at a local, state, or national professional association meeting. An individual or a group can present a poster. Poster exhibits allow for the discussion of scientific subjects, research results, clinical practice, and new technology. The **research poster** presents an original research study in which the presenter has participated. The content includes a purpose or hypothesis, statement of the problem, significance of the study, outline of methodology (design, sampling, and intervention), statistical data analysis, and results (conclusions or findings).

Posters are made from several types of material: a large photograph, several mounted boards, or a poster board displayed on a large panel. The benchmark for a poster session is a photograph poster that is placed on a foam panel board (secured by pushpins) and a 5- to 10-minute, easily repeated discussion of the content. Like a table clinic presentation, the creation of a poster session has three principal phases: preparation, presentation, and evaluation.

---

**BOX 19.6** *Typical Evaluation Criteria for Table Clinics*

| | |
|---|---|
| Innovative content | 10% |
| Organization | 10% |
| Eye-contact, mannerisms | 10% |
| Rate of speech | 10% |
| Tone and volume of voice | 10% |
| Well rehearsed | 10% |
| Enthusiasm for subject | 10% |
| Visual aids | 10% |
| Phrase variety | 10% |
| Answered questions | 10% |

Photo posters are printed on photographic paper and range in size from to 39 inches high by 55 inches wide to 4 feet high by 8 feet wide. They contain a descriptive title, presenters' names and affiliations, an abstract, research methodology, discussion, conclusions, and reference list. Photograph posters are rolled, stored in a tube, and carried to the presentation. The mounted-board format consists of multiple paper-size boards that each contain one category of content. The poster board format is assembled at the site, and smaller text and graphics are attached to a panel or easel.

A brochure or pamphlet may be created to promote discussion and dissemination of information. Poster abstracts are submitted to a committee for consideration for acceptance, as described for table clinic abstracts. The quality of the abstract determines whether the poster session is selected, so it is important that the abstract be clear and concise. The oral component of the poster presentation is 5–10 minutes long.

## PREPARATION, PRESENTATION, AND EVALUATION

As when writing any research report, the student first selects the subject matter and then gathers the needed information. For a poster session, the student must also decide on a format. The student must submit an abstract to a review board for admission into the poster competition. After writing the content, the student may present the poster session to an audience of peers.

According to the rules of competition, no brand names or manufacturer names are allowed in any of the presented information, including illustrations, photos, tables, charts, and columns. As noted earlier, the written component of the poster session should contain objectives, visual aids, rationale, valid methodology, results, conclusion, and list of references. Professional business attire is appropriate for poster presentations. Evaluation criteria are given in *Box 19.7*.

---

**BOX 19.7**  *Typical Evaluation Criteria for Poster Sessions*

Presentation
| | |
|---|---|
| Defined objectives and abstract | 10% |
| Organization | 10% |
| Explained rationale | 10% |
| Unique, innovative content | 10% |
| Conclusion | 10% |
| Eye-contact, mannerisms | 10% |
| Rate, tone, and volume of speech | 10% |
| Well rehearsed | 10% |
| Visual aids | 10% |
| Answered questions | 10% |

Research
| | |
|---|---|
| Background (describes the problem) | 10% |
| Methods (validity) | 10% |
| Results (data, statistical analysis) | 70% |
| Conclusions (clinical implications) | 10% |

## CONCEPT SUMMARY

- Public speaking involves communication between two people or between a person and an audience.
- Person-to-person communication in dental practice addresses the needs of children, adolescents, the elderly, the sensory impaired, and the learning impaired.
- Person-to-audience communication includes presenting case studies, research papers, table clinics, and poster sessions.
- Most types of public speaking require similar preparation and presentation skills.

# REVIEW QUESTIONS

1. What is the basis of client communication?
2. What techniques are used to communicate with children?
3. What techniques are used to communicate with adolescents?
4. What techniques are used to communicate with the elderly?
5. List the sensory conditions of the elderly that might alter effective communication.
6. What techniques are used in working with communication-challenged patients?
7. Why are case studies assigned?
8. When are research papers, table clinics, and poster sessions assigned?

## CASE STUDIES

1. Prepare a case study, concentrating on the evaluation criteria in the first part of *Box 19.1.*
2. Present a case study, concentrating on the evaluation criteria in the second part of *Box 19.1.*

## Communication: Practical Experience

1. Present patient education material to a client in a clinical setting. Videotape the presentation. Review the videotape to assess your communication strengths and weaknesses.
2. Create a research paper for presentation using the evaluation criteria given in *Box 19.5.*
3. Create a table clinic using the evaluation criteria given in *Box 19.6.*
4. Create a poster session using the evaluation criteria given in *Box 19.7.*

# Chapter

# 20

# Public Relations Techniques

## PUBLIC RELATIONS TECHNIQUES

The terms *image management, publicity,* and *media manipulation* are all synonymous with public relations. Good public relations means giving patients what they want and supporting their expectations for easy payments, excellent clinical skills, comfort, quality service, focused attention, evidence-based care, respect for their time, friendly team members, and a good location. Oral healthcare providers must be credible to be trusted. Patient fear and pain issues are directly related to credibility and trust. Internal and external marketing techniques are used to increase office visibility. Dental consulting firms are used in streamlining office systems, managing personnel, and making marketing decisions.

## INTERACTING WITH CLIENTS

Oral healthcare providers focused on creating a positive effect on clients are pursuing public relations. **Public relations** is the promotion of goodwill between an individual or an organization with the public. It can be achieved by promotional activities, office publications, public speaking engagements, and patient care and comfort techniques. All dental team members should actively pursue good public relations and strive to obtain good communication skills. Patients consider dental professionals to be experts; therefore, remaining credible and gaining patients' trust are fundamental to developing goodwill.

## Credibility

The consumer public has become increasingly skeptical of television and print advertising, tuning out the mass media due to a perceived lack of media credibility. Consumers do, however, respond to educational news reports and community service programs. **Credibility** in dentistry is achieved by the possession and demonstration of the following values: clinical competence, honesty, and inspiration. The dental professional who lacks any one of these values cannot win the faith and trust of patients.

A focus on patients and their dental health is the most important aspect of any dental practice. Credibility is key to successfully selling dental products and services. Clinical excellence alone will not build a loyal client base of devoted patients, who are vitally important to the success of the dental hygiene department, independent dental hygiene practice, or dental office. Having credibility absolutely requires that the dental professional have a philosophy of patient care, know what it is, and believe in it. In some practices, the office philosophy is stated orally at the daily morning huddle meeting to reinforce the purpose and beliefs of the staff. The daily affirmation of the office philosophy keeps each staff member performing in a consistent manner and communicating a similar message.

When using the marketing tools or implementing the marketing strategies outlined here, the oral healthcare provider must emphasize and cite the practice's philosophy. For example, whether the basic philosophy is comprehensive oral healthcare, treating the individual holistically, or serving the underserved, it should be communicated to help the patient understand why procedures and recommendations are made. Relate this information in a positive manner, inform patients of practice and procedure updates, and thank them for their cooperation during care. This type of teaching helps the provider affirm the shared values of trust and credibility to patients and empowers them to take ownership in their own health. Office philosophy is addressed further in Chapter 23.

## Building Trust

The public is increasingly skeptical of healthcare providers, thus, building trust with patients is vital. Once trust is established, it will yield long-term benefits. Many strategies can be used to build trust, beginning with the first impressions made by the appearance of the facility (clean and inviting) and staff (well groomed and friendly). The dental staff earns patients' faith and allays their fears by being friendly, listening attentively, paying attention, and being consistent and predictable in all actions. Spending quality time and effectively communicating with the patient and building the relationship help establish a good rapport. The dental professional can document personal conversations in the clinical record as useful reminders of shared discussions.

Just as some behaviors build trust, others erode trust. Impersonal, mechanical, and superior attitudes or appearing too busy to give the patient focused attention will cause the patient to lose faith in the dental practice.

## FREEDOM FROM FEAR AND PAIN

Pain and anxiety are critical issues in oral healthcare delivery and are at the core of public relations. Freedom from fear and pain are basic needs that must be foremost in the mind of oral healthcare providers when establishing trust and credibility. One survey found that half of all Americans dislike and distrust the dentist, and the fear of pain is frequently stated as the number one reason why people postpone and avoid dental visits. The cost of fear is the canceled and broken appointments that directly affect daily production totals. Patient fear is easy to detect if the dental professional pays close attention and observes and listens to the patient. Objective symptoms of fear include increased heart rate, respiration, blood pressure, perspiration, and muscle tension, as well as trembling and guarded body language. The patient fears pain, death, helplessness, the unknown, ridicule/embarrassment, and body mutilation.

### Pain and Anxiety Therapy

A variety of therapies are used to treat pain and anxiety, such as physical forces, spiritual and psychological treatment, and drug and biological treatment. **Physical forces** are manipulative forms of therapy used to decrease pain and muscle spasms, such as massage, chiropractic manipulation, and physical therapy. Chiropractors, osteopathic doctors, massage therapists, physical therapists, and dental professionals trained in massage can deliver this treatment. **Spiritual and psychological therapies** improve energy flow and facilitate the mind's capacity to affect bodily functions. Examples of such therapies are acupuncture, acupressure, and desensitization therapies such as controlled breathing, relaxation, guided imagery, rehearsal, biofeedback, hypnosis, prayer, and divination. **Drug and biological therapy** use medications and chemicals to relieve fear and pain. The dental professional can prescribe pain relievers, sedative drugs, nitrous oxide analgesia, and local anesthesia. Painless dental injections, needleless injections, Valium premedication, nitrous oxide–oxygen analgesia, and medications such as ibuprofen manage pain and fear, giving the patient the feeling of control. Promotion of goodwill in the dental practice by alleviating fear and pain affirms shared values of trust and credibility.

## MARKETING

Public relations activities are meant to inform, promote, and convince the public about the value of dental practice. **Marketing** in dentistry is the development and implementation of plans to disseminate healthcare information to promote the purchase of oral healthcare services and products. Marketing communications focus on telling patients about products and services, not selling them. The consumer is well educated, skeptical of healthcare providers, and will not be "sold" owing to the constant bombardment of advertising in the media. Good marketing is getting the patient to trust, agree to necessary treatment, enjoy the process, and refer friends and family. Trust helps a patient understand his or her needs, prioritize treatment, find the financing, ignore insurance issues, and overcome fear.

Marketing plans describe actions to take, timelines for completion, coordination of efforts, and the evaluation of results. A marketing plan should be developed yearly and be based on the office mission statement. (Mission statements are discussed in Chapter 23.) A marketing plan determines the target audience in need of a dental service or product, sets the fee for service, and outlines promotional activities. For example, suppose the dental practice wants to advertise that it is now offering a new "invisible" orthodontic technique. The target audience is the client with malposed teeth, the service needs are tooth straightening, and the fee is preset with financing options available. Or suppose the dental office wants to publicize the delivery of chemotherapeutic injectable antibiotics. The target audience is clients with active periodontal disease, the service needs are management of disease, and the fee is preset.

After the marketing objectives are identified, the promotional activities are planned and timelines are developed. The success of the promotional program is determined after the marketing activities end. Success is determined from a production report generated by the dental practice software system based on the American Dental Association (ADA) insurance procedure code for orthodontics or chemotherapeutics.

## Internal Marketing

Marketing to improve public relations can be conducted through a variety of internal or external methods (*Box 20.1*). **Internal marketing** promotes the office to potential prospects inside the practice. It is an ongoing system of activities designed to identify and satisfy consumer needs and wants. Practice management consultants have mixed opinions regarding asking the patient to refer family and friends. It may be better to tell clients that the office is taking new patients. When a patient of record refers new patients, a reward is usually given, such as a hand-written thank-you letter with a $10 gift certificate (which could increase in amount with each referral). Sending a computer-generated thank-you note for the referral is not enough reward for promoting the practice, nor is it good customer service.

---

**BOX 20.1** *Internal and External Marketing*

**Internal Marketing**

Birthday letters or cards
Brochures and pamphlets
Business letters with logo and catch phrase
"Care to share" referral appointment cards
Contests
Convenient appointments
Free samples
Mailing postoperative photographs
Marketing letters and aids

New patient welcome letters and packets
Office letterhead and personalized postcards
Patient education materials
Personnel appearance
Postoperative evening or next-day telephone calls
Postoperative letters
Referral letters
Thank-you letters and cards

**External Marketing**

Billboards and signage
Direct marketing mailings
Fundraising contributions
Media broadcast (radio, television, cable access channels)
New resident welcome letters and packets
Newsletters

Newspaper and magazine advertising
Office website and Internet advertising
Public service announcements
Team sponsorship
Yellow page advertising

Another powerful public relations technique is the postoperative telephone call to see how the patient is doing. Mailing a greeting card from the office staff to a patient of record when a major life event occurs builds goodwill. It has been determined that women spend the market share of money on over-the-counter (OTC) health products and drugs. As a target audience, dental offices can provide free samples to women from manufacturers and distributors to recommend OTC products. Dental novelties, such as the tooth fairy baby tooth bank, starter breathcare kits, and other samples, help exceed patient expectations. Other in-office promotional methods are the use of an intraoral camera to image cracked and damaged teeth, presented with a final postoperative intraoral photograph.

## External Marketing

**External marketing** promotes the office to potential prospects outside of the practice. It is designed to increase the patient base and revenue. External marketing tools are listed in *Box 20.1*. The new patient who accepts treatment, keeps appointments on time, returns for recare, pays promptly, and refers family and friends is the target audience. Ongoing, continuing care increases referrals and continued support of the practice. Public education via signage, mailings, media broadcasts, advertising, newsletters, and sponsorship reaches a target audience in the community, optimizing visibility. Volunteerism as a staff for community events increases public awareness of the dental office. Many dental offices produce periodic newsletters. New residents to the area can be embraced by sending welcome packets. Office staff can distribute business cards to acquaintances to help promote the dental office.

## Image

In marketing, image is everything. The look of a high-quality dental practice should reflect the high-tech, high-touch provider. Attention to detail should be given to the appearance and feel of the reception area: new magazines on display, no dental pictures, comfortable chairs, and refreshments. The grooming and physical appearance of the staff should also reflect the image of quality.

Because clients respond to factual information, certified and licensed staff credentials in the form of wall displays of legitimate diplomas, licensure, and awards should be in view. Note that some displays can be purchased and not earned, e.g., an "Outstanding Dentist Award" given for a political contribution or an advertisement. Such displays may create a loss of credibility in the eyes of clients. Tours of the office by patients with a stop at sterilization helps promote a positive image. Spa-like extras, soft music, clean air, parting gifts, refreshments, and free samples are more than expected, and customer service should exceed patients' expectations.

## Marketing Consultants and Coaches

**Dental business consultants** are practice management experts who analyze the practice management systems, personnel, and marketing efforts to advance efficiency. Business consultants and coaches work to improve office systems and communication by defining the office philosophy and goals before reorganizing systems. Organized office systems reduce stress and increase production; therefore, such consultants conduct an analysis to determine the strengths and weaknesses of the practice, which are presented by the consultant in a written report. Periodic office meetings are held by the practice consultant to implement improvement plans and follow up with a monthly report summary of the progress to the practice owner. The practice owner typically contracts with the consultant for a period of 1 year with a yearly renewal option.

## PUBLIC RELATIONS ASSESSMENT SURVEYS

To improve the quality of service and patient satisfaction, dental offices periodically conduct surveys to measure patient attitudes. Anonymous feedback from clients helps identify areas that require attention and sensitivity. Three principal types of surveys are the true–false (*Fig. 20.1*), Likert scale (*Fig. 20.2*), and open question (*Fig. 20.3*).

---

*Forever Smiles Dental Offices*
*123 Main Street, Anytown, Anystate 12345 Phone: 888-555-1515*

CLIENT SATISFACTION SURVEY

| | | | |
|---|---|---|---|
| 1. Telephone calls are answered promptly. | TRUE | FALSE | NA |
| 2. Telephone calls are answered with courtesy. | TRUE | FALSE | NA |
| 3. The dental business staff is friendly. | TRUE | FALSE | NA |
| 4. Appointments are available on short notice. | TRUE | FALSE | NA |
| 5. The office hours are convenient. | TRUE | FALSE | NA |
| 6. The office location is easy to find. | TRUE | FALSE | NA |
| 7. The office location has adequate parking. | TRUE | FALSE | NA |
| 8. The office is clean. | TRUE | FALSE | NA |
| 9. The staff is knowledgeable. | TRUE | FALSE | NA |
| 10. The staff is discreet. | TRUE | FALSE | NA |
| 11. The staff listens to my concerns. | TRUE | FALSE | NA |
| 12. The staff has educated me about my health. | TRUE | FALSE | NA |
| 13. The fees for treatment are reasonable. | TRUE | FALSE | NA |
| 14. The credit terms are agreeable. | TRUE | FALSE | NA |
| 15. The dentist explains my treatment. | TRUE | FALSE | NA |
| 16. The dentist spends enough time with me. | TRUE | FALSE | NA |
| 17. The dentist allays my fears. | TRUE | FALSE | NA |
| 18. The dentist listens to me. | TRUE | FALSE | NA |
| 19. The dentist is concerned with my well-being. | TRUE | FALSE | NA |
| 20. The dentist provides good dental care. | TRUE | FALSE | NA |

Name (optional):_____

Phone # or Email (optional):_____

---

**Figure 20.1** Sample true–false patient survey.

---

*Forever Smiles Dental Offices*
*123 Main Street, Anytown, Anystate 12345 Phone: 888-555-1515*

CLIENT SATISFACTION SURVEY

Please use the following scale to rate our service to you.

| 1 | 2 | 3 | 4 | 5 |
|---|---|---|---|---|
| Very satisfied | Somewhat satisfied | Satisfied | Somewhat dissatisfied | Dissatisfied |

- How would you rate your overall experience in our dental office?
    1    2    3    4    5
- How would you rate your experience with Dr. Drawer?
    1    2    3    4    5
- How would you rate your experience with T. Brusher, the dental hygienist?
    1    2    3    4    5
- How would you rate your experience with the dental assistants?
    1    2    3    4    5
- How would you rate your experience with the business staff?
    1    2    3    4    5
- How would you rate your experience with the facility?
    1    2    3    4    5
- Please share any comments:

  _____

  _____

Name (optional):_____

Phone # or Email (optional):_____

---

**Figure 20.2** Sample Likert-scale satisfaction survey.

## CONCEPT SUMMARY

- Public relations activities are designed to establish a loyal client base.
- Therapies to alleviate fear and pain are critical in the development of trust and credibility with patients.
- Marketing plans are designed to disseminate healthcare information by describing marketing actions to undertake, establishing timelines for completion, coordinating efforts, and evaluating results.
- Internal marketing techniques promote the office to patients and staff.
- External marketing techniques promote the office to potential prospects outside of the practice.
- Dental practice consultants analyze practice management systems, personnel, and marketing efforts to advance office systems and communication.
- Patient satisfaction surveys are conducted to measure patient attitudes.

*Forever Smiles Dental Offices*
*123 Main Street, Anytown, Anystate 12345 Phone: 888-555-1515*

CLIENT SATISFACTION SURVEY

What was the best part of your experience here?
_____

What was the worst part of your experience here?
_____

What would you change about the office?
_____
_____

What would make you feel more comfortable here?
_____

How would you describe your experience with:

- Dr. Drawer_____
- T. Brusher, the dental hygienist_____
- The dental assistants_____
- The business staff_____

How were your needs met?
_____

How were your financial questions handled?
_____

How would you rate the level of technology used here?
_____

What is your overall assessment of the care you received?
_____

Name (optional):_____

Phone # or Email (optional):_____

**Figure 20.3** Sample open-question survey.

# R E V I E W   Q U E S T I O N S

1. What is the basis for establishing good public relations?
2. What are barriers to good public relations?
3. Why are trust and credibility important?
4. Why is freedom from fear and pain a significant aspect of trust and credibility?
5. What is marketing and how does it affect public relations?
6. What is the difference between internal and external marketing?
7. What are the differences among a true–false, Likert-scale, and open-question survey?
8. Why do practice owners hire dental consultants?
9. Why would directing free samples to women clients be beneficial for dental product sales?

# CRITICAL THINKING ACTIVITY

- Determine ways to create a positive image using public relations techniques.
- Discuss the three types of patient satisfaction assessment surveys. When would each be best used?
- Discuss a new dental procedure and determine a marketing plan.
- Select one marketing technique and discuss how you would implement it in practice.
- Locate and investigate a dental consultant website and make recommendations for improvement.

# Office Publications

## LEARNING OUTCOMES

Upon mastery of the content of this chapter, the student should be able to:
- Categorize written office publications as public relations activities.
- Differentiate between public relations activities that require written communications and those that require audiovisual communications.
- Recognize situations in which office publications are used.

## KEY TERMS

| | |
|---|---|
| annual reports | news releases |
| broadcast media | print media |
| direct mail marketing | public service announcements |

## OFFICE PUBLICATIONS

Office publications are an extension of the practice's public relations (PR) activities. Of course, all of the many different types of office publications require writing, but some also require audiovisuals, graphics, print materials, and oral presentation. Whatever the PR activity, it should project a positive image to the public at large.

Dental practices engage in public relations writing to disseminate specific information; often such print material is used to promote the practice as well. Printed material may be developed and/or assembled by a staff member who is assigned to marketing, or the office may hire an outside graphic artist, marketing firm, product manufacturer, or other entity. Typical dental office PR activities are listed in *Box 21.1*. Before undertaking any PR activity, the dental professional must review the legal requirements and restrictions for his or her jurisdiction; some local governments dictate and/or prohibit certain types of public relations techniques. Penalties include monetary fines, licensure reprimand, and other disciplinary actions.

## ADVERTISING

Advertising public relations activities encompass two realms: broadcast and print media. **Broadcast media** disseminate information over the radio and television (cable) and

**BOX 21.1** *Office Publications*

| | |
|---|---|
| Advertising (print and broadcast media) | Flyers |
| Annual reports | News releases |
| Articles | Newsletters |
| Brochures | Public service announcements |
| Business cards | Signage |
| Direct marketing mail | Speeches and presentations |

through the Internet (websites; blogs). To engage in radio advertising, the dental practice writes scripts that are read over the airwaves. Television and cable advertising also use written scripts prepared by the dental practice; but, in addition, they require some form of audiovisual material, such as photographs, graphics, or video. Website and Internet advertising use written material that is posted on the dental practice's website or on other local websites as advertisements. Internet advertising requires print material plus photographs, graphics, and/or streaming video. All such advertising is directed to a preselected target audience.

**Print media,** such as newspapers, magazines, journals, newsletters, and the yellow pages, use written materials to disseminate information. The consumer public has learned to skim or skip print advertising; thus it may not be as effective as broadcast media. Print ads are directed to a specific issue or announcement—for example, "Open to new patients," or "Professional tooth whitening for $200."

Advertising in the yellow pages entails placing written PR material in the local telephone book. It is an accepted and common custom that has been used by dental practices for promotion. There are a variety of formats, ranging from a single line to a full page. These ads are renewed yearly and can be expensive; therefore, the office should monitor its return on investment (ROI). Each new patient should be asked how he or she heard about the practice; the clients who mention the yellow pages are counted to determine the effectiveness of this form of PR written communication.

### New Resident Welcome Packets

In some localities, new community residents receive a welcome packet of information from real estate agents, the city, or a new resident organization. Some dental practices create a welcome letter, brochure or pamphlet, flyer, newsletter, or direct mail marketing piece to be included in these welcome packets.

## ANNUAL REPORTS

**Annual reports** are federally mandated written communications that are published by publicly traded companies to divulge information describing the last 5 years of a company's performance. The report contains a 5-year analysis plus the most recent year's activities, profits, losses, and viability. Although most dental practices are privately owned businesses, a yearly report may be necessary to document ROI, to analyze a partnership, to list accomplishments, or to clarify use of allocations granted by a funding authority.

## ARTICLES

Articles are written to disseminate information in educational and editorial formats. They are published in newspapers, magazines, newsletters, and/or journals. Educational formats deliver scientific reviews of the literature, news items, features, and profile information. Articles are similar to essay papers in that they have an introduction, main body, and conclusion. Some publications, such as newspapers, publish feature sections, which included several articles concerning a specific theme to impart information. For example, a publication may print a feature on laser tooth whitening. Such a feature could include a main article on the technique of tooth whitening, a before-and-after client case study, and several informational news items on the use of lasers or tooth whitening.

Profiles generally involve a main story about a specific person, product, service, and/or organization. Many dental hygiene publications include profile stories about dental hygienists. A common profile format is the question and answer interview. These articles provide biographical information and the subject's point of view on selected topics. They also include direct quotations from the individual profiled. A profile focusing on a product or service offers a unique way to offer information to the public. Organizational profiles include interviews of several people within the entity.

Editorials are essays written to disseminate information based on a personal opinion. An editorial may be written to the editor of a publication, as a guest editorial for a publication, as a letter to the publication, or as a side story to a main article (for example, describing firsthand experience with a new product or technique). A dental practice may write an article for publication in local newspapers or magazines, in office or professional newsletters, and/or in journals for educational or editorial purposes.

## NEWS RELEASES

**News releases** are the most commonly used written format to disseminate PR material to the print and broadcast media. Press releases are written to publicize noteworthy information related to an organization or product, or may include a financial statement (in the case of public companies). A dental practice writes press releases when a provider in the office has been honored with an award, when the team it sponsors has won a championship title, when it has been recognized as a provider of care to a special-interest group such as the local heart association, or when it wishes to announce that it now offers a new high-tech procedure.

Press releases are frequently sent to local newspapers, radio, and television stations; however, because these news outlets receive many press releases every day, submission does not guarantee a release will be used. If a staff member follows up with a telephone call to the community news desk of the media organization, he or she will be able to confirm the receipt of the press release and determine whether it will be used and in what manner. News releases can be sent electronically via the Internet to media outlets, but a news release sent via the U.S. Postal Service may have a better chance of being noticed by an editor. A sample news release is given in *Figure 21.1.*

---

*Forever Smiles Dental Offices*
*123 Main Street, Anytown, Anystate 12345 Phone: 888-555-1515*

NEWS RELEASE

| | |
|---|---|
| **Contact:** | **Release Date and Time:** |
| Forever Smiles | For immediate release |
| 123 Main Street | |
| Anytown, Anystate 12345 | |
| 888-555-1515 | |

T. Brusher, RDH, has been awarded the state dental hygiene association's highest award for

a table clinic presentation at the annual state meeting of the American Dental Hygienists'

Association held in Capital City. The presentation, titled "Great Smiles," was honored at the

awards banquet. The table clinic award is the premier award for a dental hygiene

practitioner.

    T. Brusher's presentation addressed emerging technologies in dental hygiene that

enhance patient treatment, safety, and comfort.

    T. Brusher has been a dental hygienist with Forever Smiles in Anytown for more

than 20 years.

    For additional information, please call 888-555-1515.

#

**Figure 21.1** Sample dental office news release.

## NEWSLETTERS

Newsletters disseminate information to clients and the public at large about the dental practice, allied dental personnel, nonpractice information, and office policy. Newsletters consist of articles, profiles, headers and titles, announcements, and editorials. The information placed in a practice newsletter is 50–75% committed to the dental practice and the unique procedures performed. The remaining information is equally focused on employees and general dental information, such as an article titled "Who Smiles More?" Dental practice newsletters generally consist of four 8- by 11-inch bifolded pages and contain articles on new high-tech procedures, dental products, prescription medications, and office policies. As mentioned earlier, newsletters can be distributed to new residents in a welcome packet with a welcome letter; they can also be sent to new, active, and inactive patients; employees; and business associates. In addition, newsletters may be sent electronically to clients via email.

## OTHER PUBLICATIONS AND PR ACTIVITIES

Other publications used by dental practices are created in the office, professionally produced, or commercially preprinted, and include business cards, letterhead, brochures/pamphlets, flyers, and direct marketing mail. Office staff can distribute business cards to acquaintances with an invitation to come in for an examination to help promote the practice to the public. Letterhead is used when writing letters to anyone or any organization under the name of the practice; a secondary purpose is to promote the practice by name and location to active, inactive, new, and prospective patients.

Brochures and pamphlets are developed by the practice or an outside source to raise patients' dental awareness. The practice name and address are added to such brochures, which are distributed to clients according to their needs. Typical dental practice pamphlets focus on the following topics: cosmetic improvements, periodontal infection and the risk of heart attack, tooth whitening, bruxism, and mouth protection devices. Flyers are prepared within the practice to inform patients about care, products, or protocols. Desktop publishing and word-processing programs can help staff develop these materials for patient distribution.

### Direct Mail Marketing

Communication with the written word is powerful, thus, written promotional materials are powerful tools for marketing. **Direct mail marketing** is the development and distribution of marketing brochures, flyers, postcards, and newsletters to be mailed by ZIP codes found within a selected radius around the practice location. Entrepreneurs choose direct mail marketing to promote their businesses because it goes directly to the consumer and the results can be measured in terms of money spent for the activity and the results it generates. This type of PR entails an organized campaign of monthly mailings, such as postcards to new residents, promotional offers, rewards to current clients, and coupons.

### Public Service Announcements

**Public service announcements** (PSAs) are statements on a single topic that are broadcast in the media. Radio announcements involve only a written statement, but television announcements generally require some sort of supporting graphics or video. Businesses purchase airtime for their PSAs, but nonprofit organizations (such as the American Cancer Society) do not pay for airtime because their announcements are made in the public interest.

To develop a 10- to 30-second PSA, it is necessary to write a script. Often the local television networks, cable television stations, and radio stations can help in the production of the PSA. Dental practices produce PSAs on topics that concern the general public—for example, oral cancer awareness, the importance of mouth protection during sports participation, and the link between oral health and pregnancy outcome. The sponsoring organization is generally mentioned at the end of the PSA.

### Signage

Before purchasing and placing any signage, the dental office must determine what is legally allowable in its jurisdiction. In some areas, regulations define and describe in detail what is allowed, down to the letter size and font; furthermore, the local munici-pality may prohibit certain types of signage. Despite possible restrictions, dental prac-tices generally can choose from among many types of signs, including billboards, indoor or outdoor lighted signs, neon signs, portable signs, vinyl banners, vinyl graphics/decals, or lettering.

One of the most common forms of signage is the lettering placed on a building to identify the business lodged inside. Lettering can be made of steel, plastic, or foam, and may be cast, cut out, molded, or fabricated. In addition, most business have larger signs adjacent to the building. These signs may be manufactured from metal, plastic, foam, or wood, and may include electrical lighting or neon. Company logos or symbols can be placed on the signs or on plaques to publicize the business. Note that placing a logo on a sign is a customized operation that involves additional costs and time. Other forms of signage are vinyl banners and decals. Vinyl banners are used outdoors and are fastened with rods or string to the building. Decals are printed on adhesive vinyl, which is placed on a glass surface, such as the entry door or a large window.

Outdoor advertising involves the use of very large signs to promote businesses by reaching the consumer public where they commute, live, work, and shop. Outdoor advertising is found in the form of billboards, wallscapes, bus displays, transit shelter dis-plays, airport displays, and taxi advertising. Consumers are exposed to multiple forms of media, and this type of advertising cannot be turned off, discarded, or skimmed over. Bulletin billboards can be purchased individually or in quantity and can be located in a variety of locations. Some local professional associations purchase a single bulletin bill-board to advertise the profession. A single billboard costs between $2,500 and $6,000 for a month, with additional charges for design and production. Billboards capture attention, especially in high-traffic areas that may have extensive waiting times. A wide variety of unusual sizes and shapes are available to catch the eye and to establish awareness. All of these forms of advertising can be marketed toward a particular ethnic, socioeconomic, or other population group.

## SPEECHES AND PRESENTATIONS

Speeches and presentations are oral exchanges to disseminate information to a target audience. PR speeches are given to instruct, demonstrate, influence, or entertain. These speeches can be delivered at dental meetings, to special-interest groups, and at the open-ing of a new office. Usually, the office staff has the time to plan for such a presentation. Speeches should have a purpose and an effect on the audience. Once the desired out-come is defined, the speech is organized in a manner similar to an article; it should have an introduction, a body or discussion to emphasize the main points, and a conclusion to review and summarize.

Because speeches and presentations involve oral delivery, it is important for the den-tal professional to practice, to make eye contact, to avoid slang, and to stay with the time limitation. (Chapter 19 provides more tips for public speaking.) Speeches and presen-tations may have an audiovisual aspect to enhance the subject delivery. Finally, speeches and presentations may include a follow-up question-and-answer period; it is important that this period be brief.

## CONCEPT SUMMARY

- Public relations writing includes advertising, annual reports, articles, news releases, newsletters, public service announcements, signage, speeches, and presentations.
- Public relations activities require speaking and writing skills.
- Public relations writing is used for specific situations.

# REVIEW QUESTIONS

1. Why would a dental practice want to engage in public relations?
2. What types of outlets do broadcast media use?
3. Why would a dental practice use broadcast media?
4. What is the difference between print media and office publications, such as brochures and flyers?
5. What can be placed into a new resident packet?
6. How do dental practices use annual reports?
7. What are the three styles of articles?
8. How are newsletters incorporated into a marketing plan?
9. List the types of office publications commonly made within the practice.
10. Why would a dental practice write a news release?
11. Why are public service announcements (PSAs) made and used by a dental practice?
12. What are the different types of outdoor signage?

# CRITICAL THINKING ACTIVITY

- Imagine that you are an entrepreneur about to open an independent practice. Plan a marketing strategy and describe the public relations writing activities you will use.
- Of all of the office publications described in this chapter, which would be the most and the least effective to use?
- As a consumer, which of the office publications would most likely affect your decision to become a patient in a dental practice? Are there any that would not influence your decision?
- Read your jurisdiction's dental practice act to identify any language that regulates public relations activities.

# Chapter
# 22

# Client Letters and Forms

Upon mastery of the content of this chapter, the student should be able to:
- Be familiar with the focused written communication letters used by dental practices.
- Recognize and use client forms such as personal, dental, and medical histories; oral risk assessment surveys; dental and periodontal charts; treatment plans; services rendered; financial forms; informed consent; and Health Insurance Portability and Accountability Act compliance forms.

## KEY TERMS

international numbering system
Palmer notation system
sequenced writing

services rendered form
SOAP notes
universal numbering system

## CLIENT LETTERS AND FORMS

Dentistry is a heavily regulated industry in the United States. Written documentation of all financial transactions, clinical instructions and recommendations, referrals, and public relations activities are mandated by law. Client letters and forms are considered legal documents used to record legal transactions, and they serve as proof that the standard of care was implemented and followed. Letters are sent to clients, insurance companies, business associates, and other healthcare providers to document actions and share information. Client forms are a permanent record of the patient's health and financial status.

## LETTERS

Focused written communication activities and business letters are mailed every day to clients, insurance companies, other dental offices, other healthcare providers, and/or business associates. Mailed items range from client birthday letters/cards and thank-you notes to marketing letters and aids, narrative reports, new patient welcome letters, patient education materials, postoperative letters (including results and photographs), recall letters, and referral letters.

The basic supplies necessary for written business communication mailings include a quality bond paper containing the practice's logo and catch phrase and matching envelopes. Dental office staff must choose the paper quality, printing quality and type, and color. Letterhead stationery has the practice's name and address embossed on the page and can be ordered from a local print shop, local office supply company, office supply company catalog, or Web site. Acceptable stationery colors for dental businesses are plain white, cream, gray, and light blue. Once a letter is written, mailing lists, an individual label, or preaddressed envelopes can be generated by the office computer software.

## Client Letters

Perfect spelling, punctuation, and grammar are absolutely necessary for focused written communications. Letters should be typed or composed via a word processor, single spaced, and free of errors. The written content is kept to one page, centered on the page vertically with margins that take into account the space needed for the logo and catch phrase. The most common letter format is block style, used for the construction of brief and concise mailings (*Box 22.1*).

---

**BOX 22.1** *Essential Components of Block Letters*

Heading with Office Name and Address (if not on preprinted letterhead)
2 blank lines
Date line
2 blank lines
Name of recipient
Street address
City, state, ZIP code
2 blank lines
Salutation (e.g., Dear Sir:)
1 blank line
Body paragraph 1
  Purpose of letter
  Motivational sentence
1 blank line
Body paragraph 2
  Personal background
1 blank line
Body paragraph 3
  Request for action
2 blank lines
Closing (e.g., Sincerely,)
3 blank lines (for signature in ink)
Signature line
2 blank lines
Enc.

Many word-processing programs contain a template for a business block-style letter, which can be selected from the dialog box for opening new files. The following parameters are used for creating a letter. All parts of a block-style letter begin at the left margin. If not on the office letterhead, the letter begins with a heading that includes the practice's name, street address, city, state, and ZIP code. The date line is placed two lines below the heading at the left margin. Two lines below the date is the location of the recipient's name and address. Use the name and title of the specific person to whom the letter is addressed, preceded by a courtesy title (Mr., Ms); when the inside address includes a business name, use common abbreviations (Co. for company, Corp. for corporation, and Inc. for incorporated). The salutation is located two lines below the inside address and ends with a colon—for example, Dear Sir:, Dear Mr. Smith:, Dear Ms Jones:, and Dear Dr. Williams:.

The body of the letter is generally two to four paragraphs long and begins one line below the salutation. There is one blank line between each paragraph in the body of the letter. The first body paragraph should contain a strong opening statement that defines the purpose of the letter. A motivational sentence or fact follows to grab the reader's attention. The second body paragraph contains personal background information, additional pertinent information, and an explanation. The third body paragraph brings the letter to a close and contains a request for action.

Below the body of the letter is the closing. The first letter is capitalized, and the closing is followed by a comma; typically, a business letter closes with "Sincerely." The closing is two lines below the last paragraph of the letter body. Letters are signed in ink by the writer in the three-line space between the closing and the signature line. The signature line is a plain typed version of the letter writer's signature. If the letter includes an enclosure, it is indicated two lines below the signature line and is often abbreviated as "Enc." Before printing or typing the final copy, generate a draft and proofread it carefully. A copy or photocopy of every business letter is filed; client letters are filed with the patient records.

## Addressing the Envelope

Business letters are mailed with first-class postage in a standard #9 or #10 business-size envelope ($3\frac{7}{8} \times 8\frac{7}{8}$ inches or $4\frac{1}{8} \times 9\frac{1}{2}$ inches, respectively). The return address is typed or printed in the upper left hand corner (or a return-address label can be used). Return addresses are single spaced and located two lines below the top of the envelope and three spaces from the left side. The return address lists the practice name on the first line; street address on the second line; and city, state, and ZIP code on the third line.

The mailing address, which is single spaced, is placed 2 inches from the top edge and 4 inches from the left side of the envelope. Mailing addresses consist of the name of the person or company on the first line; title or department on the second line (e.g., Office Manager, Repair Department); street address on the third line; and city, state, and ZIP code on the fourth line. Correspondence may also be mailed in a "window" envelope, in which the address on the letter shows through a transparent panel on the envelope.

Finally, there is a proper method for folding business letters into thirds: Bring the bottom up first; then the top edge down, leaving a $\frac{1}{2}$-inch margin at the bottom, and crease it.

## Birthday Letters/Cards

Many dental offices send birthday letters or cards to their active patients as a public relations activity. Such cards can be obtained preprinted from an office supply company and labels can be generated by the dental software management program.

## Collection Letters

Statements are sent, telephone contact is made, and a series of three collection letters are mailed to patients who have delinquent accounts. After these attempts to recuperate balances due have been exhausted, those who owe money to the practice are pursued in small claims court or by a collection agency. All attempts to contact the responsible party are documented in the patient's record. A sample final collection letter is given in *Figure 22.1*.

---

*Forever Smiles Dental Offices*
*123 Main Street, Anytown, Anystate 12345 Phone: 888-555-1515*

March 13, 2006

Mrs. Sunny Day
111 Any Avenue
Anyvillage, Anystate 12345-6789

Dear Mrs. Day:

We have received your letter dated February 21, 2006, in which you assert you have no financial responsibility for the balance on your account. Enclosed you will find a detailed listing of account transactions for your family, including charges and payments. Also enclosed are copies of all processed insurance claims from your insurance company, with the payment amounts highlighted in yellow. Using this information, we have determined that you have an outstanding balance on your account of $520.00.

The statement concerning your dissatisfaction with the quality of care received is unfortunate; we try to provide quality service as comfortably as possible. We cannot remedy a problem if we have not been informed that the problem exists. Continued bleeding in the gums after nonsurgical periodontal therapy can mean the infection is gradually worsening and that continuing care is needed. Although the gums were treated, the disease is not necessarily gone; a chronic condition requires regular maintenance.

This letter represents our final attempt to clear this outstanding balance from your account. If full payment is not received within fourteen days from receipt of this certified letter, your account will be sent to a collection agency, which will report the delinquency to the major credit bureaus.

Sincerely,

T. Brusher, RDH

Enc.

---

**Figure 22.1** Sample final collection letter.

## Continuing Care Letters

Some patients are under the misconception that once they agree to treatment, their condition will not require continuing care. Continuing care letters inform the patient of the need for maintenance (*Fig. 22.2*).

## Recare Letters

Recare tracking includes a series of letters sent when the patient is 1, 3, 12, or 18 months past the recommended appointment time. Each letter documents that the office attempted to schedule recare; some people may be more inclined to save a letter to schedule an appointment than to return a telephone call. A final recare notice is shown in *Figure 22.3*.

## Insurance Letters

Dental hygienists correspond with insurance companies in the form of narrative reports and letters (*Fig. 22.4*). This correspondence concerns the need for clients' treatment, filing claims, and determining why claims were rejected.

---

*Forever Smiles Dental Offices*
*123 Main Street, Anytown, Anystate 12345 Phone: 888-555-1515*

July 8, 2006

Mr. and Mrs. Showers
444 Rain Street
Anycity, Anystate 11111

Dear Mr. and Mrs. Showers:

Our records indicate that your daughter, April, has multiple dental infections; this letter is being sent because you were not present at her last appointment and we would like to avoid the necessity for emergency dental care. When she was here for periodontal reevaluation on July 7, 2006, we indicated that we wanted her to seek a medical consultation with your physician to rule out any possibility of systemic illness. Her periodontal disease did not improve after nonsurgical periodontal therapy. After providing the scaling and root planing periodontal treatment, we believe a referral to a periodontal specialist is necessary because of the advanced nature of April's periodontal disease.

Several of April's teeth are a source of oral infection and must be removed by an oral surgeon; bacterial decay must also be removed and remaining tooth structure restored with composite fillings. Please call the office to schedule any appointments or to talk further about April's oral healthcare needs.

Sincerely,

Don Flossi, RDH

---

**Figure 22.2** Sample continuing care letter.

*Forever Smiles Dental Offices*
*123 Main Street, Anytown, Anystate 12345 Phone: 888-555-1515*

September 14, 2006

Patty Wagon
675 Cart Lane
Anycity, Anystate 11111

Dear Ms Wagon:

It has been more than a year and a half since your last dental appointment for periodontal maintenance. This concerns us because we know the nature of periodontal disease and its episodic progression. As you know, regular periodontal maintenance is necessary for oral health and systemic health. Recent research links periodontal disease to an increased rate of heart disease, stroke, diabetes, and respiratory disorders, and preterm, low birthweight babies.

Your periodontal maintenance appointment includes an oral cancer screening, head and neck examination, periodontal examination, scaling and polishing of the teeth, individualized home care instructions, radiographs to find hidden problems, and take-home items (such as a toothbrush, floss, and toothpaste). This level of individualized care helps you maintain your oral and physical health.

Many people delay dental care for economic reasons, yet a small investment in minimally invasive procedures costs less than treating disease. Please call our office to schedule an appointment for this needed care.

Sincerely,

I. M. Flossi, RDH

**Figure 22.3** Sample final recare letter.

## NARRATIVE REPORTS

A narrative report is written and submitted with each periodontal procedure performed by the dental hygienist. This report documents the necessity of care to avoid delays in insurance claim processing (*Fig. 22.5*). A general outline is given in *Box 11.4*.

# Manufacturer Letters

Letters are sent to manufacturers to comment on products, request information, or to return items. The letter in *Figure 22.6* concerns the return of merchandise for repair.

# New Patient Welcome Letters

As mentioned in Chapter 21, many communities send a welcome packet to new residents to the area. Dental offices often participate in this public relations activity to promote the practice and to increase their client base (*Fig. 22.7*).

---

*Forever Smiles Dental Offices*
*123 Main Street, Anytown, Anystate 12345 Phone: 888-555-1515*

May 2, 2006

Big Insurance Company
8888 Any Street
Anycity, Anystate 33333

RE: patient Spike B. Sharp
D/O/S: 02/02/2006

To Whom It May Concern:

It has been over 30 days since we submitted a claim for Mr. Spike B. Sharp for the above date of service and we have not received reimbursement. After repeated attempts to contact your company by telephone with no response, we are sending this letter. We have complied with the usual requirements of sending a copy of the radiographs, periodontal charting, and narrative report. The patient's coverage has been verified, yet we have not had any response regarding this claim.

A copy of this letter and our paperwork has been sent to the state insurance commissioner for investigation. We are aware of the state law requiring payment of claims within thirty days and hope our complaint to the insurance commissioner will be motivation to settle this claim.

Please contact our office with any additional information. Your cooperation in this matter is appreciated.

Sincerely,

U. R. Flossi, RDH

---

**Figure 22.4** Sample insurance letter.

## Referral Letters

When a patient's diagnosis or prognosis requires the intervention of another healthcare provider, the dental office provides a referral letter. An example of a referral letter is given in *Figure 22.8.*

## Thank-You Letters and Cards

Thank-you letters, cards, and rewards are public relations activities directed to a patient of record who has referred a friend or family member. For each referral, the office sends a gift certificate with a hand-written thank-you letter, which is more personal and more effective than a computer-generated letter.

---

*Forever Smiles Dental Offices*
*123 Main Street, Anytown, Anystate 12345 Phone: 888-555-1515*

| | |
|---|---|
| Report date: | December 13, 2006 |
| Narrative report for: | Sandy Beach, DOB 02/25/1955 |
| Patient chief complaint: | Bleeding gums and a bad taste in the mouth |
| Objective clinical findings: | Attached are periodontal chart and full-mouth radiographs |

| Date | Activity |
|---|---|
| 2-22-06 | Sandy Beach presented to our office after 20 months of oral neglect. The medical history was normal. Upon clinical, periodontal, and radiographic evaluation, type II periodontal disease was diagnosed with localized areas of type III and type IV periodontal disease. Periodontal probing depths of 4–8 mm were measured. Patient admitted to not flossing regularly. Treatment recommended was periodontal quadrant scaling and root planing owing to generalized chronic adult periodontal disease. Prescribed chlorhexidine gluconate rinse. |
| 2-28-06 | Right quadrant scaling with local anesthesia performed using a piezo scaler and hand instrumentation. Light tenacious, dark calculus was removed with moderate bleeding and suppuration. Oral hygiene instruction was given in flossing and interproximal tooth cleaning techniques. |
| 3-7-06 | Left quadrant scaling with local anesthesia performed using a piezo scaler and hand instrumentation. Light tenacious, dark calculus was removed with moderate bleeding and less suppuration than the right side. However, more granulation tissue was present and removed. Redemonstrated interproximal cleaning using an interproximal brush, floss holder, and floss. |
| 3-9-06 | Full-mouth series radiographs and periodontal probing chart were submitted with the insurance claim. |
| 3-31-06 | At this follow-up reevaluation visit, periodontal probing was performed. Placed disclosing solution to reveal moderate to heavy plaque along gingival margin and interproximal tooth surfaces. Redemonstrated tooth brushing using the Bass technique and interproximal cleaning. Coronal polished teeth and dispensed toothbrush, waxed floss, interproximal brush. Prescribed 1.1% neutral sodium fluoride due to caries and future caries risk. Next visit is a 3-month periodontal maintenance appointment. |

| | |
|---|---|
| Prognosis: | With regular maintenance and improved oral hygiene, the periodontal disease should stabilize. |
| Enclosures: | ADA insurance form, narrative report, periodontal chart, and full-mouth radiographs. |

CC: Sandy Beach

---

**Figure 22.5** Sample narrative report.

## CLIENT FORMS

Client forms consist of clinical, financial, consent, and Health Insurance Portability and Accountability Act (HIPAA) documents. Clinical forms are stored in the patient's file, creating a paper record of the patient; common forms are the personal, dental, and medical histories; oral risk assessment surveys; dental and periodontal charts; treatment plans; services rendered; informed consent; and HIPAA compliance. Today's dental prac-

March 17, 2006

Dental International
1234 Smile Way
P.O. Box 002
Anytown, Anystate 12346-5789

To Whom It May Concern:

Enclosed you will find one ultrasonic/powder polishing unit, hoses, attachments, and four polishing inserts. The polisher is clogged and does not spray powder. Please estimate the time and cost to repair and call our office and speak to the hygienist, Ms Brusher, for approval to proceed with the repairs. We can be reached at the phone number and address at the top of this letter. Thank you for your help with our unit.

Sincerely,


Hugh Flossi, DDS

**Figure 22.6** Sample manufacturer letter.

October 3, 2006

Rose R. Lovely
111 Thornbush Drive
Anytown, Anystate 12345

Dear Ms Lovely:

This packet is our way of welcoming you to our neighborhood. We want to invite you to come and visit our practice when you are seeking the care of a local oral healthcare provider. As a new resident in our area, you should know we are accepting new patients and that you can count on our practice to provide a thorough evaluation of you and your family's oral healthcare status. We see many of your neighbors as patients and hope that you will join our practice family.

The healthcare providers here are highly skilled, knowledgeable in the latest advances in dentistry, and work together as an effective team to deliver the highest quality of dentistry to maintain your health, appearance, comfort, ability to chew, and sense of taste, as well as to protect your speech. Our goal is to offer care and comfort for your oral healthcare needs, and we welcome the opportunity to meet you in our office. Please call to schedule your new patient examination and receive a 50% discount.

Sincerely,


Dew U. Flossi, RDH

**Figure 22.7** Sample new patient welcome letter.

---

*Forever Smiles Dental Offices*
*123 Main Street, Anytown, Anystate 12345 Phone: 888-555-1515*

August 24, 2006

Rosy Blush
555 Any Street
Anytown, Anystate 22222

Dear Ms Blush:

This referral is written after making a radiographic, periodontal, and clinical evaluation of
your records because the following findings were noted:

　　　　1. Moderate periodontal disease.

　　　　2. Possible carotid occlusion.

　　　　3. Possible bone density decrease.

See your physician to evaluate your overall health and to make further recommendations
regarding your health status.

Sincerely,

U. R. Flossi, RDH

---

**Figure 22.8** Sample referral letter.

tices are interested in reducing paperwork whenever possible and some are relying more
on electronically generated information (email, websites, online forms, telephone appointment confirmation) and storage (radiographs and other images, insurance processing).

## Personal, Dental, and Medical Histories

Personal history forms may document the patient's personal data: name, guardian name
(for children), address, phone numbers, place of employment, sex, birthdate, Social
Security number, dental insurance number, drivers license number, and valid credit
card number (*Fig. 22.9*). Documentation of this information is used for clinical and
financial record keeping and for collection activities. A relatively new protocol used by
some dental practices is to charge the patient's credit card for any unpaid balances after
co-pays and insurance payments have been met.

The dental history form contains screening questions about the patient's chief complaint related to comfort, function, breath malodor, and appearance. In patient-centered
care, the dental office addresses the chief complaint, meeting the patient's care and comfort needs and human need deficits. Dental history questions related to previous dental
experience collect information on attitudes, such as apprehension and frequency and
value of dental care. These forms generally include questions about headache, facial

## PATIENT INFORMATION

DATE _____

NAME _____    ☐MARRIED ☐SINGLE ☐MINOR ☐MALE ☐FEMALE
               LAST              FIRST              M

SOCIAL SECURITY #_____

ADDRESS _____
               STREET           APT. #        CITY          STATE          ZIP

BIRTHDATE_____ TELEPHONE _____
          MONTH    DAY    YEAR                 HOME          WORK          CELL          E-MAIL

NAME OF EMPLOYER_____ ADDRESS _____

IF FULL TIME STUDENT, SCHOOL NAME_____ GRADE _____

PERSON RESPONSIBLE FOR ACCOUNT - PLEASE CHECK ONE:  ☐PATIENT ☐GUARDIAN ☐SPOUSE ☐FATHER ☐MOTHER

## INSURANCE INFORMATION

MINOR CHILD - MAY NEED TO COMPLETE BOTH BLOCKS FOR PARENT INFORMATION
ADULTS - COMPLETE PRIMARY INSURED
DUAL COVERAGE? ALSO COMPLETE SECONDARY INSURED

| PRIMARY INSURED / IF NO INSURANCE COMPLETE FOR RESPONSIBLE PARTY | | | | SECONDARY INSURED | | | |
|---|---|---|---|---|---|---|---|
| LAST | FIRST | | M | LAST | FIRST | | M |
| STREET | CITY | STATE | ZIP | STREET | CITY | STATE | ZIP |
| HOME | WORK | CELL | E-MAIL | HOME | WORK | CELL | E-MAIL |
| BIRTHDATE (MO/DAY/YEAR) | | RELATIONSHIP TO PATIENT | | BIRTHDATE (MO/DAY/YEAR) | | RELATIONSHIP TO PATIENT | |
| EMPLOYER | | DENTAL INS. CO | | EMPLOYER | | DENTAL INS. CO | |
| SS# | | SUBSCRIBER # | GROUP # | SS# | | SUBSCRIBER # | GROUP # |

## PERSON TO CONTACT IN CASE OF EMERGENCY

Name _____

Address _____

City/State/ZIP _____

Telephone # _____

## AUTHORIZATION

I hereby authorize payment directly to the Dental Office of the group insurance benefits otherwise payable to me. I understand that I am responsible for all costs of dental treatment. I hereby authorize the Dental Office to administer such medications and perform such diagnostic, photographic and therapeutic procedures as may be necessary for proper dental care. The information on this page and the dental/medical histories are correct to the best of my knowledge. I grant the right to the dentist to release my dental/medical histories and other information about my dental treatment to third party payors and/or other health professionals.

X _____
        Patient or Responsible Party

_____
Date                    State Driver's License #

Has any member of your family ever been treated in our office?

☐Yes    ☐No

Whom may we thank for referring you to our office?

_____

## METHOD OF PAYMENT

Responsible party currently has an account with this office
☐Yes    ☐No

☐Payment in full at each appointment (cash or personal check)

☐Payment in full at each appointment (☐VISA ☐MC ☐OTHER)

Card # _____ Exp. Date _____

☐I wish to discuss the Dental Office's Financial Policy

**SERVICE CHARGE**
If I do not pay the entire new balance within _____ days of the monthly billing date, a service charge will be added to the account for the current monthly billing period. The service charge will be a periodic rate of _____% per month (or a minimum charge of $_____ for a balance under $_____) which is an annual percentage rate of _____% applied to the last month's balance. In the case of default of payment, I promise to pay any legal interest on the balance due, together with any collection costs and reasonable attorney fees incurred to effect collection of this account or future outstanding accounts.

C-114L STEPPING STONES TO SUCCESS™ 1-800-548-2164
www.steppingstonestosuccess.com © 1987, 1991, 1992, 1995, 1997, 1998, 1999, 2003, 2004

**PATIENT INFORMATION**

**Figure 22.9** A patient information form. Courtesy of Stepping Stones to Success, Pueblo, CO.

pain, ulcers, numbness of the face or jaw, difficulty chewing and swallowing, digestive disorders, missing teeth, sleep disturbances, and gingival-related symptoms.

Evidence-based care depends on a comprehensive medical history. The medical form collects data pertaining to medical conditions, systemic disease, medication/drug use, lifestyle, and psychosocial expectations. The dental history may be combined with the medical history, as shown in *Figure 22.10*.

## Oral Risk Assessment

An oral risk assessment survey is a form used to identify the risk factors that increase the probability of oral disease from environmental, behavioral, or biological conditions (*Fig. 22.11*). Information recorded on this form is used for treatment planning, and case presentation; it is also submitted with insurance claims to support the need for treatment and for postpayment review. Some insurance carriers verify the necessity of treatment, and the provider who uses early interventions to treat disease findings will be prepared for these review procedures by keeping an accurate oral risk assessment survey.

## Dental and Periodontal Charts

The dental chart form is used to document and identify the patient's oral condition and consists of a graphical representation of the teeth and periodontium. A variety of graphics and tooth numbering systems are available to keep a complete record of the patient's condition and progress, to plan treatment, to protect the office during legal action, and to identify postmortem remains. The three common methods used to identify primary and permanent teeth are the **universal numbering system**, **Palmer notation system**, **and international numbering system**. The periodontal chart documents information regarding periodontal conditions found during patient assessment procedures, as seen in *Figure 22.12*.

## Treatment Plan

A treatment plan form organizes the sequence of dental appointments and documents procedure recommendations and options. Treatment plans are available in a number of designs and can be generated by dental computer software programs. Some forms contain procedure names with insurance codes. See *Figure 22.13* for a sample treatment plan form.

## Services Rendered

The **services rendered form** is where progress notes for each contact with the patient are recorded and may be written in ink, dictated onto audiotape to be transcribed onto this form, or typed into the patient's computer records (*Fig. 22.14*). Many different types of services and goods are documented on the services rendered form, such as treatment, materials used, all oral and written communications, and missed appointment information. The techniques used to record services rendered are sequenced writing and SOAP notes. **Sequenced writing** is the documentation of treatment listed in the order in which it was given and includes everything from patient comments to next-visit information.

**PATIENT NAME** _____ **DATE** _____

Primary reason for this dental appointment: ☐ Examination   ☐ Emergency   ☐ Consultation

**Dental History**                                                                                    *Please Circle*

| | |
|---|---|
| Do you have a specific dental problem? Describe_____ | Yes  No |
| Do you have dental examinations on a routine basis? Last visit_____ | Yes  No |
| Do you think you have active decay or gum disease?_____ | Yes  No |
| Do you brush and floss on a routine basis? Discuss_____ | Yes  No |
| Do your gums ever bleed? Discuss_____ | Yes  No |
| Do you like your smile? Why?_____ | Yes  No |
| Does food catch between your teeth? Any loose teeth?_____ | Yes  No |
| Do you want to keep your remaining teeth?_____ | Yes  No |
| Do you ever have clicking, popping or discomfort in the jaw joint? Do you brux or grind?___ | Yes  No |
| Have your past experiences in a dental office always been positive?_____ | Yes  No |
| Do you smoke or chew? Any sores or growths in your mouth? Discuss_____ | Yes  No |

Name of previous dentist (optional):_____

Date of last full mouth x-rays (16 small films or panoramic):_____

**Medical History**

| | |
|---|---|
| Are you under a physician's care now? Why?_____ Who?_____ Phone_____ | Yes  No |
| Have you ever been hospitalized or had a major operation? Discuss_____ | Yes  No |
| Have you ever had a serious injury to your head or neck? Discuss_____ | Yes  No |
| Are you taking any medications, pills or drugs? What?_____ | Yes  No |
| Are you on a special diet? Discuss_____ | Yes  No |
| Are you allergic to any medications or substances? Please check box below_____ | Yes  No |

☐ Aspirin  ☐ Penicillin  ☐ Codeine  ☐ Acrylic  ☐ Metal  ☐ Latex Rubber  ☐ Other_____

*Women (Please check):* ☐ Pregnant/trying to get pregnant  ☐ Nursing  ☐ Taking oral contraceptives  Discuss_____  Yes  No

Do you now have or have you ever had any of the following? Please check appropriate boxes.

*If yes to any of the starred conditions, please call prior to your appointment... premedication may be required.*

| | Yes No | | Yes No | | Yes No | | Yes No | | Yes No |
|---|---|---|---|---|---|---|---|---|---|
| Heart Disease/Surgery * | ☐ ☐ | Bruise Easily/Blood Disease | ☐ ☐ | Emphysema | ☐ ☐ | Night Sweats | ☐ ☐ | Cold Sores | ☐ ☐ |
| Heart Murmur * | ☐ ☐ | Anemia | ☐ ☐ | Tuberculosis | ☐ ☐ | Yellow Jaundice | ☐ ☐ | Fever Blisters | ☐ ☐ |
| Irregular Heart Beat | ☐ ☐ | Excessive Bleeding | ☐ ☐ | Cancer | ☐ ☐ | Kidney Problems | ☐ ☐ | Herpes | ☐ ☐ |
| Angina/Chest Pain | ☐ ☐ | Sickle Cell Disease | ☐ ☐ | X-Ray Treatments (Radiation) | ☐ ☐ | Renal Dialysis | ☐ ☐ | Stroke | ☐ ☐ |
| Heart Attack/Failure | ☐ ☐ | Hemophilia (Bleeding Problem) | ☐ ☐ | Chemotherapy | ☐ ☐ | Thyroid Disease | ☐ ☐ | Convulsions | ☐ ☐ |
| Congenital Heart Disorder | ☐ ☐ | Leukemia | ☐ ☐ | Aredia I.V. | ☐ ☐ | Parathyroid Disease | ☐ ☐ | Epilepsy or Seizures | ☐ ☐ |
| Mitral Valve Prolapse * | ☐ ☐ | Recent Blood Transfusion | ☐ ☐ | Zometa I.V. | ☐ ☐ | Arthritis/Gout | ☐ ☐ | Fainting or Dizziness | ☐ ☐ |
| Scarlet Fever | ☐ ☐ | Swelling of Limbs | ☐ ☐ | Stomach/Intestinal Disease | ☐ ☐ | Rheumatism | ☐ ☐ | Glaucoma | ☐ ☐ |
| Rheumatic Fever * | ☐ ☐ | Lung Disease | ☐ ☐ | Ulcers | ☐ ☐ | Pain in Jaw Joints | ☐ ☐ | Tumors or Growths | ☐ ☐ |
| Artificial Heart Valve * | ☐ ☐ | Breathing Problem | ☐ ☐ | Recent Weight Loss | ☐ ☐ | Cortisone Medicine | ☐ ☐ | Nervousness | ☐ ☐ |
| Heart Pace Maker * | ☐ ☐ | Shortness of Breath | ☐ ☐ | Frequent Diarrhea | ☐ ☐ | Artificial Joint * | ☐ ☐ | Psychiatric Care | ☐ ☐ |
| Pulmonary Shunt | ☐ ☐ | Frequent Cough | ☐ ☐ | Diabetes | ☐ ☐ | Venereal Disease | ☐ ☐ | Alzheimer's Disease | ☐ ☐ |
| High Blood Pressure | ☐ ☐ | Hay Fever | ☐ ☐ | Excessive Thirst | ☐ ☐ | AIDS | ☐ ☐ | Allergies (Medicines) | ☐ ☐ |
| Low Blood Pressure | ☐ ☐ | Sinus Trouble | ☐ ☐ | Hypoglycemia | ☐ ☐ | HIV Positive | ☐ ☐ | Allergies (Pollen / Dust) | ☐ ☐ |
| Bacterial Endocarditis | ☐ ☐ | Asthma | ☐ ☐ | Liver Disease | ☐ ☐ | Genital Herpes | ☐ ☐ | Hives or Rash | ☐ ☐ |
| Unexplained Fever | ☐ ☐ | Bloody Sputum | ☐ ☐ | Hepatitis A (Infectious) | ☐ ☐ | Drug Addiction/Alcoholism | ☐ ☐ | Need Premedication? | ☐ ☐ |
| | | | | Hepatitis B or C | ☐ ☐ | Tattoos/Body Piercing | ☐ ☐ | Ever taken fen-phen? * | ☐ ☐ |

Have you ever had any other serious illness not checked above? Discuss_____  Yes  No

Do you wish to talk to the dentist privately about any problem?_____  Yes  No

*To the best of my knowledge, all the preceding answers are correct. If I have any changes in my health status or if my medicines change, I shall inform the dentist and staff at the next appointment without fail.*

X_____  Date_____

PATIENT SIGNATURE (PARENT OR GUARDIAN)

Reviewed By Doctor_____  Date_____  BP_____  Pulse_____

History Review and Significant Findings_____

_____

**Medical Updates**

I have read my MEDICAL HISTORY dated_____ and confirm that it adequately states past and present conditions.

| DATE | EXCEPTIONS | | PATIENT'S SIGNATURE | BP | PULSE | REVIEWED BY |
|---|---|---|---|---|---|---|
| _____ | _____ | None ☐ | _____ | ____ | ____ | Dr._____ |
| _____ | _____ | None ☐ | _____ | ____ | ____ | Dr._____ |
| _____ | _____ | None ☐ | _____ | ____ | ____ | Dr._____ |
| _____ | _____ | None ☐ | _____ | ____ | ____ | Dr._____ |
| _____ | _____ | None ☐ | _____ | ____ | ____ | Dr._____ |
| _____ | _____ | None ☐ | _____ | ____ | ____ | Dr._____ |

C-113LSTEPPING STONES TO SUCCESS™ 1-800-548-2164
www.steppingstonestosuccess.com © 1987, 1991, 1992, 1995, 1998, 2001, 2004, 2005

**DENTAL AND MEDICAL HISTORIES - UPDATES**

**Figure 22.10** A combined dental and medical history form. Courtesy of Stepping Stones to Success, Pueblo, CO.

## Periodontal Risk Assessment Questionnaire

Name_____ Date_____

### Tobacco Use
Tobacco use is the most significant risk factor for gum disease.

**Do you now or have you ever used the following:**

| | Amounts per day | Used for how many years | If you quit, list what year |
|---|---|---|---|
| ❑ Cigarette | _____ | _____ | _____ |
| ❑ Cigar | _____ | _____ | _____ |
| ❑ Pipe | _____ | _____ | _____ |
| ❑ Chewing | _____ | _____ | _____ |

*Blood Sugar*

### Diabetes
Gum disease is a common complication of diabetes. Untreated gum disease makes it harder for patients with diabetes to control their blood sugar.

**IF YOU ARE A PATIENT WHO HAS DIABETES:**

Is your diabetes under control?                ❑ Yes      ❑ No
Are you prone to diabetic complications?     ❑ Yes      ❑ No
How do you monitor your blood sugar?     _____
Who is your physician for diabetes?       _____

**IF YOU ARE NOT A PATIENT WHO HAS DIABETES:**

Any family history of diabetes?        ❑ Yes      ❑ No
    Have you had any of these warning signs of diabetes?
        ❑ frequent urination            ❑ excessive thirst
        ❑ excessive hunger              ❑ weakness and fatigue
        ❑ slow healing of cuts          ❑ unexplained weight loss

### Heart Attack/Stroke
Untreated gum disease may increase your risk for heart attack or stroke.

**Do you have any risk factors for heart disease or stroke?**

❑ Family history of heart disease      ❑ Tobacco use      ❑ Obesity

❑ High cholesterol                     ❑ High blood pressure

*If you have any of these other risk factors it is especially important for you to always keep your gums as healthy as possible.*

### Medications
A side effect of some medications can cause changes in your gums.

**Are you taking or have you ever taken any of the following medication:**

❑ Antiseizure medications. (such as Dilantin®, Tegretol®, Phenobarbital, etc.)
                ❑ Yes                ❑ No
    If you answered yes, are you still taking the anti-seizure medication?
                ❑ Yes                ❑ No
    Other Medication:_____

❑ Calcium Channel Blocker blood pressure medication. (such as Procardia®, Cardizem®, Norvasc®, Verapamil®, etc.)
    Other: _____

❑ Immunosuppressant therapy (such as Prednisone, Azathioprine, Cyclosporins, Corticosteriods (Asthma-Inhalers), etc.)
    Other: _____

### Family History/ Genetics
The tendency for gum disease to develop can be inherited.

**Is there an immediate family member(s) who currently has or had gum problems in the past?** (e.g. your mother, father, or siblings):
    ❑ Yes            ❑ No

**COLLAGENEX**
pharmaceuticals

**Figure 22.11** An oral risk assessment form. Courtesy of CollaGenex Pharmaceuticals.

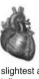

## Heart Murmur, Artificial joint prosthesis

If you have even the slightest amount of gum inflammation, bacteria from the mouth can enter the bloodstream and may cause a serious infection of the heart or joints.

**Do you have a heart murmur or artificial joint?**

❏ Yes          ❏ No

**If so, does your physician recommend antibiotics prior to dental visits?**

❏ Yes          ❏ No

Name of physician? _____

*If you answered yes, it is especially important to always keep your gums as healthy and inflammation-free as possible to reduce the chance of bacterial infection originating from the mouth.*

## Females

Females can be at increased risk for gum disease at different points in their lives.

**The following can adversely affect your gums.  Please check all that apply:**

❏ Pregnant          ❏ Nursing          ❏ Menopause

❏ Taking birth control pills

❏ Infrequent care during previous pregnancies

## Women

Women with osteoporosis have a greater risk for periodontal bone loss.

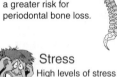

**Females:**

**Do you take any of the following:**

❏ Estrogen Replacement Therapy/Hormone Replacement Therapy (such as Prempro®, Premarin®, Premphase®, Fosamax®, Actonel®, Evista®, Fortéo®, etc.)

Other: _____

## Stress

High levels of stress can reduce your body's immune defense.

**Are you under a lot of stress?**

❏ Yes          ❏ No

## Nutrition

Your diet has the potential to affect your periodontal health.

**Do you find it difficult to maintain a well-balanced diet?**

❏ Yes          ❏ No

*All patients please complete the following:*

**Have you noticed any of the following signs of gum disease?**

❏ Bleeding gums during toothbrushing

❏ Red, swollen or tender gums

❏ Gums that have pulled away from the teeth

❏ Persistent bad breath

❏ Pus between the teeth and gums

❏ Loose or separating teeth

❏ Change in the way your teeth fit together

❏ Food catching between teeth

**Is it important to keep your teeth for as long as possible?**          ❏ Yes   ❏ Not really

**If you have missing teeth, why have you not had them replaced?**_____

_____

**Do you like the appearance of your smile?**          ❏ Yes   ❏ No

**Do you like the color of your teeth?**          ❏ Yes   ❏ No

**Do your teeth keep you from eating any specific food?**          ❏ Yes   ❏ No

PER 10371

**Figure 22.11** (Continued)

PATIENT NAME _____ DATE _____ DR. _____

Exam Dates & 1. _____ 2. _____ 3. _____ 4. _____ 5. _____ 6. _____
History Review

Medical History Alerts: _____ Pre-Medication _____

Comments: _____ Case Type (I-V) _____

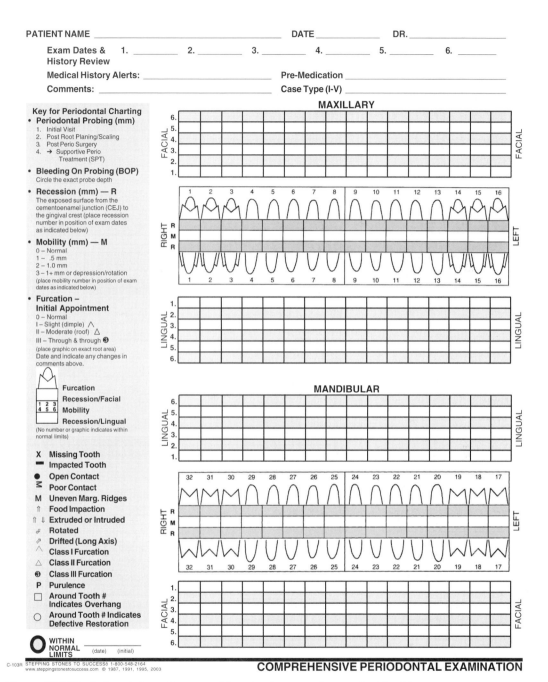

**Key for Periodontal Charting**
• **Periodontal Probing (mm)**
1. Initial Visit
2. Post Root Planing/Scaling
3. Post Perio Surgery
4. → Supportive Perio
   Treatment (SPT)

• **Bleeding On Probing (BOP)**
Circle the exact probe depth

• **Recession (mm) — R**
The exposed surface from the cementoenamel junction (CEJ) to the gingival recession crest (place recession number in position of exam dates as indicated below)

• **Mobility (mm) — M**
0 – Normal
1 – .5 mm
2 – 1.0 mm
3 – 1+ mm or depression/rotation
(place mobility number in position of exam dates as indicated below)

• **Furcation –**
**Initial Appointment**
0 – Normal
I – Slight (dimple) ∧
II – Moderate (roof) △
III – Through & through ❸
(place graphic on exact root area)
Date and indicate any changes in comments above.

Furcation
Recession/Facial
Mobility
Recession/Lingual
(No number or graphic indicates within normal limits)

X   Missing Tooth
▬   Impacted Tooth
●   Open Contact
≋   Poor Contact
M   Uneven Marg. Ridges
⇑   Food Impaction
⇑⇓  Extruded or Intruded
↻   Rotated
↗   Drifted (Long Axis)
∧   Class I Furcation
△   Class II Furcation
❸   Class III Furcation
P   Purulence
☐   Around Tooth # Indicates Overhang
○   Around Tooth # Indicates Defective Restoration

◯ WITHIN
NORMAL     (date)   (initial)
LIMITS

**MAXILLARY**

**MANDIBULAR**

**COMPREHENSIVE PERIODONTAL EXAMINATION**

C-103R STEPPING STONES TO SUCCESS® 1-800-548-2164
www.steppingstonestosuccess.com © 1987, 1991, 1995, 2003

**Figure 22.12** Periodontal chart. Courtesy of Stepping Stones to Success, Pueblo, CO.

**TREATMENT ESTIMATE FOR** _____ **DATE** _____ **ACCT. #** _____

**DENTIST** _____ **INSURANCE\*/DENTAL PROGRAM** _____

## FINANCIAL ARRANGEMENTS

I consent to and authorize the indicated dental services to be performed. I understand that at any time I may terminate or postpone such treatment. I agree to pay the fees for dental treatment as indicated:

☐ Payment in full at each appointment (cash or personal check)

☐ Payment in full at each appointment (☐ MC  ☐ VISA )

 # _____
 Exp. Date _____

☐ Payment in accordance with Dental Office's financial policy

 _____
 _____
 _____
 _____

## SERVICE CHARGE

If I do not pay the entire new balance within _____ days of the monthly billing date, a service charge will be added to the account for the current monthly billing period. The service charge will be a periodic rate of _____ % per month (or a minimum charge of $_____ for a balance under $_____ ) which is an annual percentage rate of _____ % applied to the last month's balance. In the case of default of payment, I promise to pay any legal interest on the balance due, together with any collection costs and reasonable attorney fees incurred to effect collection of this account or future outstanding accounts.

## DENTAL INSURANCE\*

I understand that my dental insurance is a contract between the insurance carrier and me and not between the insurance carrier and the dentist; therefore, I am still responsible for all dental fees. I understand that I will be charged for all dental treatment and that any payments received by the Dental Office from my insurance coverage will be credited to my account or refunded to me if I have paid the dental fees incurred.

## INFORMED CONSENT

I have been informed of my dental ailments, treatment options, benefits, substantial risks and consequences of limited or non-treatment.

Patient Signature _____ Date _____

C-112L STEPPING STONES TO SUCCESS 1-800-548-2164
www.steppingstonestosuccess.com © 1987, 1991, 1992, 1995, 1997, 1998

| | TREATMENT RECOMMENDATIONS | FEE SCHEDULE | INSURANCE\*/ ALTERNATE COVERAGE | ADJUSTMENTS | PATIENT PORTION/ COPAYMENTS |
|---|---|---|---|---|---|
| Examinations, X-Rays, Tests, and Preventive Services | Oral Examination | | | | |
| | X-Rays | | | | |
| | Diagnostic Casts/Photographs | | | | |
| | Prophylaxis (Routine Cleaning) | | | | |
| | Fluoride | | | | |
| | Disease Prevention Program (OHI) | | | | |
| | Sealants | | | | |
| Periodontal Treatment | Debridement Prior to Exam | | | | |
| | Palliative (Emergency) Perio Trmt | | | | |
| | Root Planing and Scaling (Perio) | | | | |
| | Re-Evaluation of Perio Therapy | | | | |
| | Periodontal Maintenance (SPT) | | | | |
| | Desensitizing Medicament | | | | |
| | Soft Tissue Surgery | | | | |
| | Osseous (Bone) Surgery | | | | |
| | Occlusal Adjustment | | | | |
| | Localized Therapeutic Medicament | | | | |
| Endodontic Treatment | Pulp Vitality Test | | | | |
| | Pulpotomy | | | | |
| | Palliative (Emergency) Pulpectomy | | | | |
| | Root Canal Therapy | | | | |
| | Apicoectomy/Periradicular Services | | | | |
| Oral Surgery | Routine Extractions | | | | |
| | Surgical/Impacted Extractions | | | | |
| | Biopsy | | | | |
| | Alveoloplasty | | | | |
| | Incision/Drainage of Abscess | | | | |
| Restorative Treatment | Amalgam Fillings # Surfaces | | | | |
| | Resin Fillings # Surfaces | | | | |
| | Retention Pins | | | | |
| | Inlay/Onlay Restorations | | | | |
| | Cast Metal Crowns | | | | |
| | Porcelain Veneer Crowns | | | | |
| | Stainless Steel Crowns | | | | |
| | Sedative Fillings | | | | |
| | Core Build-Ups | | | | |
| | Labial Veneers | | | | |
| | Temporary Crowns | | | | |
| Prosthetic (Replacement) Treatment | Fixed Bridges | | | | |
| | Core Build-Ups | | | | |
| | Removable Partials | | | | |
| | Complete Dentures | | | | |
| | Repair or Replace | | | | |
| | Condition/Reline/Rebase | | | | |
| | Interim (Temporary) Appliances | | | | |
| Miscellaneous Services/ Treatment | Cosmetic Services | | | | |
| | Implants | | | | |
| | TMJD Therapy | | | | |
| | Orthodontics | | | | |
| | Consultation | | | | |
| | Office/House/Hospital/After Hours Visit | | | | |
| | Other Drugs/Medicaments | | | | |
| | Sterile Pack Set-Ups Per Appointment | | | | |

There will be a charge for each broken appointment if 24 hours notice is not given.

**TOTALS**

This estimate is guaranteed for only 90 days from the above date.

Initial Payment

Balance Due

**TREATMENT ESTIMATE**

**Figure 22.13** Treatment plan form. Courtesy of Stepping Stones to Success, Pueblo, CO.

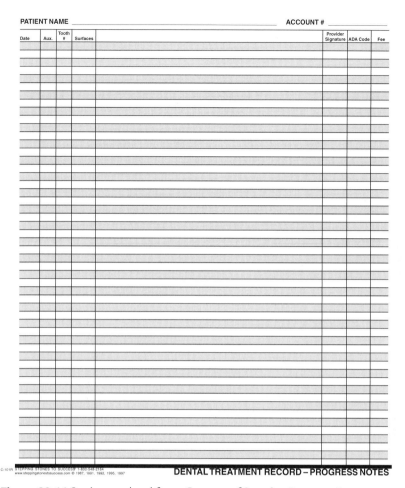

PATIENT NAME _____     ACCOUNT # _____

| Date | Aux. | Tooth # | Surfaces | | Provider Signature | ADA Code | Fee |
|------|------|---------|----------|--|--------------------|----------|-----|

C-101R  STEPPING STONES TO SUCCESS  1-800-548-2164
www.steppingstonestosuccess.com © 1987, 1991, 1992, 1995, 1997

**DENTAL TREATMENT RECORD – PROGRESS NOTES**

**Figure 22.14** Services rendered form. Courtesy of Stepping Stones to Success, Pueblo, CO.

**SOAP notes** are another record keeping system for documenting treatment. SOAP stands for subjective, objective, assessment, and planning, and each category is listed separately. The subjective section gathers information about the patient's dental and medical histories, lifestyle, and psychosocial emotions and attitudes. The objective section includes data based on the dental professional's observation, examination, and treatment. The assessment section contains the problematic findings as well as goals and a summary. In the planning section, the clinician records the actions necessary to meet the goals set in the assessment.

## Informed Consent

Informed consent is given by the patient to the healthcare provider after information regarding treatment risks, outcomes, and options has been given. A sample of an informed consent form is found in Chapter 5 and another example is shown in *Figure 22.15*.

> *Forever Smiles Dental Offices*
> *123 Main Street, Anytown, Anystate 12345 Phone: 888-555-1515*
>
> INFORMED CONSENT
>
> I, _____, have been informed that I have type ____ periodontal disease. I have been informed that this disease infects the soft tissues, ligaments, and bone in the absence of obvious symptoms. Contributing factors in periodontal disease are genetics, systemic factors and disorders, hard deposits on the teeth, and bacterial biofilm on the teeth with bacterial infiltration into the soft tissue. As the disease progresses, the infection may cause bleeding gums, swelling, bad breath, tooth sensitivity, recession, loose teeth, and loss of teeth. Studies associate oral infection to an increased rate of heart disease, stroke, diabetes, respiratory disorders, and preterm and low birth weight babies.
>
> 1. Several nonsurgical soft tissue management therapies were discussed and recommended:
> - Gross débridement to remove debris and then irrigation.
> - Periodontal scaling and root planing by quadrant to remove bacterial plaque, calculus (tartar), and soft granulation tissue.
> - Site-specific antibiotic chemotherapy.
> - Oral hygiene, dietary, and habit-modification instruction.
> - Reevaluation after 21 days to determine treatment success. If improved, a periodontal maintenance program to monitor tissue health will be implemented. If limited or no improvement is seen, additional treatment is required.
> - After all nonsurgical therapies have been performed with limited to no improvement, referral to a periodontist for evaluation and periodontal surgery to remove infected tissues will be necessary.
>
> 2. Oral hygiene home care is necessary for improvement, and failure to follow tooth cleaning techniques may cause continued infection, progression of the disease, and/or poor results.
> 3. I have been informed of all risks, benefits, and treatment alternatives for the above procedures by Dr. Drawer/staff.
> 4. I understand that no guarantees have been made.
> 5. I have been given the opportunity to ask questions regarding the treatment, and all of my questions have been answered to my satisfaction. I wish to proceed with the above procedures.
> 6. I understand that a basic cleaning of my teeth does not constitute periodontal treatment to correct this disease process or to prevent it from progressing.
>
> _____    Date_____
> Signature of patient/consenting party
>
> _____    Date_____
> Signature of witness

**Figure 22.15** Sample informed consent for periodontal procedures.

## HIPAA

To comply with HIPAA regulations, patients must be given a number of forms. For example, patients sign a HIPAA form titled "Notice of Privacy Practices" after being apprised of the office policy and implementation of privacy procedures.

## Financial Forms

All business transactions are documented on the appropriate form, according to labor, business, corporate, and tax laws. All account activity is recorded on a form, whether it is an accounts receivable, accounts payable, or insurance transaction.

**CONCEPT SUMMARY**

- Client letters and forms are legal documents of legal transactions maintained as permanent records of the patient's health and financial status.
- Letters are sent to clients, insurance companies, business associates, and other healthcare providers for a variety of reasons.
- Clinical forms include personal, dental, and medical histories; oral risk assessment surveys; dental and periodontal charts; treatment plans; and services rendered.
- Financial, informed consent, and HIPAA compliance forms are also maintained in the client's permanent record.

# REVIEW QUESTIONS

1. Why is the information collected on clinical forms necessary?
2. What information is recorded on the services rendered form?
3. What supplies are necessary for business mailings?
4. Why is the business letter photocopied? Could it be saved electronically to save paper or should it remain in the file for reference?
5. What types of letters are commonly generated in the dental practice?
6. How are an envelope and letter prepared for mailing?

## Assignment: Mailings

Compose a business letter for each of the following situations and type an envelope for mailing.

- The 9-year-old child of Mr. and Mrs. Brian Harris, Kevin, had several extractions last year. Kevin is now past due for his 6-month recall and orthodontic evaluation.
- Robert Games underwent nonsurgical periodontal therapy more than a year ago and requires a periodontal maintenance appointment.
- Dr. David Hunt referred a patient, Charles Givens, to the office for nonsurgical periodontal therapy. After a 6-month regimen of care, Mr. Givens has become asymptomatic. Thank Dr. Hunt for the referral.
- Mrs. Kurt Emery had a white lesion on the right lateral border of her tongue that was discovered at her last recall appointment. A biopsy was performed to determine its composition. The laboratory report diagnosed a benign leukoplakia lesion. Inform her of the findings.
- Last week you interviewed a potential employee, Susan Yee. Write a letter requesting a second interview.
- A supply order was incorrectly shipped. Write a letter to be faxed informing the dental supply company that the 1.1% neutral sodium fluoride foam was not shipped and that no backorder slip was found.
- John Sundberg has failed to show for a third consecutive appointment. Write a letter informing him that the practice will no longer provide treatment. Tell him that only emergency care will be provided during the next 30 days. Suggest that Mr. Sundberg contact the local dental society or dentist referral agency to find a new dental provider.

## Chapter 23

# Office Policy and Procedure Manuals

## LEARNING OUTCOMES

Upon mastery of the content of this chapter, the student should be able to:

- Describe the components of the office policy and procedures manual.
- Differentiate between vision, mission, and philosophy statements.
- Identity office policy, office treatment, and personnel protocols.
- Determine how salary, wages, and benefits all contribute to an overall compensation package.
- Recognize the importance of job descriptions.
- Identify disciplinary action forms and performance appraisal criteria.
- Create an office policy and procedures manual.

## KEY TERMS

goals
grievance procedures
merit review
mission statement
office policies

personnel information
philosophy statements
policy and procedure manuals
vision statements

## OFFICE POLICY AND PROCEDURE MANUALS

Office policy and procedures manuals contain many components. The vision, mission, and philosophy statements are used to direct and lend meaning to the dental practice's goals. The office policy, protocols, and personnel forms found in the office manual are meant to provide structure by outlining the business systems. Dental personnel are a significant aspect of any practice, and employee job descriptions and guidelines allow for improved communication and operations. Structured business systems related to employees permit fair and impartial performance appraisals, disciplinary action, collaborative partner contracts, and employment contracts.

**Policy and procedure manuals**, found in businesses, professional organizations, and government, outline operational information for employees. Sometimes called an office manual, the policy and procedure manual defines the vision, philosophy, and/or mission statement of the group; goals; office policy; business office and treatment protocols; personnel information; client information; and office maintenance schedule. Office manuals provide facts to new employees about the manner in which business is conducted in that particular setting. *Box 23.1* lists the typical contents of an office manual. The first page of the manual usually contains a disclaimer noting that it is subject to change and is not a contract.

## VISION, MISSION, AND PHILOSOPHY STATEMENTS

**Vision statements** are short written declarations of an ideal and a unique image of the future. Vision statements are shorter in length than philosophy and mission statements. They are meant to be clear and concise, inspiring, empowering, and asking for the best of the people involved to prepare for the future (*Box 23.2*).

Once the vision is identified, it is expressed as a mission statement. A written **mission statement** states what the practice wants to accomplish, whom it serves, and what makes it unique based on its strengths and weaknesses. It is an inspiring statement that is exclusive to the practice, concise, and future oriented. Printed public relations materials such as pamphlets, brochures, flyers, and newsletters may contain the mission statement. Such material may also contain office policy statements regarding office hours, missed appointments, financial matters, and procedure protocols.

Written **philosophy statements** expand on the mission statement, reflect core values, and direct progress in the dental practice. Philosophy statements contain elements of the services provided, who will be served, and the benefits to society. Mission and philosophy statements are compared in *Box 23.3*.

## GOALS

**Goals** are statements or objectives that describe how the mission statement will be achieved. Dental practices may have goals to increase production, deliver certain

**BOX 23.2** *Dental Practice Vision Statements*

This dental practice strives to:

- Serve the underserved.
- Help the handicapped.
- Promote health and wellness.

**BOX 23.3** *Mission and Philosophy Statements Compared*

| | |
|---|---|
| Mission Statement | • To promote health and wellness and improve patient quality of life through education, minimally invasive therapy, and regular healthcare maintenance |
| Philosophy Statements | • To provide comprehensive oral healthcare service to clients through the highest degree of clinical excellence and care and comfort. |
| | • To communicate information regarding oral healthcare procedures using a variety of media. |
| | • To recommend and render minimally invasive therapy as a first choice. |
| | • To promote regular healthcare maintenance by providing advanced appointments, and through actions and advertising. |

procedures, increase internal referrals, improve recare scheduling, upgrade facilities and technology, promote the practice externally, and build and nurture client relationships. Goals are further defined by assigning the responsibility for a task to a specific individual, setting a date for meeting the goal, and providing details on how to accomplish the task.

## OFFICE POLICY

**Office policies** are administrative rules set by the employer to describe how business is to be conducted. They are written to document office hours for staff and patient scheduling, lunch hour coverage, closing procedures, routine days off, staff conferences, and emergency coverage.

### Office Hours

Normal business hours are set by the employer and vary for each employee based on the individual's work schedule for the week. Office hours are usually preset up to 6 months in advance because of appointment scheduling for patients. The U.S. Fair Labor Standards Act regulating labor defines what constitutes work, full-time and part-time employment, compensation, work conditions, lunch hours, and breaks. Lunchtime and breaks are mandatory, according to this act.

In many dental practices, employees report to the office 15–30 minutes before the expected arrival of the first patient. Scheduled times out of the office are preset and stated in the office policy. Overtime for wage earners begins after 40 hours in a single week have been worked, and a policy statement regarding overtime authorization may be in effect. Often all overtime worked must be preapproved, and unauthorized overtime may not be reimbursed. End-of-the-day or closing activities are described in the office policy section, as is emergency coverage when an employee must be out of the office.

## STAFF POLICY

The payroll date is set on a weekly, every other week, or twice a month schedule. Payroll, hiring practices, staff meetings, safety issues, dress requirements, grooming, personnel records, and confidentiality issues are some of the many staff policy items. Staff meetings are held whenever necessary to discuss system changes. Attendance at morning meetings (held before the first patient arrives) and staff meetings is emphasized.

Occupational Health and Safety Administration issues are matters of office policy. Accident prevention and accident reporting are outlined, and the location of material safety data sheets is stated in the office policy section. Personal protective equipment is mandatory, and a statement of instruction that personal protective equipment must be worn during clinical or laboratory procedures is included. Clothing must be clean and pressed, and shoes worn in the office should stay in the office per the Occupational Safety and Health Act (OSHA) recommendations. Another safety issue policy statement may be found regarding the use of tobacco, as many dental offices are smoke-free environments for employees, patients, and visitors.

Another important aspect of worker safety is personal appearance and grooming. Guidelines set by the Centers for Disease Control and Prevention (CDC) state special consideration of personal hygiene is necessary. Personal hygiene issues such as body odors, hair care, fingernails, jewelry, and gum chewing may be covered by policy statements, including avoiding foods such as garlic and onions before or during the workday.

A confidential personnel record is maintained for each employee, and any changes of address, telephone numbers, marital status, or number of dependents must be reported. Employees have a right to view their file by request. Confidentiality also extends to patient records. Health Insurance Portability and Accountability Act (HIPAA) privacy laws are clearly stated in regard to patients' rights to privacy. Conversations, confidential papers, and information about a patient are all private and confidential matters that must be enforced by office policy.

## BUSINESS AND PROCEDURE PROTOCOLS

Protocols are procedures that are followed in a certain set of circumstances. The business office protocol sections of a dental practice office manual contain information on business office systems, such as telecommunications, reception procedures, new patients, laboratory requirements, accounting, insurance, credit and collections, records management, appointment scheduling, production, recare, and inventory. Procedure protocol sections of an office manual contain information on general dentistry and specialty dentistry procedures. Examples of protocols are the preparation and steps to follow when performing a composite restoration, porcelain fused to metal crown, and periodontal therapy. *Box 23.4* gives an example of a soft tissue management protocol for type I gingivitis.

## PERSONNEL INFORMATION

**Personnel information** sections of an office manual contain information regarding attendance, workload, compensation, benefits, obligations, selection of new personnel, and grievance procedures. Attendance policy is important to employers, and most employers have clear rules regarding late arrival, absenteeism, chronic absenteeism, scheduled time off, vacations, and holidays. New employees undergo a probationary period, which ranges from 1 to 3 months. It is possible that the employee will receive no employment benefits during the probationary period. Most dental practices are "at-will" employers, which means that either party may terminate employment at any time.

---

**BOX 23.4**  *Protocol: Managing and Treating Type I Periodontal Disease*

Protocol for Type I Gingivitis Diagnosis
↓
Prophylaxis will be performed and a neutral sodium fluoride 2% rinse prescribed; a 6-week reevaluation appointment is made for a periodontal evaluation, another prophylaxis, and a prescription refill
↓
A 3-month recare appointment with periodontal evaluation
↓
Oral health condition determines the next appointment time interval or
↓
Oral health condition results in a referral to a periodontist

---

## Benefits

Vacation time is accumulated over time during the year based on negotiated employment terms. The number of vacation days generally ranges from none to 1 or 2 weeks for the first 5 years, progressing in 5-year increments to 3 weeks and then 4 weeks, after 10 years of employment. Policy statements may include provisions that vacation time must be preapproved, is not accrued from year to year, and is not paid if not taken. For some practices, if additional time off is required, it can be arranged without pay.

National holidays are paid based on a regular work day and include New Year's Day (January 1), Memorial Day, Independence Day (July 4), Labor Day, Thanksgiving Day, and Christmas Day (December 25). Policy may state that the employee must work the day before and the day after a holiday to receive holiday pay. Those who observe religious holidays usually must provide due notice and use their vacation or other time off, or take the time without pay. Policy statements also specify procedures for time off for bereavement, voting in local and national elections, jury duty, maternity/medical leave, personal days, and sick days. A leave of absence is an extended absence from work owing to illness or a personal reason. Office policy may further define leave of absence in regard to temporary replacement, lay off, and documentation.

Bonus pay may be earned according to office policy and job employment negotiation and is paid monthly. Many dental practices have bonus incentive programs based on production, employment anniversaries, and collection procedures. Performance review or appraisal is a private personal interview conducted by the employer quarterly, semi-annually, or yearly to discuss skill development, attitude and work habits, communication skills, and professional development (*Box 23.5*). Cost-of-living salary increases are not the norm in private dental practice, whereas merit raise increases are prevalent. A **merit review** includes an assessment of the employee's salary and benefits (*Box 23.6*). Performance review is discussed further in Chapter 30.

### INSURANCE BENEFITS

Insurance benefits may consist of medical, dental, short- and/or long-term disability, life, and workers' compensation. Frequently, full-time employees request medical insurance coverage, and the payment of premiums are shared by the employer and employee.

**BOX 23.5** *Performance Review Criteria*

**Skill development**
  Eager to learn
**Attitude and work habits**
  Accepts criticism
  Appearance and grooming
  Assists other staff members
  Enthusiastic
  Efficient use of time
  Follows directions

**Communication skills**
  Active team member
  Participates in staff meetings
  Verbal skills
  Credible
  Trustworthy
**Professional development**
  Attends continuing education courses

Coverage can begin the first day of employment or after a 90-day grace period. The estimated employee share is deducted before taxes, and the employer contributions are made concurrently. After leaving employment, the individual is eligible for Consolidated Omnibus Budget Reconciliation Act (COBRA) benefits for up to 18 months. Dental benefits are frequently delivered at no charge to the employee, and family members (spouse and minor dependents) receive dental benefits at cost. Laboratory services may be provided at no charge or at cost to the employee and/or family members. Short- and/or long-term disability and life insurance are not automatically available and must be negotiated as a benefit of employment. Workers' compensation is a mandatory insurance coverage provided by the employer to pay for loss of wages or salary and medical expenses as the result of an injury on the job.

## OTHER BENEFITS

Many other types of employment benefits may be offered as part of the personnel policy. Educational expenses, uniform allowance, paid parking, commuting expenses, and professional association memberships may be paid by the dental practice. Required continuing education courses may or may not be paid for by the office, or the office may

**BOX 23.6** *Salary, Wage, and Benefit Components*

Assigned workload
Salary/wage compensation per year
Bonus pay
Commission pay
FICA withholding
Accidental death/Life insurance
Commuting reimbursement
Dental insurance
Education expenses
Malpractice insurance

Medical insurance
Paid time off (vacation, national holidays,
  bereavement, election day, jury duty, maternity/
  medical leave, personal, sick days)
Parking reimbursement
Pension/profit-sharing contributions
Professional association dues
Short- and/or long-term disability
Uniform allowance
Workers' compensation

grant an additional personal or vacation day for attendance at such courses. Uniform allowances are paid per OSHA requirements for personal protective equipment; the uniform usually includes scrubs, barrier jackets, and clinic shoes (that should remain in the office). In many places of employment, parking must be initially paid by the employee; however, he or she may negotiate this during a merit review, asking the employer to pay.

## Job Descriptions

Job descriptions are occupational definitions and expectations outlined by an employer. A job description identifies the tasks necessary for meeting or exceeding the employer's needs and can be used to determine any missing skills. Job descriptions for the office manager and dental business assistant were given in Chapter 7. In the independent practice, the dental hygienist is the employer. Components of the job descriptions for the employer, dental hygienist, and dental assistant for the dental hygienist are given in *Boxes 23.7, 23.8, and 23.9.*

## Employee Code of Conduct

An employee code of conduct outlines the expectation of professional behavior in the dental practice. It may be a list of behaviors or may identify contractual items that, if breached, could be grounds for immediate dismissal. Codes of conduct usually address negligence, breach of contract, technical assault/battery, misrepresentation, deceit, breach of confidentiality, permitting a hazard, insubordination, and attendance issues. Some dental offices go so far as to limit personal telephone calls; define which phone line to use; and outline long distance call procedures, Internet access, and computer use.

---

**BOX 23.7**  *Components of the Employer Job Description*

Leadership
   Inspire staff.
   Determine office policy.
   Set tone, vision, philosophy, and mission of practice.
Recruit, interview, and select new staff members with the assistance of others
   Set goals and action plans.
Public relations
   Create goodwill.
   Promote the practice.
   Provide excellent clinical care.
   Attend to the care and comfort needs of clients.
   Implement technology.
   Incorporate educational programs.
Management
   Monitor all office systems.
   Keep current of institute government regulations.
   Praise and evaluate staff.

**BOX 23.8**  *Components of the Dental Hygienist Job Description*

Assess patient, plan for treatment, implement
    treatment, and evaluate patients.
Assist in recare activities.
Communicate with clients.
Document patient care, recommendations,
    discussions, referrals.
Educate patients.

Maintain the soft tissue management system.
Participate in morning meeting.
Prescribe schedule VI medicaments.
Provide comprehensive oral hygiene services.
Provide excellent clinical patient care.
Schedule advanced appointments.
Write narrative reports.

## Grievance, Discipline, and Termination

Office conflict can be unpleasant for all staff, and office policy is established to minimize conflict and guide combatants toward a peaceful settlement of issues. **Grievance procedures** are protocols that outline the chain of command and appropriate actions to take when a conflict occurs. Disciplinary notices are forms that are completed when an infraction of the employee code of conduct occurs or when another unfortunate event happens. Disciplinary notices are meant as a warning to the employee to improve job performance or face employment termination (*Fig. 23.1*). Usually, employment termination is the last resort, taken only when multiple disciplinary notices have been documented. Because most dental practices are at-will employers, employment termination may occur at any time for any reason. Employees may be fired or given a 2-week notice to leave the practice. Employees customarily give the practice a 2-week notice when resigning.

## Contract Employees

Contractors enter into legal agreements to perform a legal act in which there will be payment by an expressed oral or written agreement. Independent contractors are self-employed people who provide specified services in the course of employment. Self-employed contractors experience profit and loss, may work in multiple settings, pay for their own expenses, provide their own instruments and materials, and are paid by

**BOX 23.9**  *Components of the Dental Assistant Job Description*

Assist during procedures.
Assist in recare activities.
Attend morning meeting.
Attend to patient care and comfort needs.
Educate the patient in oral hygiene and
    postoperative care.
Maintain equipment and inventory.
Maintain instrument processing system.
Open and close office.

Prepare and maintain darkroom.
Prepare and operate sterilization equipment.
Prepare operatories.
Receive and seat patients.
Restock and replenish operatories.
Schedule advanced appointments.
Take radiographs.
Update medical and dental history.

```
┌─────────────────────────────────────────────────────────────────────┐
│                     Forever Smiles Dental Offices                     │
│         123 Main Street, Anytown, Anystate 12345 Phone: 888-555-1515  │
│                                                                       │
│                       DISCIPLINARY ACTION FORM                        │
│                                                                       │
│   Date of Incident_____                       │
│                                                                       │
│   Description of incident:_____ │
│                                                                       │
│   _____ │
│                                                                       │
│   Goals for improving employee behavior:                              │
│                                                                       │
│   1. _____ │
│                                                                       │
│   2. _____ │
│                                                                       │
│   3. _____ │
│                                                                       │
│   4. _____ │
│                                                                       │
│   Plan to implement goals:                                            │
│                                                                       │
│   1. _____ │
│                                                                       │
│   2. _____ │
│                                                                       │
│   3. _____ │
│                                                                       │
│   4. _____ │
│                                                                       │
│   I acknowledge receipt of this disciplinary action notice and have been informed of the │
│   reasons for this warning.                                           │
│                                                                       │
│   Employee signature_____      Date_____    │
│                                                                       │
│   Employer signature_____      Date_____    │
└─────────────────────────────────────────────────────────────────────┘
```

**Figure 23.1** Disciplinary action form.

the job in a lump sum. Contract samples are available from the American Dental Hygienists' Association website (www.adha.org).

## Client Information

Client information sections of an office manual contain policies and protocols regarding telecommunication, communication procedures, new patients, appointment control, late-arriving patients, broken appointments, preventive maintenance, recare appointments, patient dismissal, financial procedures, and medical emergency protocols.

## OFFICE MAINTENANCE SCHEDULE

Office maintenance sections of an office manual contain information regarding building and equipment maintenance schedules and daily, weekly, monthly, and yearly tasks. The operatory, equipment (e.g., handpieces, suction), sterilization area, darkroom, and laboratory require daily, weekly, monthly, and yearly maintenance. Communication procedures for OSHA rules and right-to-know chemical safety rules are found in this section of the manual. Infection-control protocols, instrument processing, the use of personal protective equipment, and inventory procedures are also outlined here and must follow CDC, OSHA, and right-to-know guidelines. Office maintenance schedules list general housekeeping duties by day, week, month, quarter, and year.

Office security issues may be addressed in this section as well. Personal items, keys, and the alarm system are described. Policies regarding the investigation and access of strangers (including inspectors, visitors, and doctors) entering the facility are defined.

## CONCEPT SUMMARY

- Office policy and procedures manuals direct the dental practice, contain office policy, define protocols, outline office systems, provide job descriptions, include personnel forms, and offer guidelines for communications and operations.
- Office manuals outline the vision, philosophy, and/or mission statement of the group.
- Office manuals provide facts to new employees about the manner in which the business is conducted.
- Salary, wages, and benefits all contribute to the overall compensation package.
- Job descriptions define employer expectations and identify tasks necessary to meet and exceed employer needs.
- Forms and contracts are found in policy and procedures manuals.

## REVIEW QUESTIONS

1. What is the function of the office policy and procedures manual?
2. What are the differences among vision, mission, and philosophy statements?
3. Why are procedure protocols necessary for a well-managed practice?
4. Describe the four major criteria of a performance review or appraisal.
5. What are the components of a compensation package?
6. Why is it necessary to have a written job description?
7. How are employment contracts used in dental practices?

## CRITICAL THINKING ACTIVITY

- Identify the practice norms for your jurisdiction in terms of salary, benefits, and working conditions.
- Role-play reviewing the office's policy and procedure manual during an interview.
- Evaluate the job components found in Boxes 23.7, 23.8, and 23.9.

### Assignment: Office Manual

Prepare an office manual to be used as a reference for staff that contains the items listed in *Box 23.1*.

# Applied Communications

*Dental Hygiene Domain Competencies*[1]

## PROFESSIONALISM AND ETHICS

### Professional Behavior

- Assume responsibility for dental hygiene services.
- Provide accurate documentation when serving in professional roles.
- Communicate effectively using verbal, nonverbal, written, and electronic skills.

### Ethical Behavior

- Integrate the American Dental Hygienists' Association (ADHA) code of ethics in all professional endeavors.
- Adhere to federal, state, and local laws.
- Apply principles of risk management to prevent legal liability.

### Critical Thinking

- Analyze published reports of oral research and apply that information to dental hygiene services.

### Professional Commitment

- Advance the values of the profession by affiliation with professional and public organizations.
- Assume the role of clinician, educator, researcher, change agent, consumer advocate, and administrator as defined by the ADHA.
- Assume responsibility for lifelong learning.
- Evaluate scientific literature to make evidence-based decisions that advance the dental hygiene profession.

## ORAL HEALTH PROMOTION AND COMMUNITY HEALTH

### Education and Communication

- Identify the goals, values, beliefs, and preferences of the patient during oral and general wellness promotion, prevention, and maintenance.

---

[1]Adapted from American Dental Education Association. Competencies for Entry into the Profession of Dental Hygiene (as approved by the 2003 House of Delegates). Reprinted by permission of *Journal of Dental Education*, Volume 68, Issue 7 (July 2004). Copyright 2004 by the American Dental Education Association.

- Communicate effectively with individuals and groups from diverse populations both orally and in writing.
- Participate in service activities and community affiliations using the human needs model of patient care to advance oral healthcare.

## Community Health

- Screen, educate, and refer services that allow patients to access the resources of the healthcare system.
- Facilitate patient access to oral healthcare services through a variety of healthcare settings as a member of a multidisciplinary team.

# DENTAL HYGIENE PROCESS OF CARE

## Patient Assessment

- Assess client concerns, goals, values, and preferences to guide client care.
- Obtain, review, update, and interpret medical and dental histories, radiographs, and vital signs.

## Patient Diagnosis

- Analyze and interpret data to formulate a dental hygiene diagnosis.
- Obtain consultations as appropriate.
- Refer clients to other healthcare providers as needed.

## Implementation

- Educate clients to prevent or control risk factors that contribute to oral disease.

## Evaluation and Maintenance

- Determine the outcomes of dental hygiene services using indices, instruments, examination techniques, and client self-reports.
- Compare outcomes to expected outcomes and reevaluate goals, diagnoses, and services when expected outcomes are not achieved.
- Develop and maintain a periodontal maintenance program.
- Determine client satisfaction with care received and oral health status achieved.

### REFERENCES AND RESOURCES

**Organizations**
International Committee of Medical Journal Editors (www.icmje.org)
McKenzie Management (www.mckenziemgmt.com)
Miles and Associates (www.dentalmanagementu.com)

**Online Resources**
Dental forms and marketing (www.pattersondental.com; www.steppingstonestosuccess.com; www.medicalarts press.com/dental_supplies.asp; www.smilemakers.com; www.practicebuilders.com; www.henryschein.com)

Dental pictures in the public domain (www.nlm.nih.gov/ hmd/index.html)

Direct mail marketing information (www.postcardbuilder. com)

Giving a speech (www.speechtips.com)

Ideas on creating papers, table clinics, and posters (www. adha.org, www.cdc.gov, www.iadr.com, www.who.ch)

Poster session requirements (www.adea.org)

Sample case studies (from Procter and Gamble) (www.dentalcare.com)

Signage (www.hellersigns.com, www.onlinesignshop.com, www.classicletters.com)

Spanish to English chairside translators (www.hdassoc.org/ site/epage/32854_351.htm)

Mission statements (www.franklincovey.com)

Employment terms and contracts (www.adha.org)

### Pamphlets, Dissertations, and Papers

Board of Trustees of Community College District No. 532 and the County of Lake and State of Illinois and College of Lake County Federation of Teachers Local No. 2394 AFT. 2004–2007 Agreement.

Brennan M. Marketing: An idea whose time has come.

California DHA office manual outline (rev.).

Gehrke K. Diagnosis and treatment planning *Power Point* lecture presented at the UIC College of Dentistry, November 2002.

Judging standards for table clinics. Michigan Dental Assistants' Association, 1992.

Levin R. Partnership for growth series, section I, 5. Procter & Gamble, 1998.

McCallister L. Communication style. Paper presented at the Old Dominion University Dental Assistants Symposium, September 1994.

Pacer L. Recycling. Table clinic presented at the Michigan Dental Assistants Association Student Day, Detroit, 1993.

Semple LG. Empowerment through communication. Paper presented at the American Dental Assistants Association and American Dental Association Annual Session, Las Vegas, October 1995.

Stroud S. Presentations plus. Paper presented at the 269th Conference of Professional Development for Women, Old Dominion University, Norfolk, VA, June 12, 1995.

Table seminar guidelines. Grand Rapids Community College, Dental Auxiliary Programs, 1989.

Tolle-Watts L. Table clinic grading criteria handout. Old Dominion University, Dental Hygiene Program, 2000.

### Articles

Bale-Griffeth D. The willies. RDH Aug 1997:32–34, 36, 38, 40.

Barsh LI. 7 tips for effectively marketing a practice's Web site. Dent Prod Rept 1999: 57, 58, 60, 62, 64–66.

Blitz P, Wright V. It takes two. RDH 1994:18, 21, 23, 25.

Davidhizar R. Eye to eye. RDH 27–28.

Dorfman WM. Mailing to your patients: find the gold in your practice. Dent Prod Rept 1997:50, 52.

Forrest JL. Quality assurance—Integrating it into private practice. Dent Hyg News 9(1):12, 13, 16.

Ganssle C. Marketing oral healthcare. The Dental Hygienist's Role. Dent Hyg News 1997;10(8).

George P. Preparing a table clinic. Dent Hyg News 8(1): 20, 23.

Homoly P. Educating patients on choice. J Pract Hyg 2004:34.

Homoly P. The hygiene handoff. J Pract Hyg 2004:30.

Jones HE. Let your voice be heard. RDH 1995:36, 38, 40, 41.

Ketchum C. Freedom from fear. RDH 1995:14, 15, 17, 19.

Majeski J. Phobias. Facts on fears. Access 1993:25–31.

Meldrum H. Communicating difficult news. RDH 2005:56, 58, 59.

Miles LL. Attitudes and the bottom line. Dent Teamwork 1990.

Miles LL. Patient's dental misconceptions. J Dent Asst May/Jun 2004.

Miles LL. The eight phases of a dental visit. Dent Asst 1985:8–10.

Miles LL. The value of staff. J Dent Asst 2003:4–5.

Miller L. Presenting your case. RDH 26, 28, 30, 58.

Nanne SM. Finding the right answers. RDH 2004:62, 64.

Nesbitt-Sceviour D. Practice management and clinical research. Part 3: presenting technology solution to practice owners. Contemp Oral Hyg 2004:16.

Nunn PJ. SOAP for whiter, brighter notes! Access 1994: 26–32.

Odell D. Managing your staff: don't underestimate the power of the job description. J Dent Asst 2002:6–8.

Palenik CJ, Miller CH. Creating the position of office safety coordinator. J Dent Asst 2002:10–14.

Perich P. Practice marketing: whose job is it? Dent Teamwork 1990:55–58.

Poindexter SM. Crossed signals: communication across gender lines. Access 1993:10, 12–15.

Pollack RD. Helping the practice take flight. Dent Teamwork 1988:89–93.

Pollack RD. Hygiene partnering: optimizing the use of a hygiene assistant. J Pract Hyg 2001:53, 56, 57.

Rusack L. What desktop publishing can do for you . . . and your patients. RDH 1995:20–21.

Sklar B. Mind over matter. RDH 1995:13, 15, 32.

Smela D-M. Interacting with the hearing impaired. Dent Hyg News 7:11–12.

Sulik JE. Words of wisdom. RDH 1996:32–33.

Treating the non-English speaking patient. Neb Dent Assoc Newslett 2005.

Whitacre HL. The poster session: designing a successful presentation. Dent Hyg News 8:23–24.

Wilde J. The talking connection. RDH 14–16, 18.

**Books**

Anderson KN, Anderson LE. Mosby's Pocket Dictionary of Medicine, Nursing and Allied Health (3rd ed.). St. Louis: Mosby, 1998.

Bivins T. Handbook for Public Relations Writing (3rd ed.). Lincolnwood, IL: NTC Business Books, 1995.

Bullock R. The St. Martin's Manual for Writing in the Disciplines. A Guide for Faculty. New York: St. Martin's Press, 1994.

Colwell Systems. Dental Charting Workbook. Champaign, IL: Author

Emig J. The Web of Meaning: Essays on Writing, Teaching, Learning and Thinking. Portsmouth, NH: Boynton/Cooke, 1983.

Etzel MJ, Walker BJ, Stanton WJ. Marketing (12th ed.). Boston: McGraw-Hill Irwin, 2001.

Evans JR, Berman B. Marketing (7th ed.). Upper Saddle River, NJ: Simon & Schuster, 1997.

Fitzgerald SS. Schaum's Quick Guide to Great Business Writing. New York: McGraw-Hill, 1999.

Fulwiler T. The Journal Book. Portsmouth, NH: Boynton/Cooke,. 1987.

Geffner AB. How to Write Better Business Letters. Woodbury, NY: Barron's, 1982.

Harris TL. Value Added Public Relations. Lincolnwood, IL: NTC Business Books, 1998.

Kouzes JM, Posner BZ. Credibility. San Francisco: Jossey-Bass, 1993.

Moss A, Holder C. Improving Student Writing. Pomona: California State Polytechnic University, 1982.

Reid JM, Wendlinger RM. Effective Letters (2nd ed.). New York: McGraw-Hill, 1973.

Torres H, Ehrlich A. Modern Dental Assisting. Philadelphia: Saunders, 1980.

Wolfe D, Reising R. Writing for Learning in the Content Areas. Portland, ME: Weston Walch, 1983.

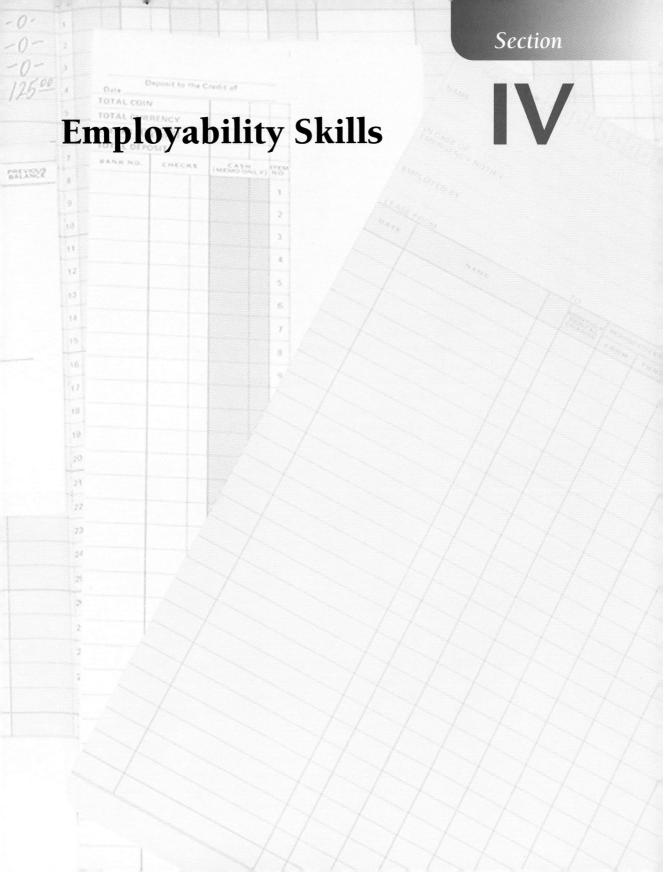

# Employability Skills

# Chapter

# 24

# Job Performance

Upon mastery of the content of this chapter, the student should be able to:

- Conceptualize the notion of the changing workplace.
- Classify personal values by completing a self-assessment.
- Develop a personal vision and mission statement.
- Establish personal goals in the five life areas using brainstorming, problem solving, and action planning.
- Recognize that academic skills, personal management skills, and processing skills are what employers want.
- Use methods to improve self-esteem.
- Develop positive behaviors to display good work habits.

## KEY TERMS

academic skills
action plans
brainstorming
goal setting
mission statement
personal management skills
problem solving

processing skills
self-assessment
self-esteem
values
vision statement
work habits

## JOB PERFORMANCE

With more than 15 million people looking for work at any given time, the number one factor to consider in a job search is the competition. Several qualified candidates will apply for any given dental hygiene job; thus, to be the successful job applicant—the one who is offered employment—it is logical to have a plan. To beat the competition, the job applicant should take the time to establish personal values, make self-assessments, develop personal vision and mission statements, set goals, and create action plans. Employers need employees with academic, personal management, and processing work skills. In addition, employers are looking for candidates who have good work habits.

Many people define themselves by the type of work they perform. The workplace is a constantly changing environment in which a large portion of the day is spent. How a worker performs on the job and how he or she is perceived by others is based on values and attitudes. **Values** are the conscious or unconscious feelings of what is correct or incorrect to do. Personal values influence an individual's behavior and give meaning to life. Attitude and feelings also determine whether information is assimilated in any given situation.

The ability to adapt to the changing work environment may well determine employment and life success. Challenges in the evolving workplace require the technical and ethical ability to perform and grow on the job, good work habits, and good communication skills. A plan to succeed involves having knowledge of personal strengths and weaknesses, setting personal goals, reaching beyond personal limits, learning new tasks for cross-training, and having a career plan. Before starting a job, a self-assessment confirms the best work environment for personal growth and attainment.

## SELF-ASSESSMENT

To become a valued employee, the student should assess his or her personal strengths and weaknesses and identify personal desires. **Self-assessment** is an individual's questioning about needs and values. Self-assessment is used to develop a strategic life plan and ascertain the situations and relationships needed to flourish in the working environment. *Box 24.1* highlights some self-assessment questions.

As graduation time nears, students think coursework and assignments are completed and may believe that they will quickly find a job. Yet the most important assignment lies ahead: getting and keeping a good, satisfying job. Job satisfaction comes with planning ahead and seeking the type of work environment that best suits personal preferences and goals. Compatibility with an employer and staff improves the likelihood of job satisfaction. When applying for a job, the student should keep in mind his or her personal conditions for job satisfaction—for example, the practice's philosophy, the staff's friendliness, the dental office's cleanliness and ergonomics, the protocol for sterilization, and the type of equipment in use. Finding the best job depends on personal preferences and a job search strategy.

### Vision and Mission Statements

A personal **vision statement** is a declaration of what an individual wants to accomplish. It is an inspiring statement that is unique, concise, and future oriented. Vision statements

---

**BOX 24.1** *Self-Assessment Questions*

| | |
|---|---|
| What do I value? | What have been my failures or disappointments? |
| What do I believe in? | What do I enjoy doing the most? |
| What are my personal strengths? | What do I enjoy doing the least? |
| What are my personal weaknesses? | What do I do well? |
| What are my interests? | What do I do poorly? |
| What are my successes? | What should I stop doing? |
| What kind of future do I seek? | What am I critical of? |

---

**BOX 24.2**  *Personal Vision and Mission Statements*

**Vision**
I will seek to promote oral health and wellness.
**Mission**
To bring meaning to my life, I will lead my life with honesty and integrity to serve my patients' needs, to continue to learn, and to strive for humility.

---

are shorter in length than mission statements. For example, you may want to serve the underserved, to help the handicapped, or to promote health and wellness. An example of a personal vision statement is given in *Box 24.2*. A personal **mission statement** addresses how to meet the personal goals based on personal strengths and recognizing personal weaknesses. An example of a personal mission statement is given in *Box 24.2*.

## GOAL SETTING

**Goal setting** is the process of mapping out a life direction. This process begins with a positive outlook, high self-esteem, and thoughts of success. People who have self-confidence and positive self-esteem are top performers on the job. People set career goals for three reasons: personal attainment, job-related attainment, and learning or performance.

Personal attainment goals include developing a career plan and locating, obtaining, and maintaining employment. (Career planning is discussed further in Chapter 25.) A job-related attainment goal may be the setting and/or exceeding of production totals. Learning or performance goals are intended to improve achievement and may include continuing education coursework, such as head and neck massage.

It has been said that goals plus actions equal reality. To set goals, individuals must know themselves and what they want to do. Goal setting involves brainstorming, valuing, and problem solving. People set goals throughout their lives—for example, before starting senior year of high school; before graduating high school, technical school, college, or university; after marriage; and after becoming a parent. Whatever the reason, goal setting helps focus energy and sets a path to follow. For many individuals, the ideal way to live a life with balance is to define their personal goals in the five life areas: financial, intellectual, physical, social, and spiritual.

Financial goals are related to the acquisition and management of money. Intellectual goals are related to learning and use of the mind to grow mentally. Physical goals are related to physical health and establishment of daily routines of physical exercise, rituals, or grooming. Social goals are related to positive interactions with other people. Spiritual goals are related to the life principle that humans have a spirit or soul that can be refined and improved. Goals direct the action one can take in these five life areas. Goals can be established at intervals of 6 months, 5 years, or throughout life. Goal setting is not a static process; it continues throughout a person's lifetime.

When brainstorming and constructing lists of tasks to accomplish during the next 6 months, 5 years, or throughout life, some individuals find it helpful to use worksheets for goal setting. It is important to first determine all the things the heart and mind want to accomplish and not evaluate what is written. The next step is to rate the listed items by numbering them in the order of importance. If problems must be solved before any of the goals can be met, the problem-solving model can help one form an action plan.

## Problem Solving

Problem solving is one of the tasks most frequently performed by dental healthcare team members. **Problem solving** is a tactic used for systematically finding an answer to a proposed question. *Box 24.3* lists the four components of the problem-solving model, which can be applied to any problem.

## Brainstorming

One technique used to problem solve is brainstorming. **Brainstorming** is a method used to generate many ideas in a short amount of time. When brainstorming, there are no right or wrong answers. Ideas can be simple, complex, wild, or wishful; the more ideas generated, the better. All ideas should be said out loud, then written down. Rating or eliminating ideas is not allowed during brainstorming because the objective is to generate ideas; only after all ideas have been generated can they be rated or eliminated.

## Action Plans

**Action plans** contain lists of activities, with timelines, to complete for short- and long-term goals. Goals are prioritized, specific dates for completion are selected, and the activities are scheduled. The action plan identifies what is known, the obstacles to overcome, and the people needed to help, and outlines a plan to achieve the goal. Completion of long-term goals is achieved by completing short-term goals within the established time frame.

## EMPLOYEE WORK SKILLS

Job openings are not always filled by the most clinically qualified applicant. Employers look for employees who can follow directions, learn new tasks, suggest improvements, and demonstrate positive values. Doing the best job also means behaving in a way that demonstrates productive work habits and basic skills. In today's workplace, the basic

---

**BOX 24.3**  *Problem-Solving Model*

1. Define the problem.
2. Develop a plan.
3. Carry out the plan.
4. Evaluate the solution.

Adapted from the state of Michigan's employability skills.

skills required are academic skills, personal management skills, and processing skills. **Academic skills** are necessary when preparing for prospective training and education and to acquire, keep, and progress in a job. **Personal management skills** are necessary for developing responsibility and dependability. **Processing skills** are necessary for using knowledge and learning new concepts.

## Academic Skills

Academic skills prepare workers for future training so they can continue to improve on the job. Academic skills include applied communication, mathematics, science, and the use of computers and other technology. Employers want employees who understand the spoken and written language in which business is conducted. Applied communication skills are used when reading package inserts, charts, and labels, and when following written, oral, or graphical instructions. Computers are used for a variety of job-related functions, such as periodontal probing and appointment scheduling.

Basic mathematics is used daily in the dental office whenever a calculation is needed, an estimate is made, something is measured, three-dimensional shapes are handled, ratios and proportions are used, or problems are solved. Applied science fundamentals are used to understand the principles of radiation or to prepare dental materials.

## Personal Management Skills

Students who have personal management skills develop the attitudes needed to progress in a job. These skills include maintaining positive self-esteem, having maturity, being committed to the job, showing enthusiasm on the job, taking pride in working, making decisions, acting honestly, and exercising self-control and good work habits.

## Self-Esteem

Open communication and positive messages are key elements of self-confidence and self-esteem. Communication is basic to all relationships and includes listening skills, talking, and having self-confidence. Self-confidence is the belief in one's ability. **Self-esteem** is the belief in and respect for oneself. There are many ways to increase self-confidence and improve self-esteem. For example, make a list of events or relationships that create a positive feeling. Self-assessment questionnaires are another method of identifying feelings of self-esteem. By completing a self-assessment, individuals are able to recognize their inner and unique talents, which strengthens their self-esteem. Friends and family members can help point out one's strengths.

Just as important is recognizing those events or relationships that produce negative feelings. Try to change these situations by finding and listing positive alternatives. A significant way to instill positive self-esteem in others is to use praise and encouragement. Another way to change negative thoughts is to stop sending negative messages. Replace negative self-talk such as "I'm stupid" or "I'll never understand this" with "I'm better using my hands than engaging in written work" or "I'll get better with practice." Accepting things that cannot be changed focuses attention on the situation instead of the lack of ability. Finally, when feelings are low, do something healthy and positive to help someone else.

## Decision Making

Employers want employees to develop responsibility and dependability. These are personal management skills that include setting and accomplishing goals, making decisions, acting honestly, and using self-control. Decision making is a tactic for systematically choosing a course to follow among a set of alternatives. If the solution to the problem will affect the whole team, it is the employer's responsibility to make the final decision after listening to input from staff. Decision making requires commitment, and the dental team should stand behind the solution. The five steps of decision making are given in *Box 24.4.*

## Work Habits

An employee's daily attitudes and behaviors at work are called **work habits.** Employers want employees with a positive attitude because a positive attitude makes a pleasant coworker. An appropriate personal appearance, in terms of clothing and grooming, represents a positive work habit. Employees must be properly dressed each day in fluid-resistant barrier gowns, surgical scrubs, safety glasses, gloves, masks, shields, and hair bonnets for worker safety. Complying with these standards demonstrates a positive work attitude. Acting in a safe and healthy way is another example of a good work habit. Employees with good work habits confine their eating and drinking to designated areas for health and safety reasons.

Respecting the rights of others is a good work habit. Disruptive behavior, such as shouting or loud, boisterous laughter, may affect the employer's ability to conduct business in a professional manner. Discussing patients outside the dental office is irresponsible and is an infringement of the patient's right to privacy according to the law. Poor work habits include sleeping on the job, engaging in horseplay, being tardy, being unproductive, applying makeup during work, and refusing to perform assigned or delegated tasks. Employers appreciate the demonstration of good work habits. Successful, secure employees are prepared to exhibit these work attitudes.

## Processing Skills

Processing skills involve using knowledge and learning new concepts. These skills involve teamwork, problem solving, and decision making as well as recalling, comprehending, applying, analyzing, synthesizing, and evaluating knowledge. Processing skills

---

**BOX 24.4** *Decision-Making Process*

1. Define the problem.
2. Brainstorm alternative solutions.
3. Evaluate and rank the alternatives.
4. Select the best option.
5. Assess the effect of the decision.

also include attention control, deep processing, memory frameworks, and study skills. Attention control is the ability to change the level of focus, depending on the activity. Deep processing generates mental pictures about information, physical sensations, feelings, and oral information heard by the mind's ear. Memory frameworks cluster information for later retrieval.

Study skills related to knowledge and awareness include reading technical text and identifying important ideas. Dental professionals are expected to learn from reading. The word *student* means "one who studies"; the student who knows how to study knows how to learn. Many students study only to review the material needed to pass a test. But employees study to learn about new products, procedures, or operations so they can perform their jobs effectively. Rapid changes in technology force workers to continually learn on the job to best serve their clients.

## CONCEPT SUMMARY

- Job performance is based on three principles: self-assessment, good work skills, and communication skills.
- Self-assessment includes vision and mission statements, goal setting, brainstorming, problem solving, and action plans.
- Employees must possess academic skills, personal management skills, and processing skills.
- Personal management skills needed to progress in a job include self-esteem, decision making, and good work habits.
- Work habits consist of personal appearance, acting in a safe and healthy way, respecting the rights of others, and taking responsibility.

## REVIEW QUESTIONS

1. What are the academic skills that employers want?
2. What are the personal management skills that employers want?
3. How can you instill positive self-esteem in others?
4. What methods can be used to improve negative thoughts?
5. What is a self-assessment?
6. Why do people set and achieve goals?
7. What are the processing skills that employers want?
8. What are positive behaviors that lead to good work habits?

## Assignment: Self-Assessment

1. Create a list of events or relationships that give you a positive feeling.
2. Create a list of or ask a trusted person about your strengths and weaknesses.
3. Create a list of events or relationships that give you a negative feeling.

4. Create a list of alternatives that can be used to change negative situations or relationships into positive ones.
5. Complete the items in the list that follows to establish personal goals.

- Brainstorming: List the goals you want to accomplish during the next 6 months and 5 years and throughout your life in the following areas:

  Financial
  Intellectual
  Physical
  Social
  Spiritual

- Rating: Number the goals according to their importance to you.
- Problem solving: Use the problem-solving model given in *Box 24.3* to determine a plan to meet these goals.
- Action planning: List the steps to complete along with a timeline.

# Chapter

# 25

# Job Search Process

## JOB SEARCH PROCESS

Happiness and success on the job require thought and planning even before starting a job search. Once a course of study is completed, new graduates must face the challenge of finding a job. As noted in Chapter 24, the foundation of any job search is determining life values and goals through self-assessment and creating an action plan. The job search entails the following steps: targeting sources of employment, preparing a résumé or vita, assembling a portfolio, completing an application form and cover letter, performing well in an interview, and negotiating the terms of employment.

Most workers change jobs several times during their life, often because of the desire for a life change. According to the U.S. Bureau of Labor Statistics, the average American changes careers at least three times as a result of job dissatisfaction or a change in life expectations. The likelihood for change depends on the level of education of the worker. Americans hold any particular job for an average of 5–8 years.

## CAREER PLANNING

One personal marketing skill used to structure a job search is the development of a career plan. **Career plans** are career options based on personal interests. Aptitudes, values, interests, and achievements affect job planning and career choices. Most people begin career planning by assessing their interests, often as early as junior or senior high school. Aptitude and ability assessment tests are administered before students select a course of study. One type of assessment test is the Armed Services Vocational Aptitude Battery (ASVAB) administered by the U.S. Armed Services to high school students. These tests are often used to identify interests and aptitudes related to various work disciplines. Assessment testing itemizes career areas based on the responses to the questions.

Career planning is an ongoing process that occurs throughout an individual's lifetime as personal interests and environment change. People are changed by attending school, life experience, and personal contacts and allegiances. Environments are changed by technology and sociological progress. As part of career planning, individuals who define goals and design action plans using decision-making skills are able to plan a life direction and are prepared to cope with the changes and choices ahead. By gathering information and rating the options, they are able to make good choices and to live according to their plan. The prudent dental professional is prepared to reevaluate his or her career plan when life's unexpected situations arise and life-altering events occur. Furthermore, the expectations of peers, family, other adults, and society can affect decision making. Most people find that planning for change makes the transition easier, something to keep in mind because it is estimated that workers completely change careers at least three times.

## MARKETING

### Direct Marketing Methods

A successful job search using direct and indirect marketing methods identifies various sources of employment to ultimately find available jobs. Direct marketing methods include targeted communications and networking. **Targeted communications** are focused on select mailings, email, and telephone calls. Direct marketing to potential employers via select mailings is recommended for long-distance job searches. Such mailings contain a résumé or vita with a cover letter. Marketing through email includes an email message with an attached cover letter and résumé. Telephone contacts are appropriate for both local and long-distance job searches. Although calling unknown people can set the applicant up for rejection, it does work. Using the telephone improves the chances of success when networking.

#### NETWORKING

**Networking** is asking all of the people you know for their advice and support on how to find employment. Finding a great job by accessing the hidden job is accomplished by personal referral. Although many people don't like the thought of "using" people to find work, the majority of job seekers find employment in this manner. The common phrase

**BOX 25.1** *Networking Script*

Call the contact person
  Hello, June? This is Reese Entgrad. I am one of the customers of your shop.
Ask for their help
  June, I am graduating and need your help. I am looking for a full-time job as a dental hygienist.
    Do you know anyone who needs a hygienist?
Record conversation highlights
  Dr. D. Kaye is looking for a hygienist? What can you tell me about the practice?
Ask permission to use them as a reference
  Would you mind if I tell him that you suggested that I call? Thank you for your help.

"It's not what you know but who you know" sums up the rationale for this approach. There are four domains in which to seek information during networking: personal networks, career networks, business networks, and electronic networks. *Box 25.1* provides a sample networking script.

The best people to start networking with are those in your immediate circle. **Personal networks** are groups that include family members, friends, and former teachers; fiscal, legal, medical, and spiritual advisors; and family acquaintances. The number one goal of networking is to ensure the cooperation of contacts, which comes from the development of friendly relationships within your personal network.

**Career networks** are groups that include current and former coworkers, professional association members, community groups, continuing education contacts, mentors, clients/patients, vendors, business consultants, and recruiters. Joining and maintaining membership in a professional association is an excellent way to meet people in the industry. Dental personnel are frequently aware of job openings in the area.

**Business networks** are groups that include similar businesses, adjunct business networking organizations, and business-related organizations. A business network job search strategy is going door-to-door making what are called "cold calls." This involves visiting offices and asking about any job openings. This technique may lead to some rejection but it can be another way to network and locate unadvertised potential job openings. Electronic networks include job search engines, and trade and research websites.

## Indirect Marketing Methods

Indirect marketing methods include school/college placement offices, printed or posted want ads, state employment offices, employment agencies, and mass mailings. School or college career placement offices have access to prospective employers and their available job postings. Many local areas hold job fairs once or twice a year that enable job seekers to speak with representatives from business and industry. Schools and employment agencies have résumé referral services and job listings. Résumé referral services are businesses that prepare and print résumés for a fee. Bulletin boards, which often contain job notices, are located in post offices, libraries, union offices, and personnel offices.

## JOB RESEARCH

Researching a career in the dental industry makes managing the job search easier. Individuals who are informed with research data have improved interviewing skills. Solid research into employment opportunities is divided into three areas: occupational, business, and organizational. **Occupational research** is the investigation of job descriptions, employment statistics, education and credentialing requirements, and employment outlook. Access to reading materials about occupations is available from schools, public library resources, and the Internet. General references available at libraries on career information include the *Occupational Outlook Handbook, Dictionary of Occupational Titles, Career Opportunities Index,* and *Occupational Outlook Quarterly.* An investigation of job descriptions entails finding out what people with a specific job title do on a daily basis. For example, interviewing a working allied dental professional will reveal information about his or her daily tasks. Ask questions about what the job encompasses, how much time is spent on tasks, which skills are important, and how to find an entry-level position. The interview also is a way to develop contacts in a particular area of interest. *Box 25.2* lists typical interview questions.

Employment outlook statistics are available for educating potential workers about job stability and job growth in a geographical location. Employment statistics provide information regarding salaries and benefits. Education and credentialing requirements in the healthcare industry are based on federal and state regulations. These rules must be investigated before taking employment, as a protection against unnecessary litigation.

**Business research** is an investigation of the healthcare industry in general to enable the job seeker to respond to questions and demonstrate a broad knowledge base. To prepare for job interviews, the applicant should discover what common practices are, what it is like to practice in the healthcare industry, what professional organizations and publications are available, and whether the economy affects this industry. The occupations of dental assisting and dental hygiene share common job tasks with other healthcare professions and options for employment extend outside the realm of dentistry; for example, jobs may be available in veterinary science or medicine.

**Organizational research** is an investigation into a particular place of employment. The job seeker learns about the age of the dental practice, the location of the office and satellite offices, whether the dental staff is fully credentialed, and business growth potential, to better prepare for an interview and to stand out from other interviewees. Knowing the answers to these questions before the interview leads to better performance during the interview.

---

### BOX 25.2 *Interview an Allied Dental Professional*

How long have you been employed here?

How did you get your position?

What advice do you have for someone seeking an entry-level position?

What are your daily tasks?

How much time is spent on these tasks?

Which skills are important on the job?

Why did you choose a career in dentistry?

What is the most satisfying aspect of your job?

What is the most frustrating aspect of your job?

In what other related occupations would you work?

## Sources of Employment

Employment opportunities can be gleaned from a number of sources (*Box 25.3*). The more sources an applicant contacts, the better the chances he or she has of getting an interview. The area of greatest change in the job search process over the last decade is the availability of the Internet to find jobs. Internet job searches are done by accessing many different sites. Local professional associations, colleges, and newspapers as well as state employment commissions maintain websites that list job openings. National or regional job openings may be located via job search engines or the websites of national professional associations and the federal government. Job openings in dental manufacturing or product sales companies are posted on company websites.

Sometimes, employers advertise job openings when there is no position to be filled. This is done for many reasons. Some employers have already selected a candidate for the position but must interview other candidates to meet equal employment opportunity requirements. Employment agencies advertise to collect résumés of potential employees to show there are plenty of qualified people needing work in the industry. One business strategy is to interview employees in other dental practices as a way of finding out information on wages, benefits, policies, and procedures available in other dental offices. Another business strategy is to advertise a position to determine whether current staff is seeking another position.

Unscrupulous advertising may be placed to collect information on people in the field to use for targeted market research or to sell products or services pertaining to dentistry. Another more sinister form of advertising is used to identify people with high-income jobs to target for identity or home theft. As a rule of thumb, remember that most people are hired by word of mouth and networking; focus on these areas.

Employment agencies basically operate in two ways: as temporary agencies or as private businesses. A trend in the job market is that new available jobs are temporary or part-time. Many dental healthcare workers are employed by temporary agencies. **Temporary agencies** are businesses that provide employment opportunities on a short-term basis. Short-term jobs include seasonal work (e.g., summer jobs), part-time work, and task work lasting several hours to several months. These agencies can be found in the yellow pages under the heading "Employment Contractors—Temporary Help." Some temporary agencies require documentation of credentials and education. Some also require grammar, spelling, reading, or math tests before job placement and may require

---

**BOX 25.3**  *Sources of Employment Leads*

| | |
|---|---|
| Bulletin boards | Networking |
| Computerized and clearinghouse systems | Newspapers |
| Government agencies | Private employment agencies |
| Job placement offices | Professional association publications |
| Job and career fairs | Radio and television |
| Résumé referral services | Recruiters |
| Self-employment or entrepreneur | Volunteerism |
| Temporary agencies | Websites |
| U.S. employment service | Yellow pages |

signing an employment contract. Frequently, temporary work leads to full-time employment at the place of assignment.

**Private employment agencies** are private businesses licensed by the state that charge a fee to the worker or employer for job referral services. The fee may be a fixed amount or a percentage of a month or year's salary. Be sure to discuss this fee before signing any document or paper to determine who pays the fees. These agencies are found in the yellow pages under the heading "Employment Agencies." Long-distance job searches can be handled by private employment agencies. Civilian employment on military bases is contracted by private employment agencies.

**Computerized/clearinghouse systems** are computer databases accessed by job market research organizations. These databases contain information about job openings that can be matched to the qualifications and needs of job seekers. There is a fee associated with these services, and this technique is appropriate for nationwide job searches. Advertised job openings in virtually all major media throughout the United States can be tracked via computer.

Recruiters, sometimes called "headhunters," are individuals seeking job applicants for corporate clients who earn a fee from the employer when a job opening is filled. In dentistry, recruiters frequently seek applicants for sales positions for manufacturers of dental products.

Some allied dental professionals choose to become self-employed by seeking temporary employment with many different dental practices. These entrepreneurs enjoy the freedom of selecting their hours of work and interact with staff at a variety of practices. Some entrepreneurs end up starting their own temporary agency.

Professional associations hold regular meetings, and networking efforts at those meetings can reveal hidden jobs and provide support and motivation during the job search. Throughout the year, organizations mail newsletters, publications, and trade journals that may offer additional information on available employment opportunities. Often, state professional associations have Web sites that members can access to view and post job openings.

**Volunteerism** is donating time and skills to an organization to gain insight and experience. Many geographical areas have dental clinics that are operated by private groups, such as the American Red Cross. By volunteering to serve the underserved, the dental professional can make a difference in society while gaining a feeling of satisfaction. Some oral healthcare professionals donate time and perform services in these settings to make valuable contacts.

Perhaps one of the most frequently used avenues for finding employment is reading the want ads in local newspapers. Job advertisements are listed alphabetically or may be sorted under a heading for medical or dental jobs, or healthcare professions. Larger metropolitan areas have many competing newspapers, and the savvy job seeker will check them all and then access their websites for additional employment opportunities.

**Civil service** jobs are in government-funded agencies. Government agencies have a policy and procedure to follow when screening job applicants. Each state's Employment Security Commission is a government agency with the primary goal of helping people find jobs. Federal government agencies secure employees for veterans' hospitals or military installations.

In some locations, local access cable television channels display job opening advertisements. Similarly, local broadcast radio stations announce job openings during cer-

> **BOX 25.4** *Why People Change Jobs*
>
> Assigned additional tasks without a raise
>    in salary
> Being fired
> Company goes out of business
> Desire for a life change
> Dissolution of partnerships
>
> Economic downsizing
> Illness or accident
> Job obsolete as a result of improved technology
> No chance for advancement
> Poor communication with coworkers
> Retirement

tain times or show segments. The more sources of employment the applicant becomes familiar with, the greater the chances of scheduling an interview.

## CHANGING JOBS

Fortunately, the health professions offer the largest number of career options through 2007. Unfortunately, jobs can change profoundly overnight. The job that was wonderful yesterday can become not so wonderful today. Recall that the most common reason people change jobs is because of poor communication with the employer or fellow workers.

People change employment settings for a variety of other reasons as well. The desire for a life change is frequently cited as the motivation for seeking a new place of employment. An individual may want to relocate to be closer to family or to move to a new state. For this person, a life change is necessary for personal happiness. Employees may be forced to change employment settings owing to economic downsizing. **Economic downsizing** means the employer is reducing the number of employees because of financial reasons. An individual may need to relocate when his or her job is eliminated and no other comparable work is available in the area. Additional reasons for a life change include dissatisfaction with an employer who assigns additional tasks without a raise in salary, a new employee who is difficult to get along with, or a change in marital status.

Improvements in technology may eliminate some jobs—for example, a transcriptionist is replaced by voice-actuated computer software. Workers are fired when they do not meet job requirements. Dental practices go out of business as a result of death, retirement, or dissolution of partnerships. A worker may be unable to do the same work he or she was hired to do because of illness or injury. When there is no chance for advancement, the employee may change jobs. *Box 25.4* lists these and other reasons people change jobs.

## CONCEPT SUMMARY

- The average individual changes jobs every 5–8 years and changes careers three times.
- The job search includes career planning and job research strategies to identify sources of employment.
- Career planning entails direct and indirect marketing methods.
- Networking is a highly effective way to find employment.
- There are many reasons to change jobs; having a plan helps manage these changes.

**BOX 25.5** *Log Form for Tracking Networking Efforts*

Source       _____

Name        _____

Title         _____

Business     _____

Address      _____

Phone        _____

Fax           _____

Email        _____

Date contacted   _____

Conversation highlights   _____

_____

_____

_____

Action taken    _____

_____

_____

_____

# REVIEW QUESTIONS

1. How often does the average worker change jobs throughout his or her lifetime?
2. Why is career planning an important personal management skill?
3. List job search strategies that relate to finding sources of employment.
4. What is networking?
5. Who are the best people to network with?
6. What is occupational research and how does it help you to find employment?
7. What is business research and how does it help you to find employment?
8. What is organizational research and how does it help you to find employment?
9. What is likely to occur when you use various sources of employment?
10. What are the three main reasons people change jobs?

## Assignment: Job Research

1. Use the questions listed in *Box 25.2* to interview two working dental hygienists.
2. Use the log form provided in *Box 25.5* to track your networking efforts.

## Chapter 26

# Personal Marketing Tools

## PERSONAL MARKETING TOOLS

To be a successful job seeker and stand out from the competition, it is necessary to sell an important commodity—yourself. Personal marketing tools are used to promote job applicants for interview selection. Some job searches necessitate the use of several personal marketing tools. Each personal marketing tool involves specific preparation to meet particular job search requirements.

Marketing of personal and professional skills requires tools for direct and indirect personal marketing methods. Some of these methods were discussed in Chapter 25. Marketing tools include résumés, reference lists, curriculum vitae, portfolios, application cover letters, and job application forms. A **résumé** is a one-page history of personal information, education, experience, accomplishments, and other qualifications. A **reference list** is a one-page listing of people who will give a positive recommendation about the applicant's character. A **vita**, sometimes called the curriculum vita (plural = vitae), is a multipage biographical and historical summary emphasizing professional background, qualifications, and accomplishments. A **portfolio** is a collection of academic and credentialing documents, achievement awards, certificates, and other records that can be used to document accomplishments. When a résumé or vita is sent to an employer, an **application cover letter** is written to accompany it. This letter is also called a **letter of application.** An **application form** is an information-gathering method created by the employer to learn about the job applicant.

## PREPARING A RÉSUMÉ

Résumés are personal advertisements used to sell an individual, to distinguish him or her from other job applicants, and to convince the people capable of hiring to schedule an interview. Usually, résumés are requested before a job interview to help the interviewer screen the applicants. Therefore, a carefully prepared résumé must clearly and succinctly verbalize personal strengths and demonstrate how they will be valuable to the prospective employer. Résumés summarize skills, accomplishments, background, and strengths to show the potential employer the benefits of hiring the applicant. Employers generally take 10–20 seconds to scan each résumé, and as few as 2 résumés out of 100 result in an interview. Just as immediate judgments are made when meeting new people, employers quickly judge résumés on neatness and appearance.

There are many reasons to create an effective résumé. First, most prospective employers expect to receive a résumé from each applicant. It is submitted with an application cover letter in response to a request for job applications or an announcement of a vacancy or is submitted with the job application form to provide supplemental information.

Résumés can be used for networking and given to friends, family members, classmates, alumni, former employers, and professional association members to help in the job search. Résumés are helpful when completing job applications because they list specific information such as dates, addresses, telephone numbers, and email addresses. Employment agencies and temporary staffing and placement offices include the résumé in the job seeker's personnel file for reference.

There are three styles of résumés: chronological, functional, and combination. Job seekers should study the description of each type of résumé before deciding which style is most appropriate for their personal characteristics and the requirements of the jobs being sought.

The chronological résumé furnishes dates of all employment experience and education and arranges them in a time sequence beginning with the most recent. Interviewers are accustomed to this style of résumé, and it is the easiest to write. This style highlights steady employment and provides a guide for the interview process. However, chronological résumés can reveal gaps in employment that may hinder the applicant who has not been working regularly or who is changing careers.

The functional résumé emphasizes skills, achievements, and accomplishments rather than dates of employment. In this type of résumé, job titles are not emphasized; instead, transferable job skills are accentuated. The person who is changing careers or has gaps in employment should use this style. Recent graduates with limited work experience can point to newly acquired skills that are in high demand. Functional résumés do take longer to read than chronological ones, however, and the person screening them may not give the document proper attention. This could be significant for jobs with a good deal of competition.

Combination résumés are, as expected, a combination of the previous two styles. This style emphasizes the applicant's qualifications and grabs the reader's attention. The employment history is included in a separate section. In addition, this style of résumé does not emphasize employment gaps. Combination résumés also take longer to read than chronological ones, and the application screener may not give the document adequate attention.

## Collecting Résumé Data

Résumé data collection begins by completing a résumé fact sheet (*Fig. 26.1*). This form organizes résumé information and helps in the preparation of the final document. The most recent and important information is listed first. The typical categories used to organize information on a résumé are given in *Box 26.1*.

In formatting the document, the word *résumé* is typed in capital letters and placed above the heading. The heading provides information on how to contact the job applicant and includes name, address, telephone numbers, and email address. The location of the heading on the page depends on the format followed. Capitalize the first and last names and set them in boldface type to call attention to them. Do not use a courtesy title (Ms, Mrs., Miss, Mr.) in front of your name. Spell out the words in the street address (street, avenue, boulevard), use the U.S. Postal Service's abbreviation for the state, and be sure to include the ZIP code. For telephone numbers, include the area code even if job hunting within a small local area.

The career objective statement is optional, although it does specify the type of work being sought and suggests a directed job search. If using a career objective, the content of the résumé should support the objective. Objectives are stated in work-specific terms, such as occupational designation or occupational designation within a specialty area. For example, the occupational designation for the field of dental hygiene is dental hygienist. An occupational designation within a specialty area could be stated as "dental hygienist in a prosthodontic practice." Avoid using the pronoun *I*, and eliminate the use of full sentences, such as "I am seeking a part-time dental hygiene job." Use short, concise phrases that are not vague or confusing, such as "Willing to relocate for a full-time dental hygiene position in a periodontic practice."

Specific job-related skills can be substituted for the objective or can be placed in the next section. This section may also be called "areas of strength." Use nouns or action verbs in this section to showcase abilities (e.g., maintain inventory, instruct patients in home care, sustain good interpersonal relations, submit insurance claims, administer local anesthesia, place sealants).

The education information section lists the highest completed level of education first; any additional degrees follow in descending chronological order. List universities, colleges, community colleges, vocational/technical schools, and high schools attended whenever possible. Be sure to include the name of the school, the address, graduation date, major area of study, minor area of study, grade point average (if good), and type of degree or certificate earned. This section can be pared down or eliminated when space is an issue. Delete any incomplete schooling and the name of the high school attended, for example.

Work experience is listed next in descending chronological order and includes all former employers with addresses, employment dates, job titles, duties, tasks, and name of supervisor. This is a section in which the job seeker can stand out from other applicants. Emphasize the skills that are in demand or that can transfer from one environment to

(Heading) RÉSUMÉ

Name: _____
(First name, middle initial, last name)

Address: _____
(Street address, city, state, and ZIP code)

Phone numbers: _____
(Home and cellular with area codes)

Email address: _____
(Primary and alternate)

**Career Objective**     _____
(State the position)

**Skills**     _____
(List a skill and how you used it [use an action verb])

_____
(List a skill and how you used it [use an action verb])

_____
(List a skill and how you used it [use an action verb])

**Education**     _____
(List most recent degree with year completed)

_____
(Provide school name and address)

_____
(List two courses relevant to job)

_____
(List next most recent degree with year completed)

_____
(Provide school name and address)

_____
(List two courses relevant to job)

**Work Experience**     _____
(Most recent place of employment with dates)

_____
(List job title, place of work, and address)

_____
(List best accomplishment)

_____
(Next most recent place of employment with dates)

_____
(List job title, place of work, and address)

_____
(List best accomplishment)

**Military/Other Service**     _____
(List branch and years)

_____
(List rank, rate, and relevant duties)

**Special Recognition**     _____
(Decorations, awards, special assignments, campaigns)

**Personal Information**     _____
(Talents, languages, professional memberships, volunteerism)

**Figure 26.1** Résumé fact sheet.

**BOX 26.1** *Résumé Organization*

Heading with personal identifying information
Career objective or skills
Educational background
Experience

Military or other service
Personal information such as awards, special
    skills, and pertinent activities

another. This section also highlights internships, clinical rotations, and significant volunteerism. Complete sentences are unnecessary; if possible, begin statements with an action verb (*Box 26.2*).

Personal information at the end of the résumé can include activities or interests to help project a positive image for a good first impression. When space is limited, this section can be minimized. However, list at least three areas of interest such as hobbies, activities, awards, personal accomplishments, and honors, and keep the résumé clear

**BOX 26.2** *Résumé Action Verbs*

| | | |
|---|---|---|
| accelerated | focused | produced |
| accomplished | formulated | promoted |
| administered | gathered | qualified |
| analyzed | generated | recognized |
| arranged | guided | recommended |
| assessed | handled | recruited |
| assisted | illustrated | reorganized |
| attained | implemented | researched |
| awarded | improved | resolved |
| budgeted | incorporated | scheduled |
| cataloged | initiated | serviced |
| chaired | innovated | simplified |
| collaborated | instructed | started |
| completed | launched | strengthened |
| controlled | licensed | structured |
| coordinated | located | supervised |
| created | managed | targeted |
| delegated | monitored | taught |
| designed | motivated | trained |
| developed | negotiated | treated |
| directed | observed | used |
| earned | organized | volunteered |
| established | participated | worked |
| expanded | performed | wrote |
| expedited | planned | |
| facilitated | prepared | |

Adapted from *Writing an Application Letter*. Clarkston, MI: Oakland Technical Center, Northwest Campus, 1990.

and condensed. Provide activities that show leadership or initiative. Personal information regarding birth date, Social Security number, health, age, weight, eye color, religious affiliation, or marital or family status is never included. Any legally acceptable information for employment is provided after negotiations on hiring forms.

## Appearance and Format of the Résumé

The appearance of the résumé should be consistent and well balanced on the page. To project the best image possible, be sure the résumé is perfect, with no mistakes in spelling, grammar, punctuation, and formatting. Spacing and any abbreviations used should be consistent throughout the body of the résumé. Most word processing programs provide several templates for creating résumés.

As a general rule, résumés are one page long, but they can stretch to two pages. The potential employer, however, may never read beyond the first page. In some industries, the first screening of résumés and email applications is done by computers, which scan the text for specific key words.

Select a résumé format and use a computer word processing program to create a rough draft for proofreading. Critique the first draft and look at the overall appearance, contact information, organization, content, wording, and length. Mistakes in typing and errors in judgment can sabotage the chance for success, so give the résumé to several people to proofread. Select someone with good English skills and ask for his or her advice on how to improve the document.

Once the editing process is complete, the final copy is prepared and taken to a print shop, which can make high-quality copies. Quality bond paper that is 8½ by 11 inches is used for printing résumés. The paper should be white or a soft neutral color such as ivory, cream, or light gray. Purchase matching envelopes and extra paper for the application cover letters. Make several copies of the résumé to have on hand.

## PREPARING A CURRICULUM VITA

The curriculum vita is a multiple-page biographical history that emphasizes professional background and qualifications. Curriculum vitae are 3 to 10 pages long and are commonly used when applying for positions in education, medicine, research, and related fields. With a concentration on the job applicant's accomplishments, the vita chronicles the related details of scholarly pursuits, service, and research. The dental hygienist who seeks a teaching position should develop a vita. Many experienced clinical dental hygienists apply to local colleges and universities to teach and supervise students enrolled in clinical dental hygiene courses. The typical categories used to organize information on a vita are given in *Box 26.3*; *Figure 26.2* is a fact sheet that is used to create the document.

## REFERENCE LIST PREPARATION

Reference lists contain information about responsible people who will make favorable comments about the applicant's character. This information is gathered and placed on a separate piece of paper to be given to the interviewer. Select teachers, instructors, counselors, work supervisors, former employers or co-workers, older friends, and clergy or other community leaders and obtain their permission before using their name on a

**BOX 26.3** *Curriculum Vita Organization*

Heading with personal identifying information
Educational background
Work, academic appointments, teaching, and research experience
Awards, honors, fellowships, and scholarships
Publications
Conference presentations
Curriculum development
Grants and fellowships
Professional consultantships
Licensure and certification
Professional associations
Military, professional, and university service

reference list. Avoid using the names of relatives and boyfriends as references; this practice is considered unprofessional. Reference lists include the full name of three to six people along with their address, phone number, job title with affiliation, and relationship to the applicant.

Some résumés may contain the following statement at the bottom of the page: "References available on request." However, interviewers already know that names of references will be provided on a separate list; instead, use the last statement of the résumé to impress the person screening job applicants. *Figure 26.3* provides an example of a reference list; *Figure 26.4* is a fact sheet for preparing a reference list.

## PREPARING A PORTFOLIO

Portfolios have been used for years by graphic artists, fashion models, and business-people to market and promote their skills. A portfolio for the dental hygienist is a collection of academic and credentialing documents, achievement awards, and records of accomplishments. The portfolio is assembled to keep documents in one place for easy access during the interview process. The portfolio is used during the interview to reveal a "self-portrait" demonstrating a path of personal growth. As with résumés and vitae, interviewers will judge the portfolio for neatness and general appearance. Portfolio materials are placed in clear plastic sheet protectors, divided by sections, and stored in a three-ring binder. *Box 26.4* outlines the section contents of a portfolio.

### Appearance and Format of a Portfolio

The beginning of the portfolio can be arranged in a variety of ways. A table of contents that highlights the sections of the portfolio may come first or it may be preceded by a title page that contains the applicant's name, a biographical sketch, or the job objective. A copy of a résumé or vita can also be placed at the beginning. In the education section, place photocopies of school records, such as diplomas, certificates of completion, and transcripts. This section also contains licensure and credentials, such as cardiopulmonary

(Heading) CURRICULUM VITA

Name: _____
(First name, middle initial, last name)

Address: _____
(Street address, city, state, and ZIP code)

Phone numbers: _____
(Home and cellular with area codes)

Email address: _____
(Primary and alternate)

**Education Background**          _____
                                  (Years completed, degree, school name, city, state)

**Work Experience**               _____
                                  (Academic appointments, professional consultantships,

                                  teaching, research experience)

**Personal Accomplishments**      _____
                                  (Awards, honors, fellowships, and scholarships)

**Publications**                  _____
                                  (Most recent first in descending order)

**Conference Presentations**      _____
                                  (Most recent first in descending order)

**Curriculum Development**        _____
                                  (Most recent first in descending order)

**Grants and Fellowships**        _____
                                  (Most recent first in descending order)

**Licensure and Certification**   _____
                                  (Most recent first in descending order)

**Professional Associations**     _____
                                  (Most recent first in descending order)

**Service**                       _____
                                  (Military, professional, university service)

**Figure 26.2** Curriculum vita fact sheet.

B. B. Tooth, RDH
Any address
Any city and state
Phone number
Email address
Co-worker at Dr. Grin's office
Professional and personal reference

Ann T. Dote, RN
Head Nurse
Any address
Any city and state
Phone number
Email address
Co-worker at Nursing Care Facility
Professional and personal reference

Cora Spondance, RDH, MA
Dental Hygiene Program Director
Any college or university
Any address, city, and state
Phone number
Email address
Clinical Instructor
Professional reference

Petey Atrics, BS, RN
Any address, city, and state
Phone number
Email address
Assistant to the Director at Children's Hospital
Personal reference

**Figure 26.3** Sample reference list.

resuscitation (CPR), Health Insurance Portability and Accountability Act (HIPAA), or Occupational Safety and Health Act (OSHA) training certificates. Also include any continuing education certificates of attendance or completion. A minimum of two letters of recommendation from employers, teachers, counselors, or other selected people should be placed in the reference section. An extra photocopy of the reference list can be kept here until it is given to the interviewer.

Photocopies of awards, certificates of recognition, and any other achievement go here as well. Recognition may come from various organizations and people such as 4H, the Special Olympics, the National Honor Society, the Dean's list, dignitaries, and Phi Beta Kappa. Documentation of scholarships, scholastic achievement, and fellowships can also be added here.

Work samples are photographs of study models, case studies, poster sessions, table clinic handouts, research papers, and documentation of clinical skills. Valuable clinical skills are proficiency in radiology, local anesthesia, or expanded functions. Last, any authored, co-authored, or edited publications belong in this section, as does documentation of participation in research studies. Membership certificates from professional

Reference Name            _____

Address                   _____

City, State, ZIP Code     _____

Telephone Numbers         _____

Email address             _____

Job Title                 _____

Type of Reference         _____


Reference Name            _____

Address                   _____

City, State, ZIP Code     _____

Telephone Numbers         _____

Email address             _____

Job Title                 _____

Type of Reference         _____


Reference Name            _____

Address                   _____

City, State, ZIP Code     _____

Telephone Numbers         _____

Email address             _____

Job Title                 _____

Type of Reference         _____

**Figure 26.4** Reference list fact sheet.

**BOX 26.4** *Section Contents of a Portfolio*

Table of contents
Résumé/Curriculum Vita
Education (diplomas, certificates, transcripts, licenses, credentials, continuing education certificates)
Letters of recommendation
Awards, honors, scholarships
Work samples
Publications, research, association memberships

societies such as the American Dental Hygienists' Association (ADHA), the student division of the ADHA, or other professional or service groups belong here.

## PREPARING THE APPLICATION COVER LETTER

The letter of application may be the first actual contact the applicant has with a potential employer, and it is the best opportunity to market abilities to the person with hiring power. It is sent with a résumé as a means of introduction when responding to job postings, vacancy announcements, and advertisements. A letter of application can spotlight special abilities that aren't mentioned in the résumé and can emphasize how the job seeker's skills match the job requirements.

Application cover letters are written to fit the specific requirements mentioned in the job posting and should contain the most current information. Perfect spelling, punctuation, and grammar are absolutely necessary to make the best possible first impression. The letter should be typed, single spaced, and free of typing errors and obvious erasures. It is printed on paper that matches the résumé. The body of the letter is centered on the page vertically and kept to one page in length. The essential components of application letters and a suggested format are provided in *Box 26.5*. Additional details on formatting and content of the opening and closing of a letter in block style can be found in Chapter 22.

The body of the letter should target the job and encourage the reader to consider the enclosed résumé. Begin with a sentence explaining how the job opening became of interest. Catch the eye of the reader by using the name of a mutual acquaintance. If a mutual acquaintance is not available, attempt to form a bond by using a sentence to grab the reader's interest. An attention-grabbing sentence indicates knowledge about the business and how the applicant can benefit the employer. For example, "Because your dental office specializes in periodontics, my recent training in dental hygiene will be of help to you."

The next paragraph should highlight one or two points from the résumé regarding experience, abilities, or accomplishments, and should concentrate on items relevant to the position. Chose sentences such as: "My clinical skills are excellent, and I have an in-depth working knowledge of dental materials," "I type 65 words per minute, and my skills increased production by 30%," or "I volunteer at a children's clinic." The final paragraph includes a follow-up plan for further contact resulting in an interview and thanks to the reader for his or her attention. Indicate that your résumé is enclosed and remember to include your résumé.

For proofreading purposes, always make a draft copy before making the final copies. Ask someone else to proofread the letter to be sure it projects a positive business image. Keep a copy of the final copy and file it for a follow-up telephone call within a week. *Figure 26.5* provides sample application cover letters.

## PREPARING THE APPLICATION FORM

Job applications are forms provided by employers to be used by the interviewer to screen job applicants. Application forms are similar to résumés, cover letters, and portfolios, with rules for completion. Whenever possible, fill out the application form at home so you can type it. To project the best image, complete the application perfectly with no mis-

**BOX 26.5** *Essential Components of the Application Cover Letter*

Begin 1 inch from the top of the page
Heading
Sender's name (optional location)
Street address
City, state, ZIP code
2 blank lines
Date line
2 blank lines
Recipient's name
Street address
City, state, ZIP code
2 blank lines
Salutation (e.g., "Dear Sir:")
1 blank line
Body paragraph 1
   Purpose of letter
   Position title
   Announcement source
   Announcement date
   Attention-getting sentence
1 blank line
Body paragraph 2
   Personal background
1 blank line
Body paragraph 3
   Ask for interview
1 blank line
Closing (e.g., Sincerely,)
3 blank lines (for signature in ink)
Signature line
Street address (optional location)
City, state, ZIP code
2 blank lines
Enc.

takes in spelling, grammar, or punctuation. If it is not possible to take the application home to complete, use a pen with black ink and print neatly (do not use cursive writing). Take time to read the form completely before answering any questions to reduce the chances of making errors. The résumé can be used to help complete the application form so have it on hand. Remember to use action verbs, to limit abbreviations, and to use complete sentences.

Answer all the questions on the form, complete all lines, and avoid leaving blanks. When a question does not apply, write "not applicable" (or N/A) on the line or draw a straight line in the space to acknowledge that the line was read but the question does not apply to the current circumstances. These actions show the employer that the appli-

Ima Graduate, RDH
123 Silver Lake Road
Silver Lake, MI 49999

May 1, 2006

Dr. Milton Yermouth
321 Oceana Street
Hart, MI 49990

Dear Dr. Yermouth:

This letter is in response to the dental hygienist vacancy posted at the Good Community College dated April 26, 2006. Mr. John Gibbons suggested that I contact you regarding my excellent periodontal clinical skills.

Recently, I worked part-time as a chairside assistant for Dr. D. Kaye, 456 Any Street, Any town, Michigan. Dr. Kaye was my supervisor. My associates in applied science degree in dental hygiene was earned at Good Community College. Other pertinent courses that I have taken include HIPAA training, CPR, and first aid.

I am an energetic person who adapts quickly to new environments. My résumé documents other healthcare delivery experiences. Please contact me at 555-555-1234 to schedule an interview. Enclosed is a copy of my résumé for you to read at your convenience. Thank you for your time.

Sincerely,


Ima Graduate, RDH

Enc.

**Figure 26.5 A.** Sample application cover letter.

September 2, 2006

Dr. Hal O'Tosis
123 Main Street
Anytown, MN 53627

Dear Dr. O'Tosis:

This letter is in response to your announcement for the dental hygiene position that appeared in the *Anytown Times* on September 2, 2006. I was recently graduated from the dental hygiene program at Minnesota Technical Institute.

Please consider me as an applicant for this position. I feel that my abilities as a clinician make me well qualified to work for your office. In addition, my experience as a volunteer for Operation Smile for the last two summers was excellent preparation for working in private practice. My resume is enclosed for your review.

I would welcome the opportunity to meet with you to discuss this position and my qualifications. I will call your office to schedule an interview or feel free to contact me. I can be reached by telephone at 555-555-5678. Thank you for your time and consideration.

Sincerely,

Reese Entgrad, RDH
11 Up Hill Drive
Anytown, MN 53627

Enc.

**Figure 26.5** (Continued) **B.** Sample application cover letter.

cant read the question and understood it. Neatness counts, as does spelling, grammar, and punctuation. Scribbles detract from the neatness of the application form. If a mistake is made, draw one line through it and write the correction next to it.

Experts recommend writing "negotiable" or "open" in response to a question about desired salary. This signals the employer that wages are open to discussion. If the job posting has a salary range or established salary, put this information down. Protect the application form from food and drink stains. Do not staple or tear it. Read the application after completion to check for blanks and accuracy. Sign the form with your proper name on the signature line.

## Addressing the Envelope

There is a proper manner in which to address a business envelope. Application materials are mailed in a business-size envelope (3⅞ inches by 8⅞ inches) or in a first-class mailing envelope. The return address of the sender is typed in the upper left hand corner. Return addresses are single spaced and located two lines below the top of the envelope and three spaces from the left side. The return address consists of the name on the first line, street address on the second line, and city, state, and ZIP code on the third line.

The mailing address is typed single spaced, 2 inches from the top edge and 4 inches from the left side. Mailing addresses consist of the name of the person to whom the materials are being sent on the first line, the person's title on the second line (e.g., Office Manager), the street address on the third line, and the city, state, and ZIP code on the fourth line (*Fig. 26.6*).

Finally it is important to fold the materials properly. If sending a résumé, the cover letter is placed on top and the two sheets are folded together. The materials should be

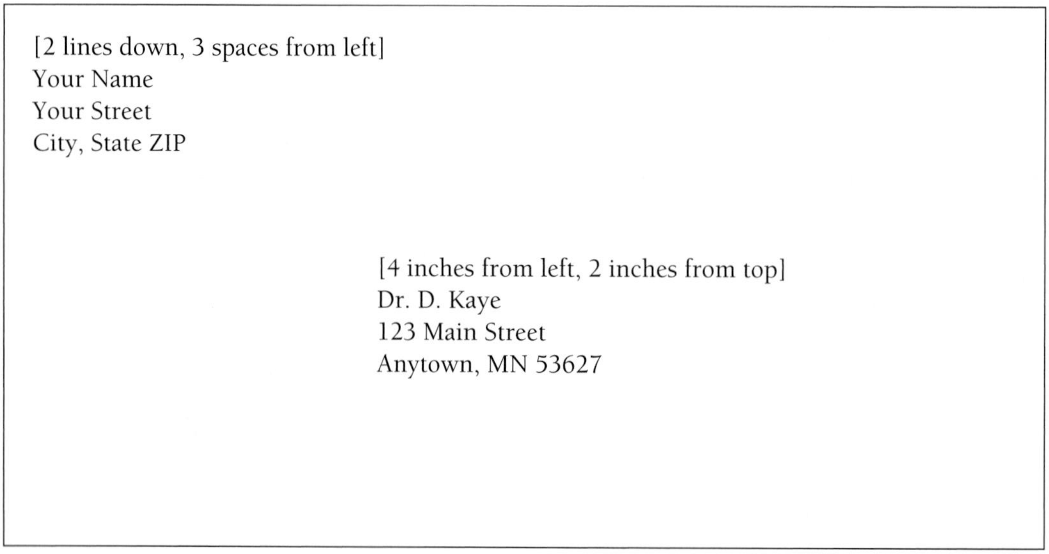

[2 lines down, 3 spaces from left]
Your Name
Your Street
City, State ZIP

[4 inches from left, 2 inches from top]
Dr. D. Kaye
123 Main Street
Anytown, MN 53627

**Figure 26.6** A properly addressed business envelope.

folded into thirds by bringing the bottom up first and folding the top edge down, leaving a ½-inch margin at the bottom.

Now it is time to schedule the interviews.

## CONCEPT SUMMARY

- Résumé formats are functional, chronological, or a combination of the two.
- A curriculum vita is used for education, medicine, research, and related fields.
- Reference lists contain contact information of responsible people who will make favorable comments about the applicant's character.
- Portfolios contain a collection of academic and credentialing documents, achievement awards, and records of accomplishments.
- Application cover letters are sent with a résumé or vita and the application to emphasize how skills match the job requirements.
- Applications are forms provided to jobseekers and are used by potential interviewers for screening.
- Business envelopes must be properly completed before application materials are mailed to prospective employers.

# REVIEW QUESTIONS

1. Describe a functional, chronological, and combination résumé.
2. How should you list employment when you have held more than three jobs?
3. If you have been involved in extra-curricular activities, where should they be mentioned on your résumé?
4. When selecting and listing references (after obtaining their permission) how many should you have?
5. What is the difference between a résumé and a curriculum vita?
6. When are curriculum vitae used?
7. What is a portfolio and how does it help the job seeker?
8. What is a letter of application and when is it used?
9. How do you sign a letter of application?
10. What should you do when completing an application if you do not have an answer to one of the questions on the form?
11. What should you do if you make a mistake when completing an application?
12. Why is it necessary to read all the instructions on an application before completing it?
13. Is the appearance of the envelope as important as the appearance of the letter of application?

## Assignment: Creating Marketing Tools

1. Prepare a résumé or vita by completing the appropriate fact sheet and preparing a draft copy. Type or print it and then evaluate it for accuracy. Ask someone to proof-read it.

2. Prepare a reference list by consulting *Figure 26.4*. Prepare a draft reference list using the information gathered. Type the reference list, then evaluate it for accuracy and ask someone to proofread it.

3. Assemble a portfolio, consulting *Box 26.4*. Prepare a table of contents and section cover page and place them in a three-ring notebook. Collect materials and place them into clear plastic sheet protectors.

4. Consult *Box 26.5* and *Figure 26.5* and write a personalized letter of application to an advertisement selected from a local newspaper. Make sure you include an attention-getting sentence in your cover letter.

5. Consult *Figure 26.6* and properly address an envelope for your letter of application and résumé.

# Chapter

# 27

# Job Interviews

## JOB INTERVIEWS

Once the preliminaries of a job search are completed and all current sources of job leads are identified, then businesses are contacted to schedule appointments for interviews and to present personal information. Some places of employment require the completion of employment skills tests. These may test speed and accuracy in typing; basic mathematics; or proficiency in reading, spelling, and grammar. In addition to skills tests, expect to complete application forms, present a professional image, and answer and ask many questions.

Before an interview, it is sensible to practice answering interview questions to increase confidence in oral communication skills. If possible, talk to any of the potential employer's current employees, patients, vendors, or other business entities to learn about the place of employment before the interview, enabling discussion of its services. Be on the lookout for commonly asked difficult and illegal employment questions, be prepared to tell personal stories to highlight unique abilities, and be aware of interview techniques. Maintaining a job search campaign report worksheet helps document all follow-up activities.

## PREPARATION

By preparing for an interview, the job applicant appears organized and professional. Dental office personnel are sophisticated, and a sound communication strategy can improve the chances that the first interview will result in a second interview. Usually, a job offer is not made during the initial interview; instead, expect a series of interviews, meetings, and/or communications. Job applicants need telephone skills and should be familiar with email and fax machines. As noted earlier, all applicants must plan their personal appearance, anticipate interview tactics, be able to field difficult and illegal questions, feel comfortable telling personal stories, and ask questions of the employer. The applicant's first contact with the dental office may be in person, by mail, or by telephone, and involves scheduling an interview.

Prospective employers use the telephone to save time, determine the interest level of applicants, and schedule interviews. Prospective employees use the telephone to save time, find information about job openings, network, save on transportation costs, and employ marketing skills. Tact and business manners are essential when making contact by telephone. Formal greetings such as "Hello" and "Good morning" are appropriate responses. The applicant should state his or her name and affiliation—for example, "My name is Ginger Vitis, a recent dental hygiene graduate. Laurie Young suggested that I call you regarding a dental hygiene position." Or, when necessary, the applicant should explain the purpose of the call, "I am calling in response to the advertisement for the dental hygienist job opening."

## GROOMING AND PERSONAL APPEARANCE

Communicating competency at a job interview begins with a **professional personal appearance**. Judgments regarding a person's character are made within the first minute of contact. It is important to do everything possible to project a positive image and stand out from the competition. Job seekers should follow basic rules for personal appearance when going to a job interview. Although it may seem obvious, grooming, personal hygiene, and cleanliness are fundamental. Applicants should shower or bathe, wear their clean hair away from the face, brush their teeth, and clean and trim their fingernails. Perfume or cologne should not be detectable. Before the interview, applicants should avoid foods that will affect breath odor, use a mouth rinse or a mint to ensure pleasant breath, and avoid exposure to cigarette smoke owing to its lingering scent.

Clothing is also an important personal appearance issue for a job interview presentation. A standard rule is to wear clothing that is one level above the job one is applying for. A uniform is not appropriate dress for an interview in a dental office because this is the attire worn on the job. Clothing should be business-like; clean; pressed; and free of spots, stains, and odors. Appropriate conservative solid colors are black, blue, gray, white, and ivory. Avoid brightly patterned clothing.

Women should wear a suit, a skirt and blouse, or a dress with a jacket. The blouse should not be shiny, revealing, or frilly. Costume jewelry, no matter what the current fashion trend, is distracting and should not be worn for the interview. Makeup should be limited to create a natural look. Men should wear a suit or slacks, dress shirt, sports jacket, and tie. Neckties should be conservative, no wider than the jacket lapels, and made of silk. Patterns should be subtle; if a striped tie is worn, it should be a uniform pattern without variation in widths and color hues.

Both men and women should wear clean and polished shoes. For women, heels should be of a sensible height.

Watches, cell phones, and digital pagers should be turned off; if an electronic device signals during the interview, it suggests that the applicant is not fully focused on the job.

## NONVERBAL COMMUNICATION

Correctly answering the interviewer's questions will not guarantee a second interview that leads to a job offer. Body language or **nonverbal communication** is just as important as appropriate personal appearance and clothing during an interview because the interviewer may believe what is seen instead of what is heard. Create a favorable positive image using body language. Good posture communicates to the interviewer interest and attention. Face toward the interviewer and smile to indicate a cheerful and friendly disposition. Frequent eye contact and a nod of the head communicates understanding and demonstrates confidence. Nervous habits detract from appearance so do not smoke, tap fingers, look at a watch, shuffle feet, look around the room, or chew gum.

## INTERVIEW TACTICS

Hidden rules of behavior or **interview tactics** exist for job interviews. There are an infinite number of ways to sabotage the success of an interview by not recognizing these hidden rules. The job interview begins when entering the door. One interview tactic is to arrive at the correct time, not too early and not too late. Applicants should arrive at the building 30 minutes early to find the office and then double-check their appearance in a public restroom. Enter the office 15 minutes before the scheduled time. This is the real time the interview starts and if you are not early, some employers will consider you tardy.

Some employers ask job applicants to wait for the interview beyond the scheduled time and observe them as they wait. Having to wait for the interview tests the job seeker's patience and composure. An observer will look at body language, nervous habits, and gestures. Other employers may ask candidates to complete an application form or skills test. The job applicant may be observed during this time for appropriate behaviors.

When going to the job interview, do not have a friend wait in the lobby or car; the presence of a support person makes the applicant appear unprofessional and not fully interested in the job. Applicants should greet the receptionist, introduce themselves, and treat this person as if he or she has the power to hire because he or she may be a future coworker. Offer a firm handshake to the interviewer and do not sit until the interviewer sits. When given a choice of seating, select the chair closest to the interviewer. Do not accept gum or a cigarette when offered, as this may be a test of character. The ensuing few minutes of small talk and conversation is preparation for a series of questions so relax, be honest, and listen carefully.

## EMPLOYMENT QUESTIONS

Application materials tell the potential employer about the applicant's education and experience. The interview tells the potential employer about the job applicant's personality. The interviewer may briefly describe the job and the business, then he or she will ask questions concerning skills, abilities, and achievements. Remember that it is appropriate for the applicant to ask questions about the job.

Interview questions fall into two categories: legal and illegal, and the prepared job seeker knows how to respond to them before going to the interview. Many interviewers know which questions are legal and illegal to ask, but other interviewers may not know. **Legal interview questions** are standard and can be easy or difficult. Easy interview questions require a short answer, and more difficult ones require an explanation. Anticipating and responding to difficult questions helps present a positive image to the potential employer. *Box 27.1* can help the job applicant prepare for an interview.

**Illegal interview questions** are those that are not directly related to the job. Such questions bring up topics that are private and are protected by federal law. *Table 27.1*

---

### BOX 27.1  *Typical Interview Questions*

**Easy Questions**
How long have you been in the dental field?
How did you get started in the dental field?
How would you describe your communication style?
Are you flexible with working hours?
What are your employment goals?
Can you describe your energy level?
How would you react to a patient's outburst of emotion?
Are you able to perform multiple tasks at once?

**Difficult Questions**
What can you tell me about yourself?
Why do you want to work here?
What are your future plans?
How would you describe your strongest asset?
Have you had any difficulties with former supervisors or teachers?
What is your grade-point average?
Why have you had so many jobs? (or Why haven't you had many jobs?)
How long do you plan to work here?
Do you plan to continue your education?
What salary do you expect?
How did you get started in this career?
Why should we hire you?
What do you do for relaxation?
Do you use tobacco, drugs, or alcohol?
Do you work best alone or in a group?
Do you have questions to ask?

Adapted from *Developing interview skills.* Clarkston, MI: Oakland Technical Center, Northwest Campus, 1990.

## TABLE 27.1 Comparison of Legal and Illegal Interview Questions

| Category | Question | Legal |
|---|---|---|
| Age | Are you 18 years or older? | Yes |
| | How old are you? | No |
| | When is your birthday? | No |
| Ancestry | Are you from Texas? | No |
| | Were your relatives from Russia | No |
| Arrest record | Have you ever been arrested? | No |
| | Have you ever been convicted of a crime? | Yes |
| Dependents | Do you have any children? | No |
| | Do you plan to have any children? | No |
| Finances | Are you in debt? | No |
| | Do you own a car? | No |
| | Do you receive alimony or child support? | No |
| Handicaps | Do you have a disability? | No |
| | Do you have any impairment that requires special accommodation? | Yes |
| Marital status | How long have you been married? | No |
| | What did you do after becoming widowed? | No |
| National origin | What languages do you speak, read, and write? | Yes |
| | What nationality are you? | No |
| | Are you a citizen of the United States? | Yes |
| | What country are you from? | No |
| Race | Are you Hispanic? | No |
| Religion | Are you Catholic? | No |
| | Do you attend church regularly? | No |
| Skin color | Do you have a suntan? | No |
| Habits | Do you smoke or drink | Yes |

Adapted from *Completing an application*. Clarkston, MI: Oakland Technical Center, Northwest Campus, 1990.

compares legal and illegal interview questions. Illegal interview questions relate to age, ancestry, arrest record, dependents, finances, handicaps, marital status, national origin, race, religion or creed, and skin color.

There are three courses of action an applicant can take when asked an illegal question:

1. Go ahead and answer it, even though it is an illegal question.
2. Respond by asking, "How does that information relate to this position?" or by saying, "I do not think that information is relevant to this job."
3. Contact the Equal Employment Opportunity Commission (EEOC) to report the employer.

Many interviewers may not be familiar with the details of the law. Applicants who are asked illegal questions and wish to pursue a claim with the EEOC must be able to prove that they did not get the job because of the questions asked.

## PERSONAL STORIES

**Personal stories** can illustrate how the applicant handled a challenging situation. They are used in interviews to describe situations, opportunities, duties, actions taken, and results. These stories can be told in response to interview questions such as "What can you tell me about yourself?" Be sure the story includes information about specific professional actions and the positive results of those actions. The savvy applicant presents results in terms of increased production, earnings, or patient satisfaction, which are measures employers readily understand. When preparing for an interview, the job seeker should practice telling personal stories as a means of presenting information in an interesting manner. An example of a personal story is given in *Box 27.2*.

## INTERVIEW THE EMPLOYER

Prospective employees need to ask questions during the interview to determine whether or not they want to work in the establishment. Asking questions shows interest and enthusiasm. Listen carefully to the oral responses of the interviewer and watch for nonverbal actions. Take notes, if necessary, about the job responsibilities and people. *Box 27.3* lists questions job seekers can ask prospective employers.

It is not uncommon to have two, three, or four interviews with the same place of employment. When that happens, the applicant should keep the focus on clinical and communication skills to be consistent. Just as there are questions to ask, there are questions *not* to ask during the interview. Questions relating to salary, benefits, and promotions are best asked at the employment negotiation meeting. These are valid questions; however, the purpose of the first interview is to screen the applicants.

Sometimes, job applicants are interviewed by a number of people in a **group interview.** Many employers have job candidates meet with the entire dental staff because they want to have everyone involved in the decision-making process. When the dental staff

---

### BOX 27.2 *Personal Story*

INTERVIEWER: What can you tell me about yourself?

APPLICANT: I am a recent dental hygiene graduate and have worked as a dental hygienist in the college clinic and in off-campus rotations. The patients were the best part of my education and training. One patient, anxious about having dental treatment, had difficulty speaking English. He was scheduled for a quadrant scaling and root planing, and I was able to help in communication by drawing on a piece of paper. We were able to communicate about what I was doing and when we would be finished. The procedure was completed in the scheduled appointment time, and the patient left pleased. My job satisfaction comes from helping people.

**BOX 27.3** *Questions to Ask the Interviewer*

What is your philosophy of dentistry?
How long have you been a dentist?
What do you like best about your practice?
What type of employee do you get along with the best?
Do you have written job descriptions for employees?
Is this a new position or am I replacing someone?
Why did the last person leave?
What type of housekeeping duties are expected?
How often are performance reviews conducted?
What are your growth projections for next year?
Have you reduced your staff in the last 3 years?

Adapted from Lathrop R. *Who's hiring who*. Berkeley, CA: Ten Speed Press, 1989.

is gathered around a conference table and the job applicant must respond to different personalities, he or she should try to be flexible or think of the interview as making a speech. The job seeker should ask questions about the dental practice when in a group interview. It is still relevant for the applicant to gather information to determine whether the environment of that practice meets his or her goals and expectations.

## CLOSING THE INTERVIEW

Sometimes the interviewer will offer the job at the conclusion of the first interview. Gracefully thank the interviewer for the offer and ask for a couple of days to make a decision. Most employers will agree to this and will negotiate the terms of employment before the applicant accepts the job. It is not advisable to accept the first job offer from the first interview attended. Job applicants who attend several interviews and can negotiation employment terms with more than one dental office will be able to find the job that offers the best chance for personal satisfaction, good compensation, and reasonable employee benefits.

The prospective employer should end the interview, and the applicant should let the interviewer stand up first. The job seeker should thank the interviewer and restate interest in the job, reinforcing the idea that his or her skills will benefit the business. While turning to leave, the applicant should comment on what impressed him or her the most. If the employer has a deadline by which to hire an employee, he or she will say so; the applicant must make sure the interviewer knows the best manner in which to make contact. A week after the interview, the job seeker may call to find out how the job search is proceeding, even if the interviewer indicated that many people had applied for the position.

## FOLLOW-UP ACTIVITIES

When attending an interview that is the result of a referral by a networking contact, let the contact know the results of the interview. Send the prospective employer a hand-written **thank-you note** for the interview, even though it is not clear whether an offer will be made. The thank-you note should be short and sent on the same day as the meeting. Alternatively, send a **follow-up letter** to ask additional questions, furnish more information, emphasize an important point, or serve as a reminder of the applicant's continued interest in the position (*Fig. 27.1*). Although a follow-up letter is not mandatory, it may provide an edge over the other applicants. Another follow-up activity is to inquire by mail or telephone if the job has been filled. Statistically, a job offer is made in one out of every four or five interviews. A key to successful interviewing is to not become discouraged, but to learn from the experience and to improve one's skills for the next time. To keep track of the job search and to evaluate interview performance, applicants should record pertinent information; a sample worksheet is given in *Figure 27.2*.

## CONCEPT SUMMARY

- The first contact with the dental practice is usually made over the telephone, thus tact and business manners are essential.
- Judgments about character and personality are made based on grooming and personal appearance.
- A favorable image can be enhanced by using nonverbal communication such as good posture, eye contact, and smiling.
- Interview tactics include arriving on time, being patient, and using appropriate body language and business manners.
- Anticipation of difficult and illegal employment questions allows the applicant to prepare a proper response.
- Personal stories told during an interview can describe situations, opportunities, duties, actions taken, and results to illustrate competence.
- Employers are asked pertinent interview questions to assess the work environment.
- Follow up includes handwritten notes, letters, and/or telephone calls and the completion of an interview data worksheet to monitor the job search process.

# REVIEW QUESTIONS

1. What preparations are made before the job interview?
2. How does grooming and personal appearance at the interview affect the situation?
3. What type of tests may be required at an interview?
4. How does the telephone affect the job interview process?
5. How does nonverbal communication affect an interviewer?
6. List four interview tactics.
7. What are the three options for responding to an illegal interview question?
8. Why do you ask the employer interview questions?
9. What is the purpose of an interview data worksheet?

123 River Road
Park City, UT 87765

October 15, 2005

Dr. Perry O'Donnell
301 Main Street
Park City, UT 87765

Dear Dr. O'Donnell:

Thank you for taking the time to meet with me today. I am very interested in the Dental Hygiene position and appreciate your considering me for it. Based on our discussion, I feel that I am qualified for this position due to my recent clinical experience and can offer knowledge in recent periodontal trends to your dental practice.

As we discussed in the interview, I am an organized and efficient worker with good communication skills. If you require any additional information, please contact me. Thank you for your time and consideration. I look forward to hearing from you soon.

Sincerely,

Ginger Vitis

**Figure 27.1** Sample "Thank-You for the Interview" letter.

INTERVIEW DATA SHEET

Employer:_____

Contact person/title:_____

Address:_____

Phone:_____

Fax:_____

First contact date:_____

Interview date:_____

Position title:_____

Source of job lead:_____

Key information:_____

Job requirements:_____

| Date | Job Search Activity |
|------|---------------------|
| _____ | Called |
| _____ | Sent résumé |
| _____ | Interview |
| _____ | Sent thank-you letter for interview |
| _____ | Second interview |
| _____ | Employment negotiation |
| _____ | Accepted employment |

**Figure 27.2** Interview data sheet.

# CRITICAL THINKING ACTIVITY

1. Discuss other interview tactics not covered in the text.
2. Do you know of any other hidden rules of interviewing not covered in the text?
3. How do you think the staff at a dental practice would respond to a job applicant who had body piercing, tattooing, and other types of body modification?
4. Prepare three personal stories, including one regarding your ability to communicate in a difficult situation.
5. What interview slip ups can you think of that may ruin the chance of being hired?

## Assignment: Difficult Interview Questions.

1. Prepare an answer to each of the difficult questions listed in *Box 27.1*.
2. Prepare an answer to each of the illegal employment questions listed in *Table 27.1*.
3. Interview a potential employer by using the questions listed in *Box 27.3*.
4. Using the sample provided in *Figure 27.2*, prepare and complete an interview follow-up worksheet to keep track of your interviewing activities.

# Employment Negotiation

## LEARNING OUTCOMES

Upon mastery of the content of this chapter, the student should be able to:
- Discuss common working conditions.
- Realize that drug testing may be required for employment.
- Recognize common employment benefits.
- Write a letter of acceptance and letter of declination.
- Describe an employment contract.
- Negotiate an employment benefit package that includes job description, working hours, salary, and employment benefits.

## KEY TERMS

| | |
|---|---|
| Americans with Disabilities Act | Employment Eligibility Verification Form I-9 |
| at-will | employment negotiation |
| child labor laws | Equal Employment Opportunity Act |
| employment contracts | |

## EMPLOYMENT NEGOTIATION

After the interview process is over and the job has been offered, employment negotiations begin. **Employment negotiation** is the determination and settlement of the working conditions, salary, and benefits for the labor to be performed. It would be unwise to accept a job without first knowing fully the conditions of employment. Before accepting a job offer, consider the job description and office policy and procedures in terms of working conditions, salary, benefits, and office location. To receive adequate compensation, an investigation of salary and benefits is necessary. The job description, working conditions, salary, and contract are determined before employment in a dental practice.

Working in a job that does not match one's interests and ability is not fulfilling in the long term, and boredom, dissatisfaction, or disinterest is likely to occur. Workers are motivated by the opportunity to grow as a person and as a professional. Working in clinical practice will be satisfying only if the environment is suited to the individual's skills and interests. The interview process settled some of the conditions of employment, and other conditions will be found in the office policy and procedure manual. Ask for a copy to read, but remember that receiving or reading the office policy and procedure manual is not an offer of employment.

Most people want to perform their job and be compensated adequately for their daily work. Negotiating the best financial package possible is not a difficult task. A basic understanding of the workplace helps one become an informed negotiator. Negotiation does require a certain attitude and presentation and the background knowledge to be successful.

## WORKING CONDITIONS

Most dental practices are "at-will" employers. **At-will** means that the employer or employee may terminate employment at any time, with or without a reason. Although most employers terminate employment for cause, a reason is not required. The U.S. Fair Labor Standards Act (FLSA) establishes the minimum wage, overtime pay, record keeping, and child labor standards for American workers in private business (*Box 28.1*). Individual states legislate the payment of wages, fringe benefits, complaint procedures, discrimination issues, civil actions, and penalties.

Full-time employment is defined as a workweek of 40 hours (*Box 28.2*). Overtime pay at a rate of $1\frac{1}{2}$ times the regular rate is required by law for any time worked over 40 hours in a workweek for nonexempt employees. Vacation, holiday, severance, and sick pay are not required benefits under the law.

## LABOR LAWS

The federal **Equal Employment Opportunity Act** protects job applicants from discrimination based on race, color, religion, sex, age, national origin, handicap, or any other

---

**BOX 28.1**  *U.S. Fair Labor Standards Act*

Federal minimum wage
   $5.15 per hour beginning September 1, 1997.
   $2.13 per hour for "tipped employees" with tips combined to equal the minimum hourly wage or
      the employer must pay the difference.
Overtime pay
   At least 1½ times an employee's regular rate of pay for all hours worked over 40 in a work week.
Child labor
   An employee must be at least 16 years of age to work in most nonfarm jobs, at least 18 to work in
      nonfarm jobs declared hazardous.
   Youths 14 and 15 years of age may work outside school hours in various nonmining, nonmanufac-
      turing, nonhazardous jobs under the following conditions:
      No more than:
         3 hours on a school day or 18 hours in a school week.
         8 hours on a non-school day or 40 hours in a non-school week.
      And:
         Work may not begin before 7 A.M. or end after 7 P.M., except from June 1 through Labor Day,
            when evening hours are extended to 9 P.M. Different rules apply in agricultural employment.

Adapted from the Fair Labor Standards Act fact sheet. Available online at www.dol.gov/dol/topic/wages/minimumwage.htm.

**BOX 28.2** *Worker Descriptions*

| | |
|---|---|
| Full-time regular employees: | Maintain 40 hours of continuous work |
| Temporary employees: | Work 40 hours or less of limited duration |
| Nonexempt employees: | Work 40 hours or less for the minimum wage |
| Exempt employees: | Work 40 hours or less and are excluded from the minimum wage standards, such as minors and vocational trainees. |

Courtesy U.S. Department of Labor, Bureau of Labor Statistics. Available online at www.dol.gov/compliance/guide/minwage.htm#who.

characteristic protected by law. This law prohibits discrimination in the hiring and promotion of workers and endorses job advancement based on merit. Title 1 of the federal **Americans with Disabilities Act** prohibits discrimination based on disability or limitations. This legislation mandates that employers make reasonable accommodations for workers with a disability. The FLSA's **child labor laws** protect the rights of minors under the age of 18 years in the workplace and prohibit conditions that may be detrimental to their health and well-being. High school students who work in the dental office are protected under these laws and are prohibited from being exposed to ionizing radiation. Minors in the dental office workplace must wear radiation monitors as outlined in the U.S. National Council on Radiation Protection and Measurements.

The **Employment Eligibility Verification Form I-9** (*Fig. 28.1*) is a U.S. Citizenship and Immigration Services, U.S. Department of Homeland Security publication used to certify that a job candidate is legally allowed to work in the United States. Employment opportunity is a strong motivation for people to risk illegal entry to the United States. Form I-9 documents that employees are U.S. citizens or aliens who are authorized to work by verifying the identity of workers. Identifying documents that establish employment eligibility may include but not be limited to a U.S. passport, INS form N-560 or N-561 certificate of U.S. citizenship, INS form N-550 or N-570 certificate of naturalization, INS form N-I-688A employment authorization card, or a Native American tribal document.

## State Dental Practice Act Interpretation

At all times, the allied dental professional is required to adhere to all laws, rules, and regulations regarding practice within the U.S. jurisdiction of employment. Difficult moral dilemmas can occur when dental professionals are asked to perform illegal duties and functions. This matter should be discussed at the beginning of employment to prevent any questionable situations. Otherwise, refusing to follow a directly stated request is considered insubordination, which can be grounds for dismissal.

## Occupational Safety and Health Issues

At all times, the allied dental professional is required to adhere to all federal and state occupational safety and health laws. This includes the use of personal protective equipment, and radiation, nitrous oxide, anesthetic, and mercury safety procedures. Many U.S. businesses are tobacco-free environments, depending on the statutes of the juris-

**Department of Homeland Security**
U.S. Citizenship and Immigration Services

OMB No. 1615-0047; Expires 03/31/07
**Employment Eligibility Verification**

Please read instructions carefully before completing this form. The instructions must be available during completion of this form. **ANTI-DISCRIMINATION NOTICE:** It is illegal to discriminate against work eligible individuals. Employers **CANNOT** specify which document(s) they will accept from an employee. The refusal to hire an individual because of a future expiration date may also constitute illegal discrimination.

**Section 1. Employee Information and Verification.** To be completed and signed by employee at the time employment begins.

| Print Name:   Last | First | Middle Initial | Maiden Name |
|---|---|---|---|

| Address *(Street Name and Number)* | Apt. # | Date of Birth *(month/day/year)* |
|---|---|---|

| City | State | Zip Code | Social Security # |
|---|---|---|---|

**I am aware that federal law provides for imprisonment and/or fines for false statements or use of false documents in connection with the completion of this form.**

I attest, under penalty of perjury, that I am (check one of the following):

☐ A citizen or national of the United States
☐ A Lawful Permanent Resident (Alien #) A _____
☐ An alien authorized to work until _____

(Alien # or Admission #)

| Employee's Signature | Date *(month/day/year)* |
|---|---|

**Preparer and/or Translator Certification.** *(To be completed and signed if Section 1 is prepared by a person other than the employee.) I attest, under penalty of perjury, that I have assisted in the completion of this form and that to the best of my knowledge the information is true and correct.*

| Preparer's/Translator's Signature | Print Name |
|---|---|

| Address *(Street Name and Number, City, State, Zip Code)* | Date *(month/day/year)* |
|---|---|

**Section 2. Employer Review and Verification.** To be completed and signed by employer. Examine one document from List A OR examine one document from List B and one from List C, as listed on the reverse of this form, and record the title, number and expiration date, if any, of the document(s).

| List A | OR | List B | AND | List C |
|---|---|---|---|---|
| Document title: _____ | | _____ | | _____ |
| Issuing authority: _____ | | _____ | | _____ |
| Document #: _____ | | _____ | | _____ |
| Expiration Date *(if any):* _____ | | _____ | | _____ |
| Document #: _____ | | | | |
| Expiration Date *(if any):* _____ | | | | |

**CERTIFICATION - I attest, under penalty of perjury, that I have examined the document(s) presented by the above-named employee, that the above-listed document(s) appear to be genuine and to relate to the employee named, that the employee began employment on** *(month/day/year)* _____ **and that to the best of my knowledge the employee is eligible to work in the United States. (State employment agencies may omit the date the employee began employment.)**

| Signature of Employer or Authorized Representative | Print Name | Title |
|---|---|---|

| Business or Organization Name | Address *(Street Name and Number, City, State, Zip Code)* | Date *(month/day/year)* |
|---|---|---|

**Section 3. Updating and Reverification.** To be completed and signed by employer.

| A. New Name *(if applicable)* | B. Date of rehire *(month/day/year)* *(if applicable)* |
|---|---|

C. If employee's previous grant of work authorization has expired, provide the information below for the document that establishes current employment eligibility.

Document Title: _____   Document #: _____   Expiration Date (if any): _____

I attest, under penalty of perjury, that to the best of my knowledge, this employee is eligible to work in the United States, and if the employee presented document(s), the document(s) I have examined appear to be genuine and to relate to the individual.

| Signature of Employer or Authorized Representative | Date *(month/day/year)* |
|---|---|

**NOTE:** This is the 1991 edition of the Form I-9 that has been rebranded with a current printing date to reflect the recent transition from the INS to DHS and its components.

Form I-9 (Rev. 05/31/05)Y Page 2

**Figure 28.1** Employment Eligibility Verification Form. Courtesy U.S. Department of Homeland Security.

diction. Tobacco smoking is prohibited in public or is limited to certain areas. Dress codes are established for health and safety reasons in addition to promoting a professional business image.

## CONDITIONS OF EMPLOYMENT

### Drug and Alcohol Testing

Many businesses require drug tests as a condition of employment or when warranted. There is a sense of concern on the part of businesses in determining illegal drug use because of its effect on absenteeism and healthcare costs. Illegal drug habits can be discovered through the preemployment testing of hair and urine. Signs of drug use evidence remains in the hair for several months, and hair testing is considered more accurate than urine testing because drug molecules are bound in the interior of the hair. If confronted with a request to give hair and urine samples as a condition of employment or when asked to do so once employed, employees must decide whether or not to comply with the request. Be aware that refusing to comply may be cause for employment termination.

### Working Hours

Employers want employees who will be there and who will be on time. Attendance is paramount in providing oral healthcare services to the public. There is a great deal of variation when it comes to working hours owing to provider preferences and patient scheduling. Work schedules are established and should remain constant. Some dental offices have evening hours and are open on Saturdays. Office policy will dictate hours of operation and requirements in instances of absence and tardiness.

### Criminal Background Checks

Criminal background checks may be a condition of employment. Notification and authorization for a criminal background check must be obtained in writing before the employer can carry out these investigations. Background checks investigate an applicant's personal history, educational background, military record, and motor vehicle and criminal records.

### Communication Policy

Electronic communication systems include computers with Internet capability, telephones, and voice or electronic mail. This technology is available in dental practices as a means to conduct business transactions, not personal matters. The inappropriate use of these systems has prompted businesses to develop policies to prevent fraudulent activities, the use of offensive or obscene materials, harassment, and the attempt to defeat security systems. New employees should check whether the employer allows personal use of the electronic systems before incurring any criticism or claims of misconduct.

## EMPLOYMENT SALARY

Information on the average wage and employment benefits for allied dental professionals changes from year to year and is based on geographical location. This information is available from several sources. Contact the American Dental Assistants Association, American Dental Hygienists' Association, American Dental Association, *Dental Management,* and *U.S. News & World Report* for current salary information on allied dental professionals. This information may also be available through the Internet.

### Salary Negotiation Tactics

Negotiating a salary for the first time can be an emotional event, and the new employee may feel uncomfortable because this is not a frequently performed task. Future success and happiness may depend on how salary is negotiated. The new employee should use assertiveness skills to keep emotions under control; be low key, sincere, and easy-going; and avoid being aggressive or emotional. If possible, avoid negotiating salary and benefits at the time of the job offer. Instead, ask for time to think it over. When this is not possible, it may be wise not to answer questions about money. The employee should try to talk around the subject by steering the conversation to the job until he or she is sure the practice is committed to hiring. By pleasantly avoiding naming a number, the potential employee lets the employer state a range. Another option is to direct the conversation to "What kind of salary range is available for this job?" If forced to give a range, the new hire should aim higher than the salary wanted because it may be a long time before any pay increases are granted, unless regular salary and/or wage increases have been specifically negotiated.

If the salary offered is too low, let the employer know how pleasing the offer is and ask for time to consider the salary. Express slight vulnerability, noting that accepting the job at that rate of pay will be difficult. Call the next day, discuss the problems with the salary, and suggest a redefinition of the job description to increase the pay. The wise negotiator will make positive statements about the position and suggest a salary figure that is 10% higher than the amount offered. Another manner in which to negotiate a higher wage is to request an early salary review after 30 or 60 days of employment.

## EMPLOYMENT BENEFITS

Salary is not the only thing to consider during the job selection process. Employment benefits are tax-free additions to salary and wages. For example, healthcare insurance coverage may be desired. This is an important benefit to negotiate; perhaps a reduced amount in salary will cover the cost of healthcare insurance. When a spouse has healthcare insurance coverage, then vacation time or paid personal days may be a more desirable substitution.

Selection and negotiation of employment benefits depends on what the employer currently offers and is willing to provide. Recall that FLSA does not require vacation, holiday, severance, or sick pay. The most commonly shared benefit is paid vacation time. *Box 28.3* contains examples of employment benefits offered in typical dental office employment packages.

**BOX 28.3** *Dental Employment Benefits*

Continuing education
Free dental care
Healthcare insurance coverage
Holiday pay
Life insurance
Long-term disability insurance
Malpractice insurance coverage
Paid parking
Paid personal days

Pension plan participation
Professional association dues
Profit sharing
Severance pay
Short-term disability insurance
Sick leave and pay
Uniform allowance
Vacation pay

## ACCEPTING OR DECLINING JOB OFFERS

When a job has been offered and the employment terms have been negotiated, the new employee should write a letter of confirmation to legally agree to the employment terms—even if he or she accepted the job orally. The new employee must file the letter for safekeeping. The letter should also confirm the starting date and time (*Fig. 28.2*).

It is proper business etiquette to notify an employer when not accepting a job offer (*Fig. 28.3*). This closes the negotiation process and allows the employer to find another candidate. When this process is conducted in a positive manner, the opportunity exists for reapplication to the same dental practice. For oral healthcare professionals living in a small community, it is important not to burn any bridges.

---

June 5, 2006

Dr. Yank M. Out
123 Main Street
La Jolla, CA 99888

Dear Dr. Out:

I received your letter in the mail today and will gladly accept the dental hygienist position. I feel that my training and skills will contribute to your business.

As we had discussed in the interview, I will need to give my current employer 2 weeks notice. I will be available to start work at your office on June 19, 2006. If you require any additional information before I start, please feel free to contact me at my home address.

I appreciate your offer of employment and your confidence in my abilities to do the job. I look forward to working with you.

Sincerely,

Anna Septic, RDH
44 Woody Trail
El Cajon, CA 97700

---

**Figure 28.2** Sample acceptance letter.

April 2, 2006

Dr. Yank M. Out
123 Main Street
La Jolla, CA 99888

Dear Dr. Out:

After careful consideration of the offer for the dental hygiene position, I must decline at this time.

As we had discussed in the interview, I am seeking a position that is close to my home to reduce commuting time. I appreciate your offer of employment and your confidence in my abilities to do the job. I wish you continued success in your endeavors.

Sincerely,


Anna Septic, RDH
44 Woody Trail
El Cajon, CA 97700

**Figure 28.3** Letter of declination.

## EMPLOYMENT CONTRACTS

A common business maxim is "get it in writing." This is a means to verify the terms of an oral agreement. An employment package is an agreement between the allied dental professional and the employer. **Employment contracts** are written legal documents of agreement that set forth the obligations and compensation pertaining to work. An employment contract protects the worker's rights and prevents any misunderstandings regarding job description, working hours, salary, interpretation of the state dental practice act, occupational health and safety issues, and other benefits.

Many workers rights in the United States are outlined in employment contracts. An attorney should prepare the employment contract for the dental hygienist and dentist relationship. Topics covered in an employment agreement are listed in *Box 28.4*.

**BOX 28.4** *Employment Contract Topics*

| | |
|---|---|
| Employment benefits | Starting date |
| Legal obligations | Termination and severance |
| Occupational health and safety issues | Worker's compensation |
| Performance review | Working hours |
| Salary | |

## CONCEPT SUMMARY

- Working conditions, salary, and benefits are negotiated employment terms.
- Labor law mandates many oral healthcare worker requirements.
- A written letter to accept or decline an offer of employment completes negotiations.
- Employment contracts are legal documents defining employer–employee duties in the employment relationship.

# R E V I E W   Q U E S T I O N S

1. Why is a clear understanding of the job description necessary?
2. What are the legal working hours and salary rate as determined by the U.S. Fair Labor Standards Act?
3. Why is it necessary to negotiate the interpretation of the state dental practice act before employment?
4. What is the allied dental professional's duty in regard to health and safety?
5. List the most common employment benefits in dental offices.

6. Why is a letter of acceptance written?
7. Why is it a good practice to write a letter of declination?
8. Is it a good idea to use an employment contract? Explain your answer.
9. How do child labor laws affect the practice of dentistry?
10. Why would an employer require drug testing before hiring?

## Assignment: Acceptance Letter

1. Write an acceptance letter using the letter in *Figure 28.2* as a guide.
2. Write a letter of declination using the letter in *Figure 28.3* as a guide.

# Healthcare Interactions

Upon mastery of the content of this chapter, the student should be able to:
- Conceptualize the tenets of authority.
- Communicate with coworkers using formal and informal oral and written techniques.
- Recognize the factors affecting communication with co-workers such as nonverbal cues, physiologic clocks, level of attention, personal issues, listening, and gender.
- Use assertion principles for proper message transfer.
- Acknowledge that teamwork skills depend on positive interdependence and the use of creative thinking, problem solving, leadership, and negotiation skills.

**KEY TERMS**

| | |
|---|---|
| aggressiveness | influence |
| assertiveness | informal communication |
| authority | leadership |
| autocrat | listening |
| co-dependence | positive interdependence |
| counterdependence | power |
| formal oral communication | teamwork |
| formal written communication | |

## HEALTHCARE INTERACTIONS

The authority figures in the dental practice may be the employer dentist, independent practice hygienist, and/or office manager with whom employees communicate. Communication among coworkers involves formal, informal, oral, and written techniques. Many factors affect healthcare worker interactions, such as physiologic clocks, level of attention, personal issues, listening, and gender. The use of assertion principles improves the likelihood of proper message transfer among coworkers. The dental team must be able to communicate; its success depends on positive interdependence.

## WORKPLACE INTERACTIONS

Healthcare interactions are the daily communication activities among the dental team. The dental professional participates on the dental healthcare team by using communication, teamwork, problem solving, and conflict-resolution skills. Team members must be able to follow and give directions, communicate with supervisors, make and respond to requests, and gather and use information. To do this, professionals use various modes of behavior in different situations. Sometimes, dental office interactions involve negative situations in which assertiveness skills are required.

### Authority

Employers may employ an office manager with whom the dental professional communicates. The staff is expected to follow directions, instructions, and directives issued by the office manager. The communication duties of the office manager are basically the same in all dental offices. Office managers apply communication skills for the daily operation of business, scheduling of employees and patients, dissemination of information on policies and procedures, and resolving conflicts.

The office manager gives directives and the employees comply. The reason an employee does so is based on three principles: power, influence, and authority. **Power** is the force one holds over another by means of coercion. The use of power supplies something of value that a person cannot obtain elsewhere or deprives the person of something valued. When an individual uses power over another, he or she does not seek consensus or agreement for compliance. **Influence** is the ability to persuade others to obtain compliance. When an individual uses influence, the other person accepts it voluntarily. **Authority** is the right to issue orders, make assignments, coordinate activities, and delegate tasks. Office managers are empowered to use authority to give instructions, directions, and suggestions on behalf of the employer.

Most dentists are male and most dental assistants and dental hygienists are female. Although these statistics are changing, males still dominate many positions of power in dentistry. Employers control conduct in the dental office, thus creating an autocratic hierarchy. An **autocrat** is a person with unquestioned power over others. Awareness of these facts helps in the understanding that male employers may communicate using power over female employees instead of authority and influence.

## COMMUNICATION SKILLS

Harmony among the dental staff is best when there is a spirit of friendship and teamwork, which in turn fosters a productive work environment. Friendly relationships with coworkers can make the time at work full of joy and fun. Good communication skills help establish and maintain good relationships with coworkers. Dental hygienists communicate with other members of the staff in a variety of ways: formally and informally, verbally and nonverbally. As mentioned earlier, appearance, physiologic clocks, level of attention, personal issues, and listening affect communication with coworkers. The dental office workspace is usually small, and more than 80% of the day is spent in that confined space. Effective communication with coworkers while in close proximity to each other takes some effort, but the rewards are immeasurable.

In the first few minutes of any interaction, each individual assesses the other following a sequenced process. Assessment begins with skin color, sex, age, personal appearance, body language, and the nature of the other's touch. At this time, first impressions will determine more than half of the meaning of the message. Because people make judgments about appearance, it is important to be aware that overall appearance is judged quickly. Few people will trust what they hear over what they see.

## Formal Communication

Formal communication can also be called "following the chain of command." Each workplace has a layered social system, and individuals have different roles and responsibilities based on power or status. **Formal oral communication** is the oral exchange of instructions, information, or ideas. A person's cultural background or the use of power can influence oral message transfer. In the dental office, formal oral communication may be established so that situations in need of attention are reported to the office manager instead of the employer. As an example, reporting to the office manager helps the dentist concentrate on patient care and comfort, which in turn reduces the workday stressors for the dentist.

**Formal written communication** is the printed or transmitted exchange of messages that follows a chain of command. For example, the office manager determines employee scheduling. When an employee needs to take a personal day off from work, a written note to the office manager may be required before the request can be considered. Another example of formal written communication is the office policy and procedure manual that outlines policy, procedures, protocols, and other job-related expectations.

## Informal Communication

**Informal communication** is the spread of information via talking and writing. It can include written directives, small talk, and office gossip. Informal communication can also be anonymous, such as an employee suggestion box. Informal communication travels quickly and can become the source of inaccurate information. Communication distance is an important aspect of informal communication and may be associated with cultural background or the use of power. Communication should occur outside an individual's personal space, usually at arm's length. This distance is reduced during conversation with friends and increased with strangers.

## Physiologic Clocks

Communication can be affected by each person's physiologic (or internal) clock. Our physiologic clocks affect such things as the time of day when our body temperature and functioning are at their highest. Some individuals are "morning people" who tend to go to bed early and are more alert and productive early in the morning. Others are "night owls," preferring to stay up late at night; they are more alert and productive in the evening. By recognizing the differences among coworkers' internal clocks, staff can improve communication in the office.

## Level of Attention

Controlling one's attention level can improve interactions with coworkers. Attention control is the monitoring and adjusting of attention level. This first begins by becoming aware of one's own attention level. Some activities require more attention than others—for example, setting up an operatory requires less attention than engaging in formal oral communication with a coworker. There are times when raising or lowering the attention level will ensure proper message transfer, prevent boredom, or help when hearing unpleasant news.

## Personal Issues

Humans bring past experiences with them to work every day. Many people have personal issues from dealing with problems at home. Although the dental professional is trained in a specific area of expertise, there are times when outside family issues may affect a coworker's performance at work. Two common issues that affect work relationships are co-dependence and counterdependence. **Co-dependence** relates to a relationship in which one person is psychologically reliant on someone who has a physical or psychological addiction, as to alcohol or drugs. **Counterdependence** relates to the behavior of a person who relies too heavily on himself or herself. These two issues can undermine the interactions of the dental team and disrupt office harmony.

## Listening

**Listening** is paying attention to what another person is saying. This is one of the most important parts of communication. Allied dental personnel spend a good portion of the day listening to patients and colleagues. It is tempting to jump to conclusions and interrupt the speaker to speed up the conversation. To be a better listener, let the speaker finish, resist interrupting, and suspend judgment to focus on the patient. Communication is a two-way process, and listening skills involve more than just hearing what is being said. Listening involves interpreting and evaluating what is heard and eventually responding to it.

Healthcare professionals are accustomed to collecting facts in conversations, but they must remember to look at body language, emotions, and attitudes. As a listener, separate the person from the words and watch for actions that may contradict what the person is saying. Body position such as crossed arms, standing rigidly, slouching, or touching sends a significant portion of message transfer. Touch is used frequently to reassure someone and includes a touch on the hand, pat on the back, firm handshake, or a hug. Touching someone is therapeutic and projects more concern for the receiver than the spoken word can. Nonverbal sounds such as a *hmm* or clearing of the throat are also ways to send messages. Ask questions when the other's body language does not support what he or she has said.

In addition, make judgments about message transfer by listening to the tone and inflection of the voice, as the tone of voice indicates emotions. Limit distractions and restate what the speaker said. This is a method of verifying that the intended message was received. The healthcare professional should have two goals when listening:

- Try to listen to the other's message.
- Determine if the person has heard and understood the message given to him or her.

## Intergender Communications

Although major research studies on gender communication in the dental office have not been conducted, information is available from studies on male–female communication, opinions, and anecdotes. In the past, society placed a higher value on male behavior, attitudes, and achievements, and females were conditioned to be subordinate. Although equal rights are legally granted, women must learn certain behaviors to earn respect in the dental office setting and to achieve and maintain job satisfaction. One such behavior is to be verbally direct. Women are focused on feelings and tend to add other elements to message transfer, which detract from the intended meaning. A technique to practice is stating exactly what is meant and avoiding any unnecessary words that may alter the message. Men have the desire to take control of situations that might force women to speak in an assertive and confident manner.

## ASSERTIVENESS SKILLS

**Assertiveness** is speaking in a positive, consistent manner to express needs, wants, feelings, thoughts, or opinions or to give praise and convey information. It is a communication skill needed when speaking to coworkers, authority figures, patients, and vendors. This skill allows an individual to gain confidence and to influence people appropriately in a business situation. The most common assertions are straightforward statements used to raise an issue with someone for the first time. Assertions are direct sentences, for example, "I need to leave by five o'clock." Repeating an assertion reemphasizes the need when the initial statement was ignored or devalued.

Assertions can have an element of empathy to allow the listener to recognize that the speaker is aware of and sensitive to the present situation. For example, the dental professional may say, "I understand that you don't like the idea of an air polisher; however, I'd like you to try it. If you can't tolerate it after I've done a couple of teeth, I'll stop." And "I recognize how difficult it is to be precise about out-of-pocket costs, but we would like to give you a rough estimate."

Assertion statements can be used when someone's undesirable behavior produces negative effects. The assertion statement should contain information on when the behavior occurs, its effect, how it feels, and what behavior is preferred. In this situation, negative feelings of hurt, anger, or resentment toward the person may occur. Making an assertive statement allows one to express feelings without an emotional disturbance and helps one take responsibility for feelings and expressions. An example is "When you schedule an extra patient before lunchtime, it involves my working during lunch. I feel annoyed about this, so in the future I'd like to have any extra patients scheduled earlier in the morning or right after lunch."

Aggressiveness is the opposite of assertiveness. **Aggressiveness** is speaking in a negative or quarrelsome manner; it is not conducive to good working relationships. Gaining assertiveness skills and confidence takes practice. Attempting to understand the point of view of the other person earns respect, which is reinforced when restating information in a positive manner.

## TEAMWORK

Employers want employees with teamwork skills. **Teamwork** is the positive interdependent functioning of a group of people. **Positive interdependence** means that people are connected within a group, and the group cannot succeed without the help of each member. This enables the individuals to become stronger people. Daily, the dental office staff works together to reach shared goals. Every team member uses many skills when participating within the group. The working environment involves frequent interaction with changing groups of people who are from a variety of backgrounds with unique personal histories. By listening to the thoughts and opinions of group members who may have minority, ethnic, or economic differences, the dental professional learns to be sensitive to their needs. Compromise helps oral healthcare workers achieve team goals.

Frequently, daily goals are discussed in the 15-minute morning meeting, at which the entire dental office staff can discuss the day's schedule of events. Many collaborative skills are needed by each team member to participate in these group discussions. An active group member should be able to identify with the goals, values, customs, and culture of the group. Collaborative skills needed for teamwork include cooperation, identifying and solving problems, leadership, decision making, and conflict management.

Cooperation is a vital component of a healthy connected group of people. It is an important aspect of participating within a group. Cooperation maximizes the dental team's potential for positive joint efforts. This interdependence makes for a positive situation. When the dental team members work against each other to achieve a goal only one or a few can attain, it is called competition. Competition is the maximizing of an individual's effort. This can have a negative effect on office harmony. Coworkers who work by themselves to accomplish goals unrelated to the others are individualistic. Individualism is considered neither positive nor negative.

Positive interdependence creates the desire to work to achieve the goals of the group. Goal accomplishment requires interpersonal skills, interaction, and accountability. Imagine that a bonus at the end of the month is the current goal of the dental team. Establishing mutual goals to complete by the end of the month allows the group to plan how it can accomplish this task. During the month, each person does the work that is necessary and interacts by helping and encouraging the efforts of coworkers, and each individual is accountable for goal achievement.

## LEADERSHIP

**Leadership** is the ability to guide others. Sometimes it is better to be a leader, but other times, it is better to be a follower. Leaders are chosen for their trustworthiness, decision-making ability, initiative, tact, dependability, and friendliness. In today's business climate, employers want independent thinkers who can identify opportunities and problems and then take action. Such independent thinkers are often chosen as team leaders. Determine when to be a leader or a follower depending on what is required to get the job done.

### CONCEPT SUMMARY

- Employees comply with directives based on power, influence, and authority.
- Skills are needed for formal oral and written communication as well as for informal communication.
- Assertiveness is a communication skill necessary for positive healthcare worker interactions.
- Teamwork interactions connect the oral healthcare workers in a positive collegial manner.

# REVIEW QUESTIONS

1. How is communication with coworkers accomplished using the following techniques: formal oral, formal written, informal oral, and informal written communication?

2. How are an individual's communication skills affected by his or her physiologic clock?

3. What happens to communication with coworkers when their level of attention is low?

4. What personal issues affect communication with coworkers?

5. How do teamwork skills depend on positive interdependence?

6. How can touch be a communication technique?

7. What skill would a person in an autocratic relationship need to use to communicate effectively in the workplace?

8. What is included in a basic assertion?

9. Why do we listen to coworkers?

10. What is an appropriate communications distance and why is it important?

# Maintaining Employment

## LEARNING OUTCOMES

Upon mastery of the content of this chapter, the student should be able to:
- Identify personality type principles.
- Recognize that lifelong learning may include creative thinking training.
- Discuss staff meetings.
- Conceptualize the effects of stress.
- Describe conflict resolution.
- Define sexual harassment.
- Participate in job performance review.
- Discuss voluntary and involuntary employment termination and recognize that everyone experiences failure.

## KEY TERMS

| | |
|---|---|
| environmental sexual harassment | quid pro quo sexual harassment |
| future envisioning | severance |
| job stress | severance pay |
| performance review | vicarious liability |

## MAINTAINING EMPLOYMENT

Whether involved in an ongoing active job search, starting a new job, or working in an established position, the dental professional must plan for continuing success and long-term job enjoyment. Performing dental hygiene duties with the other dental team members to the best of one's abilities is only one aspect of employment. There will always be competition for employment, and remaining competitive while maintaining team spirit helps one get and keep a job. The world of work has its ups and downs; this chapter serves as a guide through the inevitable tribulations of employment.

Success on the job is more than clinical excellence, good communication skills, and exemplary work habits. Job success entails dealing with coworker personalities, using creativity, participating in daily morning meetings, coping with job stress, managing conflict, preventing sexual harassment, undergoing periodic performance reviews, and accepting possible job termination and the potential for failure.

## PERSONALITY TYPES

Many public institutions and private and public businesses use assessment testing to help individuals investigate interests and aptitudes. The Myers-Briggs interest inventory assesses abilities and attitudes to determine personality types. It was developed by the military during World War II to classify people by character traits to help them be more productive. An individual's preferences are compared to those of people in fields of work who enjoy what they do. When taking this test, the individual answers questions that are associated with four principles. Once the responses are analyzed, they are grouped into four main categories: extroverted or introverted, sensing or intuitive, thinking or feeling, and judging or perceiving. From this inventory, 16 personality types are possible, each correlated to various occupations. The dental team will consist of people with a mix of these personality types. Because people are not exactly the same from day to day, communicating and working with the staff on a daily basis can sometimes be challenging.

## CREATIVITY

Lifelong learning, including creativity training, helps the professional maintain a competitive edge and long-term employment. Every person in business has clients seeking a quality product or service. Work processes are evaluated using creativity, problem solving, and future envisioning, which all improve the quality of care. Creativity and innovation improve productivity, work quality, and employee job satisfaction. In general, American companies offer their employees more creative-thinking and problem-solving courses than reading and writing courses. Creativity training has increased in the past decade, and business analysts note that training in creativity and in problem solving are frequently combined because they use similar processes. Creativity also helps when planning for the future and developing mission statements. **Future envisioning** is based on a mission statement–oriented strategic plan that guides a group into the future.

## STAFF MEETINGS

An essential component of a well-managed dental practice is the staff meeting. These meetings are used to keep the group focused on the practice's goals. They also allow the dental office staff to come together to discuss office operations. Effective communication takes practice, and the staff meeting provides a forum for everyone's input. Monthly staff meetings should be held during working hours at peak energy time, such as morning or lunchtime, to maintain a smooth and efficiently managed dental office.

Typically, agenda items are submitted, prioritized, and presented to the staff by the office manager. Agenda items are the topics to be discussed at staff meetings. Reports on production, collection, new patients, and projects are examples of agenda items. Problems and concerns that arise from the staff or management can receive attention and suggestions from all employees in an open forum situation. The use of problem-solving techniques, listening skills, and brainstorming at staff meetings facilitates resolution of staff concerns.

Announcements regarding new procedures, policies, or government regulations to be instituted by the dental practice are made at staff meetings. With the mandate of continuing education, the staff meeting is an excellent time to conduct an in-service training.

Some dental offices use one staff meeting a year to renew the staff members' cardio-pulmonary resuscitation (CPR) certification. Another form of staff meeting, often called "lunch and learn," enables the dental staff to have lunch together and receive updates on new trends or high-tech advances. A sample morning meeting agenda is given in *Box 30.1*.

## JOB STRESS

Simply stated, **job stress** is the frequent bombardment of an employee with situations that require constant adaptation. It is not labeled as good or bad, it is just a part of the work environment. What is good or bad about job-related stress is how the dental professional labels and handles these situations. There are many reasons to reduce job stress. Stress affects employment success and damages overall health, causing headaches, allergies, illness, heart problems, mental health problems, and early death.

Stress-beating strategies are important not only for good health but also for maintaining employment. These strategies include controlling, compromising, avoiding, or accepting stress. Controlling stress is achieved by identifying the causes and eliminating them, communicating anger, or dealing with problems immediately. Compromising or being ready to settle for less is a stress reducer. Avoiding stress by finding different situations or taking a break from a problem can be useful. Accepting that life will have moments of stress and using relaxation techniques can give a sense of control to help in dealing with daily stressors. Another stress-beating strategy is to talk the stress out with a good listener, either a counselor, a trusted person, or a mental health professional. Avoid or ease the physical effects of stress on the body by eating well, sleeping properly, exercising, avoiding overscheduling, using assertion skills, saying no, and laughter. Ergonomics can further reduce the physical effects of stress on the body.

## CONFLICT

Conflict is a negative aspect of working in cooperative groups. When conflict happens, everyone in the dental office feels it. Conflict occurs when there is a clash between ideas, values, or interests and the equilibrium of the group is disturbed. Because conflict has a negative effect on office harmony, conflict resolution skills help change the situation into a learning experience. There are two ways to deal with conflict: avoid it or confront it. *Box 30.2* outlines the procedural steps for conflict resolution.

---

**BOX 30.1** *Morning Meeting Agenda*

Concerns and comments regarding yesterday's schedule
Discussion of today's schedule
Open schedule time
New patient information
Financial information
Production goals
Discussion of tomorrow's schedule

**BOX 30.2**  *Conflict Resolution*

1. Study the conflict during an uninterrupted period of time.
2. Compile a list of both sides of the issue.
3. Read each list and label the positive and negative issues.
4. Compile a list of the positive and negative issues.
5. Group the issues into similar categories and rewrite the list.
6. Set the list aside for a period of time.
7. Weigh the positive and negative forces and make a decision.

## SEXUAL HARASSMENT

In the business place, employees may feel uneasy when references to sexual situations are made. The ratio of women who will experience sexual harassment before they retire is 6–9 out of every 10. Federal Equal Employment Opportunity Commission (EEOC) guidelines, based on Title VII of the Civil Rights Act of 1964, define two types of sexual harassment. **Quid pro quo sexual harassment** occurs when unwelcome sexual advances are made that affect hiring, firing, or advancement. **Environmental sexual harassment** occurs when unwelcome sexual behavior creates a hostile work environment. Sexual harassment includes sexual advances, requests for sexual favors, improper comments (sexual slur, insult, innuendo, or physical contact), and verbal or physical contacts that are sexual in nature. When submission to sexual harassment is made a condition of employment, it interferes with work performance and creates an intimidating or offensive environment.

Sexual harassment in any situation is reprehensible and subverts the working environment because victims feel degraded. Employees have the right to freedom from employment discrimination and hostile working conditions. Employers should have a written sexual harassment policy in the office procedures manual because they are liable not only for their own conduct, but also the conduct of their employees, the harassment of workers by nonemployees, and the effect such harassment may have on other employees. If benefits were granted to an employee because of acquiescence to sexual demands, other qualified employees who were denied benefits may sue for unlawful sex discrimination. **Vicarious liability** means that not knowing about a sexual harassment situation is no defense if the person is in a position to supervise (this includes the dentist or office manager).

### Steps to Take

Any staff member who has a complaint of sexual harassment about anyone at work, including supervisors, co-workers, patients, or visitors, does not have to accept the situation. *Box 30.3* outlines a course of action for dealing with sexual harassment.

## PERFORMANCE REVIEW

The **performance review** is a private meeting between the allied dental professional and the employer to discuss job accomplishment. Performance reviews are conducted pri-

**BOX 30.3** *Sexual Harassment*

1. Tell the harasser that his or her comments or advances are not welcomed.
2. Verbalize your objections when the advances begin.
3. Put your objections in writing to the harasser.
4. Request a written response.
5. Talk to colleagues.
6. Keep notes about each incident, recording when it occurred, what happened, and who was present.
7. If these efforts fail, follow the office's grievance procedures.
8. If the supervisor is the harasser, contact the U.S. Equal Employment Opportunity Commission or State Employment Security Commission.

vately and may be scheduled quarterly, semiannually, or yearly. The more frequent the employee evaluation, the more valid it is; infrequent reviews tend to substitute for routine conversation. An appraisal time is scheduled when there are no interruptions. The areas of job performance appraised are skills development, work habits, communication skills, and professional development.

The performance review begins by concentrating on the positive areas of job performance. This provides an opportunity for building a communication bridge between the employer and the employee. Areas that need improvement are then discussed, and solutions or goals are set. Performance review time may be when a conversation about remuneration or supplemental benefits is held. Be prepared to state the case for a raise based on merit and have a situational story ready to present to validate a request for salary or benefit increase. A good performance review is not a guarantee of salary or benefit increase.

Once goals are established and set for the next review period, keep track of ways they have been met. This may be done following a self-evaluation process. This provides a progress report to be presented at the next performance review. Pay raises and benefit increases are based on merit, so be sure to record any progress made toward goal achievement.

# JOB TERMINATION

## Voluntary Termination

Any worker may quit a job at any time for any reason without warning. There are many good reasons to quit a job. Experts agree that finding another job before quitting is the best course of action. Cordially plan and execute exiting from the dental office because the manner in which an employee leaves may well affect his or her ability to be hired again. Notice of intent to leave should be in writing and hand delivered to the office manager or employer. Notice of employment termination is given to the employer with enough time available to find a replacement; usually, 2 weeks' notice is sufficient.

A letter of termination may or may not contain the reason the employee is leaving the job. Citing communication problems with coworkers is not a wise action because it may hinder the dental professional's chances of receiving a good recommendation from the practice. Instead, the letter should indicate that the employee wants to make a life change. The letter should state the last date of employment and should be written in a positive manner. When leaving the office on good terms, ask the employer to be a reference in the future. A sample resignation letter is given in *Figure 30.1*. Searching for the next job should be done out of the office.

## Involuntary Termination and Severance

An employee can be terminated from the job at any time. **Severance** is another term associated with being terminated. Keep in mind that nobody owes you a job. Being terminated can be the result of performing the job satisfactorily or unsatisfactorily. Termination for unsatisfactory work must be well documented by the employer. Often, several performance review meetings are held to discuss performance before an employee is fired for such reasons. Performance goals are set with the expectation of satisfactory goal achievement.

When termination occurs, many feelings may emerge—from disappointment to bitterness, anger, and sadness. In some instances, severance pay is given to the employee. **Severance pay** is a monetary payment based on length of service given to an employee once employment is terminated. It is not a requirement for employers to disburse severance pay.

## Feelings of Failure

No one is successful all of the time. Failure happens to everyone at some point. Some professionals fail a course or the board examinations the first time around; most have

---

123 Buffalo Pass
Fog Tree, ND 54779


June 14, 2006


Dr. Pete E. Atrics
123 Northland Drive
Southfield, MN 50799


Dear Dr. Atrics:

This letter serves as official notice of my intention to resign my position effective July 1, 2006. My plans to move to another state have made it necessary to leave. Thank you for the opportunity to work in your office, and I wish you continued success in your endeavors.

Sincerely,


Ann Estesia, RDH

---

**Figure 30.1** Sample letter of resignation.

given a poor interview, and others have been fired from a job. Whatever the circumstances, the individual's self-esteem is damaged, and he or she may blame others or deny that there are any problems. Managing failure is necessary for getting back on course with a life's plan.

When a significant setback happens, an analysis of what went wrong is in order. This time to regroup is an emotional process. A loving environment is a good place to start to rebuild self-esteem. Talking about the experience with a trusted friend or family member helps restore wounded pride.

After the emotional aspect of failure has eased, a thoughtful, reflective assessment of what occurred should be conducted. At this time, reconsider the events to ascertain why failure happened. Once this reflection has occurred, it is time to reevaluate the career plan and personal goals to settle on an action plan with new timelines. Set a course for completion, whether it consists of retaking the boards at the next interval or refocusing your job search efforts. The future success of maintaining employment depends on it, so good luck!

## CONCEPT SUMMARY

- The Myers-Briggs assessment of personality principles has identified 16 personality types.
- Lifelong learning may include creative-thinking training.
- The spirit of teamwork is demonstrated by participating in staff meetings.
- Stress is inevitable but stress-beating strategies can help keep oral healthcare workers employed.
- Conflict occurs within the dental team.
- Sexual harassment may be quid pro quo or environmental.
- A good job performance review is not a guarantee of a salary or benefit increase.
- Any worker may quit a job at any time, and any employer may fire an employee at any time.
- Employment termination is not guaranteed to render a severance payment.
- Everyone experiences failure. A reflection on the emotional effects and a thoughtful analysis of the situation can make failure a learning process.

# REVIEW QUESTIONS

1. How do the personality types affect oral healthcare providers?
2. Why is creativity a frequent topic for continuing education?
3. How does participation in a staff meeting help maintain employment?
4. List stress-beating strategies.
5. How does conflict affect the dental team?
6. What are the two types of sexual harassment?
7. What is the function of the performance review?
8. When is it acceptable for an employee to sever employment? For an employer?
9. Are employers mandated to pay severance for terminated employees?
10. What are the steps to take after experiencing failure?

# CRITICAL THINKING ACTIVITY

Read each of the following scenarios of actual lawsuits and identify the type of sexual harassment that has occurred (environmental or quid pro quo). Discuss each scenario.

1. A female employee is discharged for absenteeism after the supervisor said he would "get even" for the employee's rejection of his sexual advances.
2. A temporary employee is terminated after repeatedly rejecting an employer's sexual advances, but all other employees with comparable qualifications are retained and additional employees are hired for jobs for which the dismissed employee was qualified.
3. A supervisor chooses to accept sexual favors offered by a subordinate employee and the personal relationship is terminated. The supervisor contends that the employee's work deteriorated after the affair ended.
4. An employee is passed over for a promotion in favor of a lower-level employee who is sexually involved with the office manager.
5. An employer investigating an employee's claim of sexual harassment took action to prevent further sexual harassment by interviewing employees. In a private meeting, the employer informed the employee that this conduct would not be tolerated and that he would be fired for any further misconduct.
6. The dental practice has a sexual harassment policy that is not effectively followed and seems to protect the harasser, rather than the affected employee.

## Assignment: Letter of Resignation

1. Write a letter of resignation using the letter in *Figure 30.1* as a guide.

# Employability Skills

*Dental Hygiene Domain Competencies*[1]

# IV

## PROFESSIONALISM AND ETHICS

### Professional Behavior

- Communicate effectively using oral, nonverbal, written, and electronic skills.

### Ethical Behavior

- Adhere to federal, state, and local laws.

### Professional Commitment

- Advance the values of the profession by affiliation with professional and public organizations.
- Assume the role of clinician, educator, researcher, change agent, consumer advocate, and administrator as defined by the American Dental Hygienists' Association.
- Assume responsibility for lifelong learning.

### REFERENCES

**Organizations**
American Dental Hygienists' Association (www.adha.org/careerinfo/jsearch/jsearch1.htm)
America's JobBank (www.ajb.dni.us)
Career Builder (www.careerbuilder.com)
Career Magazine (www.careermag.com)
Career Net (http://careernet.4jobs.com)
Careers.org (www.careers.org)
Eriss (www.eriss.com)
Monster Board (www.monster.com)
Monster Canada (launch.monster.ca/guide/conducting/)
The CV Doctor (chronicle.com/jobs/2003/09/2003092602c.htm)

**Online Resources**
Aggressiveness (www.wbenjamin.org/marcuse.html)
American job market and statistics (www.dol.gov)

Assertiveness (www.mentalhelp.net/psyhelp/chap13/chap13e.htm)
Authority and autocrats (www.brainydictionary.com/words/au/autocrat133746.html)
Avoiding job stress (secure.ehealthconnection.com/stress/approot/OWL/content/job_stress.asp)
Career and employability skills (www.michigan.gov/documents/Career&Employ_Standards_12_01_13760_7.pdf)
Co-dependence and counterdependence (www.relationdancing.com/Interdependence.htm)
Curriculum vitae (www.businessballs.com/curriculum.htm, jobsearch.about.com/cs/cvsamples/chronicle.com/jobs)
Employability related to academic, personal management, and processing skills (www.nwrel.org/scpd/sirs/8/c015.html)

---

[1]Adapted from American Dental Education Association. Competencies for Entry into the Profession of Dental Hygiene (as approved by the 2003 House of Delegates). Reprinted by permission of *Journal of Dental Education*, Volume 68, Issue 7 (July 2004). Copyright 2004 by the American Dental Education Association.

Employability related to work habits (www.ericdigests.org/pre-9217/fifth.htm)

Employment benefits (www.ebri.org/)

Employment contracts (www.career.vt.edu/JOBSEARC/Contracts.htm)

Employment negotiation (www.itworld.com/Career/1727/ITW2109/)

Interview advice (interview.monster.com/)

Job application cover letters (jobsearch.about.com/od/resumés/a/resumécenter.htm)

Job searches and interviewing (dmoz.org/Business/Employment/Job_Search/Interview_Advice/)

Leadership (www.leaderu.com/)

Performance review (www.employer-employee.com/performancereview.html)

Personal marketing tools (www.michigan.gov/documents/Career&Employ_Standards_12_01_13760_7.pdf)

Personal marketing website (www.paworkplace.com)

Personal mission statements (www.franklincovey.com)

Personality types (www.discoveryourpersonality.com)

Portfolios (www.teachnet.com/how-to/employment/portfolios/)

Power interviewing (www.amazon.com/exec/obidos/tg/detail/-/0471177881/002-0071082-4230449?v=glance)

Resume action verbs (www.bc.edu/offices/careers/skills/resumes/verbs; http://content.monster.com/resume/resources/phrases_verbs)

Résumé samples (http://resume.monster.com/)

Severance pay (www.dol.gov/dol/topic/wages/severancepay.htm)

Sexual harassment (www.eeoc.gov/facts/fs-sex.html)

### Pamphlets, Dissertations, and Papers

Career path: The job search sourcebook. Norfolk, VA: Old Dominion University Career Services. 1993–1994.

Completing an application. Clarkston, MI: Oakland Technical Center Northwest Campus.

Developing interview skills. Clarkston, MI: Oakland Technical Center Northwest Campus.

Employee handbook policies, practices, benefits. Rosemont, IL: Velsicol Chemical Corp., 1996.

Job Placement Services. Sources of employment. Clarkston, MI: Oakland Technical Center Northwest Campus.

Jonker N. Student portfolio: Meeting the demand for competence (draft legislation). Michigan State House of Representatives. 1992.

Michigan State Board of Education. Employability skills (working draft). January 1991.

Old Dominion University placement manual: 1993–1994. Evanston, IL: CRS Recruitment Publications, 1993.

U.S. Department of Justice, Immigration and Naturalization Service. Handbook for employers [Publication M-274 (11-24-1991)]. Available online at http://www.uscis.gov/graphics/formsfee/forms/files/i-9.pdf.

U.S. Department of Labor, Employment Standards Administration, Wage and Hour Division. Handy reference guide to the fair labor standards act. Available online at http://www.dol.gov/esa/whd.

Writing a resume. Clarkston, MI: Oakland Technical Center Northwest Campus.

Writing an application letter. Clarkston, MI: Oakland Technical Center Northwest Campus.

### Articles

Besson T. How to choose the best job. Manage Your Career 1992.

Best K. Get a job! Wordperfect Mag 1992.

Burt P. How to speak the doctor's language. RDH 1993.

Burt P. A regional analysis average hourly pay per region. RDH 1993.

Burt P. Where do benefits fit in the picture? RDH 1993.

Caplan C. Charting your flight plan for job satisfaction. Dent Asst 1983.

Cole D. Confronting the committee. Manage Your Career 1992.

Corwin W. Shark resumes for flounders. Manage Your Career 1992.

Dube L. Portfolios can be student's passport to employment. Balance Sheet 1990.

Half R. Resume goofs. Manage Your Career 1990.

Hannon K. 1994 Career guide. U.S. News & World Report, November 1, 1993.

Hayes GW. The product is you. Manage Your Career 1992.

Innis K. 10 tips: great job search advice you didn't learn in school. Manage Your Career 1994.

Jameson C. Making performance appraisals work. Dent Teamwork 1991.

Karush T. The great resume makeover. Cosmopolitan Life after College 1993.

Karush T. Six interview mistakes . . . and how to avoid them. Cosmopolitan Life after College 1993.

Karush T. Write a winning cover letter. Cosmopolitan Life after College 1993.

Lee T. Networking. Manage Your Career 1992.

Lennon SJ, Schulz TL, Johnson KKP. Forging linkages between dress and law in the U.S., Part II Dress Codes. Clothing Textiles Res J 1999;17(3).

Pride J. Employee performance problems: how to resolve them the right way. J Am Dent Assoc 1992:123.

Radica B. Developing a career strategy. Dent Asst 1988.

Richardson DB. Dress for duress. Manage Your Career 1992.

Sapp J. How to interview the dentist employer. Dent Asst 1977.

Scruggs RR, Stewart L. Marketable resumes and cover letters. Dent Asst 1985.

Semple L. Managing occupational stress in the dental office. Texas Dent J 1997:59–60.

Six steps to feel great-don't wait! Scholastic Choices 1988:7.

Speck JB. Interviewing etiquette. Manage Your Career 1989.

Swain M, Swain R. How to write letter that wins jobs. Working Woman, April 1989:120–123.

Sweet D. Successful job hunters are all ears. Manage Your Career 1992.

Thomas SE. How I spent my summer vacation . . . as a temp. Manage Your Career 1994.

Weinstein B. Ten sure ways to blow an interview. Career Futures 1991.

Wilcox J. Tough choices. Vocational Educ J 1991.

Willis DO, Utters JM. Employee benefit: how they affect staff turnover. J Am Dent Assoc 1992:123.

Willis DO, Utters JM. Money isn't everything . . . or is it? RDH 1994.

**Books**

Austin LA. What's Holding You Back? 8 Critical Choices for Women's Success. New York: Basic Books, 2000.

Bolles R. The 1994 What Color is Your Parachute, A Practical Manual for Job-Hunters and Career-Changers. Berkeley, CA: Ten Speed Press, 1994.

Channing L. What You Should Know About Getting a Job. South Deerfield, MI: Bete, 1982.

Kelley J. Dear Jean. Tulsa, OK: Atwood, 2000.

Leading Children to Self-Esteem: A Guide for Parents. Chicago: National PTA & Keebler, 1988.

McDaniels C, Knobloch MA. Developing a Professional Vita or Resume (3rd ed.). Chicago: Ferguson Publications, 1997.

Munschauer JL. The Resume: How to Speak to Employer's Needs. CPC annual, 1987–1988.

Palladino D. Vocational Resume Writing. Mission Hills, CA: Glencoe, 1986.

Pathways to Your Future! Mid-Atlantic Guide to Information on Careers. District of Columbia, MD, VA, and WV. 1997.

Salmon WA, Salmon RT. Office Politics for the Utterly Confused. New York: McGraw Hill, 1999.

Vacca RT, Vacca JL. Content Area Reading (2nd ed.). Boston: Little, Brown, 1986.

# Appendix

# Answers to Review Questions and Selected Critical Thinking Activities

## CHAPTER 1

1. The earliest written oral diagnosis dental record, found on a Sumerian clay tablet dated nearly 7,000 years ago, stated that the cause of toothache was a parasitic worm that devours the tooth. It was theorized that small gnawing tooth worms must be removed or destroyed via cautery or poisoning to relieve tooth pain. The tooth worm theory persisted until the 20th century in remote areas of Europe and Asia.

2. Records from ancient India document oral healthcare surgery and therapeutic procedures. Herbal, botanical, and mineral remedies (Ayurvedic); laxatives; emetics; scarification; medicinal pastes; and gargles were used to treat gingival inflammation and other dental problems. Information on surgical instrument designs, calculus removal, bandage instructions for fractured jaws, cauterization of tumors, and oral hygiene instructions are also found in these ancient records.

3. Chinese contributions to modern dental practice include plant and mineral combinations for oral healthcare practices, poisoning tooth worms, filling teeth with silver amalgam dough (659 AD), tooth whitening using hydrochloric acid, acupuncture procedures to cure yin and yang energy imbalances, and the modern toothbrush design (1490s).

4. The caduceus symbol of a staff with wings and a serpent coiled around it is used to represent the healthcare professions and the medical branches of the U.S. government. Greek priests, who carried large staffs and snakes, treated the ailing patients in the temples of Asclepius using massage, bathing, and exercise. The temple statues of Asclepius depict the deity holding a staff with a serpent coiled around it.

5. Galenos of Pergamon (Galen) combined all of the ancient medical texts into one Latin work that included drugs, dietary recommendations, description of diseases, and the study of human anatomy.

6. Apollonia was the daughter of an Egyptian magistrate who was arrested and told to renounce Christianity and accept pagan values, or be burned at the stake. She refused to deny her Christian beliefs and a mob seized her, broke her teeth, and lit a fire to burn her alive. She knelt, prayed, and jumped into the fire of her own free will and was martyred around 249 AD. She is considered to be the patron saint of dentistry, to whom people with toothaches prayed for relief of dental pain during the Middle Ages.

7. Around the end of the 9th century, Abu al-Qasim compiled an encyclopedia of medicine and surgery that reported the relationship between calculus and periodontal disease, and described scaling, prevention, saving teeth by cautery, setting fractures, and extracting teeth.

8. Anton van Leeuwenhoek took bacterial plaque scrapings of his teeth and viewed them under a magnification of 40–160×. He discovered microorganisms and the dentin tubules.

9. Pierre Fauchard is known as the father of modern dentistry because of the two-volume work he published, *Le Chirurgien Dentiste Oú Traité des Dentes*. This work described nearly every phase of dentistry and led the way to modern scientific instruction. Fauchard rejected the tooth worm theory and helped the French become leaders in dentistry and the use of silver amalgam restorative material and artificial porcelain teeth.

10. Paul Revere, the famous patriot, was a silversmith who studied and practiced dentistry for 7 years in

Boston. He identified the postmortem remains of Dr. Joseph Warren who was killed and buried in a mass grave at the Battle of Bunker Hill in 1776. The two-unit dental bridge Revere constructed for Warren was unique; thus, he was able to positively identify the human remains. This event is recognized as the beginning of the science of forensics in the United States.

11. Greene Vardiman (G.V.) Black learned dentistry as an apprentice in his home state of Illinois and developed many dental instruments during his years of practice before the Civil War. After the war, he taught himself chemistry, German, and cellular pathology so he could read and understand the current research. He authored more than 500 scholarly articles and several books during his tenure at Missouri Dental College and Chicago College of Dental Surgery. His contributions to dentistry include cavity classifications, operative dentistry techniques, and the use of fluoride as a caries preventive agent.

12. In 1921, Juliette A. Southard was one of the organizers of the Education and Efficiency Society, which later became the American Dental Assistants Association (ADAA). She was elected and served as its president for the first 5 years of its existence.

13. As a dental assistant to Dr. Alfred G. Fones in Connecticut, Irene Newman was trained to examine and polish teeth above the gingival margin and perform oral prophylaxis on her employer's family members as well as on patients. Fones founded and taught in the first dental hygiene educational program; 1914 saw the first graduating class, which consisted of 27 students, including Newman. Newman further contributed to the dental hygiene profession by becoming the first woman licensed in dental hygiene, forming the Connecticut Dental Hygienists Association with her classmates, and serving as the first president. Newman and the students from the class of 1917 rendered oral healthcare services to the National Guardsmen in Bridgeport, Connecticut, establishing the first organized effort to provide preventive oral healthcare services to soldiers.

14. In the late 1700s, a practice was adopted of transplanting a donor tooth taken from a living or dead human or animal into a tooth socket of a patient who had undergone tooth extraction. The recipient patient would slowly die from infection or the body's rejection of the tooth.

## CHAPTER 2

1. (A) Dentists are near the top of the step scale. (B) Dental hygienists are in the middle of the step scale. (C) Dental assistants are at the lower end of the step scale. (D) Dental laboratory technicians are at the lower end of the step scale.

2. (A) Dentists diagnose oral conditions and perform operative dentistry to restore the teeth using a variety of dental materials (metals, plastics, glasses, inorganic salts such as dental cements). (B) Dental hygienists use assessment procedures and treat periodontal diseases to maintain the patients' oral health. (C) Dental assistants serve as a second pair of hands to help the dentist clinically and perform business office functions. (D) Dental laboratory technicians fabricate fixed and removable appliances for patients in the dental laboratory setting.

3. (A) Dentists usually have completed a minimum of 6 years of education (2–4 years of undergraduate college and 3–4 years of dental school are required). (B) Dental hygienists complete programs that vary from 2 to 4 years in length. (C) Dental assistants are not required to have advanced training or earn a college degree. Dental assisting programs are found at universities, community colleges, vocational/technical schools, and private proprietary schools. (D) Dental laboratory technicians enroll in academic programs offered at the community college, vocational school, technical institute, or dental school; apprenticeship programs are available in dental laboratories.

4. (A) Dentist: doctor of dental surgery (DDS) or doctor of dental medicine (DMD). (B) Dental hygienist: registered dental hygienist (RDH). (C) Dental assistant: certified dental assistant (CDA), certified orthodontic assistant (COA), certified dental practice management assistant (CDPMA), registered dental assistant (RDA), or expanded functions dental assistant (EFDA). (D) Dental laboratory technician: certified dental technician (CDT).

5. (A) Dentist: graduate from an ADA-accredited program, pass a written and clinical examination recognized by a state or region of the United States, and pay the fees. (B) Dental hygienist: graduate from an ADA-accredited program, pass a written national board examination and a regional board examination recognized by a state or region of the United States, and pay the fees.

(C) Dental assistant: graduate from an ADA-accredited program, successfully complete a written and clinical state examination. (D) Dental laboratory technicians are not licensed.

6. (A) Dental assistant: take a DANB written national board examination after graduation from an ADA-accredited dental assisting program or be a high school graduate with at least 2 years of full-time dental office experience. (B) Dental laboratory technician: successfully complete a national board examination.

7. Group dental practices have two or more dentists. Private practices are owned by an individual dentist. For some group practices, dentists share the office space; sometimes a dentist is hired by another dentist.

8. On-the-job training is an entry-level position of employment in dentistry in which dental assistants may be trained while working.

9. A dental laboratory technician may be an apprentice.

10. The registered dental assistant (RDA) is a state-licensed dental assistant. The certified dental assistant (CDA) has successfully completed a national examination.

11. Mandatory continuing education keeps oral healthcare professionals current in technology as well as new advances, knowledge, and techniques to safeguard the public.

12. Cardiopulmonary resuscitation (CPR) certification may be required for the renewal of licensure.

13. The dental nurse.

14. Dental therapists perform dental hygiene duties plus routine restorations, extractions, pulpal therapy and placement of preformed crowns on deciduous teeth, and limited orthodontics. They make referrals and provide access to care to people in need.

15. The dental therapist is an occupational title found in other countries and is an educated dental hygienist who performs additional job tasks such as restorations, extractions, pulpal therapy and placement of preformed crowns on deciduous teeth, and limited orthodontics. The dental nurse is an occupational title found in the United Kingdom; he or she performs job tasks similar to the dental assistant. However, dental nurses are mandated to meet specific requirements before being eligible to become a dental hygienist or dental therapist. The denturist is a person who prepares removable dentures by providing oral

examination, dental impressions, jaw relation records, fabrication, and insertion. Denturists provide instruction on denture care and take care of denture repair, relines, and adjustments. The dental laboratory technician makes fixed and removable appliances.

# CHAPTER 3

1. General dentists refer patients to a dental specialist or dentist with advanced training in a concentrated subject area when the patient's condition is beyond their ability to manage.

2. The dental specialist has completed a general dentistry degree, taken postgraduate training in an accredited dental specialty program, and passed a certification board examination.

3. Dental specialties are ADA-recognized subject matter taught in accredited programs; a discipline is subject matter that is unique in scope. A discipline may become a dental specialty once requirements for specialty status recognition are met.

4. (A) Dental public health: public programs in preventive education, community treatment, and applied dental research funded by federal, state, and local government agencies. (B) Endodontics: the morphology, physiology, pathology, cause, diagnosis, prevention, and treatment of pulpal and periapical disease. (C) Oral and maxillofacial pathology: the origin, diagnosis, management, and research of diseases that affect the maxillofacial structures. (D) Oral and maxillofacial radiology: the production and interpretation of images created by radiant energy to diagnose and manage diseases that affect the maxillofacial region. (E) Oral and maxillofacial surgery: the diagnosis and surgical repair of injuries, defects, and diseases of the maxillofacial region. (F) Orthodontics and dentofacial orthopedics: the correction of misaligned teeth and jaws. (G) Pediatric dentistry: the treatment of children. (H) Periodontics: the prevention, diagnosis, treatment, and maintenance of the supporting structures of the teeth using preventive, surgical, and nonsurgical techniques. (I) Prosthodontics: the replacement of lost maxillofacial structures with fixed or removable prosthetic devices.

5. Dentists with the title diplomate of the board are dentists who have progressed to the furthest reaches in a field of study by completing additional education.

6. (A) Complementary and alternative dentistry: the treatment of chronic health problems using nontraditional healthcare practices. (B) Cosmetic dentistry: the aesthetics of dental treatment. (C) Forensic dentistry: the identification of postmortem human remains for legal purposes. (D) Geriatric dentistry: the treatment of the elderly. (E) High-tech dentistry: incorporating the latest technological advances into dental practice using state-of-the art, sophisticated equipment and procedures. (F) Oral anesthesiology: pain and anxiety control. (G) Oral implantodontics: the surgical and prosthodontic aspects of placing mechanical devices into or on the alveolar bone. (H) Oral medicine: the diagnosis and treatment of the oral manifestations of systemic disease or the care of the medically compromised patient. (I) Special care dentistry: caring for patients with mental, physical, or sensory disabilities. (J) Sports dentistry: the prevention and management of oral and maxillofacial sport injuries. (K) Temporomandibular joint disorder: the proper functioning and management of the TMJ.

## CHAPTER 4

1. (A) American Dental Association, Academy of General Dentistry. (B) American Dental Hygienists' Association. (C) American Dental Assistants Association. (D) National Association of Dental Laboratories.
2. Professionals join organizations for professional interaction and representation, ethics, access to resources, public awareness, and access to quality oral healthcare promotion, career advancement, promotion of education standards, advocacy, and credentialing.
3. Association membership benefits include professional interaction opportunities, communication among professionals, annual meetings, support of research, publications, educational opportunity, information resources, group insurance plans, research funding, code of ethical standards, awards, scholarships, credit card options and other discounts, and legislative representation.
4. Several hundred ADA councils study situations or problems, recommend the policies of the ADA, review all educational programs, and review products and other issues affecting dentistry.

5. ADA publications include the *Journal of the American Dental Association* and the *American Dental Directory*. ADHA publications include the *Journal of Dental Hygiene* and *Access*. ADAA publications include *The Dental Assistant*.
6. The Golden Rule is the basis of the ethical codes of the helping professions: to treat others in the manner you would want to be treated.
7. A professional code of ethics is a set of written rules of behavior based on virtues important to that profession.
8. These organizations have a code of ethics to guide their members to achieve high levels of ethical awareness and use ethical decision-making principles.
9. Violation of an organization's code of ethics can result in peer review leading to an official inquiry, local police action, disciplinary actions by the regulatory board, the loss of association membership, and the loss of the respect of others in the profession.
10. Issues related to clothing and grooming can become an ethical problem. Employers have the legal right to regulate workplace dress even though there are no laws about what is allowed. They do this because patients make judgments about appearance, because there are health standards for worker protection, because personal odors can be offensive, and because sanitary fingernails are necessary and jewelry may harbor microorganisms.
11. Ethics are standards of conduct that apply attitudes and values. Etiquette is behavior related to customs and rituals. Protocol is a procedure to be followed in a certain set of circumstances. Virtues are values that include honesty, tolerance, patience, lawfulness, charity, responsible behavior, justice, and kindness.

## CHAPTER 5

1. Ethics are standards of conduct that apply attitudes and values. Jurisprudence is a system of laws.
2. Federal laws affect all U.S. jurisdictions. State laws apply within the boundaries of a jurisdiction. Judicial law (common law) applies to an area in which a judge presides, and fills in the gaps of state laws.
3. Practicing dentistry without a license is a violation of state criminal law. Dental personnel

should perform only those functions legally allowable within their jurisdiction. Performing illegal dental procedures places the allied dental professional in the situation of practicing dentistry without a license, which is a serious criminal offense.

4. The dentist–patient relationship is based on an implied or expressed contract.

5. The two divisions of civil law are contract law and tort law.

6. Dental licensure requires good moral character with no criminal convictions, successful completion of an ADA-accredited educational program, successful completion of required examinations, CPR certification, and payment of licensure fees.

7. Supervision is the level of management that allows one to perform one's job duties. The level of supervision is defined differently in each U.S. jurisdiction.

8. Each jurisdiction has its own supervision rules and language, such as lists of job duties that may or may not be performed. A jurisdiction may have a statement such as "all duties that are reversible" to control the practice of allied dental personnel.

9. Dentists who undergo peer review may receive a formal reprimand that is announced to the profession via the Internet and may have their licensure suspended or revoked.

10. Risk management is the understanding and following of legal principles to prevent legal liability and responsibility.

11. (A) Breach of contract: the dentist must notify the patient in writing of his or her intent to withdraw from the dentist–patient relationship. (B) Technical assault: the education of the patient is followed by the completion of standardized consent forms. (C) Technical battery: the education of the patient is followed by the completion of standardized consent forms. (D) Misrepresentation: inform the patient of his or her treatment status. (E) Deceit: do not guarantee results or create unrealistic expectations; perform only those procedures for which you qualified, educated, experienced, or licensed. (F) Maligning a patient: do not defame patient character by slander or libel or perform unnecessary dental treatment. (G) Breach of confidentiality: do not violate the confidential relationship between the patient and healthcare provider. (H) Permitting a hazard: fol-

low all local, state, and federal workplace safety regulations. (I) Negligence: do not breach or fail to perform a legal duty through neglect or carelessness, resulting in damage or injury.

12. The three elements of negligence are (1) the existence of a duty and the breach of that duty, (2) proximate cause, and (3) damages.

13. Malpractice lawsuits arise from: a foreign object being left in the body; failure to diagnose and treat diseases and disorders; failure to obtain informed consent and to keep the patient informed; failure of a dental implant; failure to sterilize; failure to refer a difficult case to a specialist; failure to identify medically compromised patients or drug allergy; failure to take precautions to protect a patient; fracture of the jaw; and improperly fitting dentures or bridges.

14. Accurate, organized dental record documentation regarding patient treatment is the best defense against a malpractice claim. Properly maintained and organized dental records provide evidence of appropriate diagnosis, treatment, and billing and lessen the likelihood of treatment error.

15. Public relations is defined as the promotion of goodwill between an organization or individual with the public. The quality of the relationship between the dentist and the patient has a direct bearing on malpractice claims. Patients are more likely to file malpractice lawsuits when they feel they have been overcharged, when there has been a failure to diagnose, or when adequate care is not provided. Office staff can have a positive or negative effect on clients and should attempt to pursue good public relations.

16. If you receive a summons or subpoena, immediately contact your liability insurance carrier by telephone and follow-up by sending a letter, certified mail, return receipt requested, with a copy of the summons or subpoena.

17. A deposition is a sworn written testimony in which a series of questions are answered under oath before the case goes to trial.

18. Mediation is the settling of differences before a case goes to trial and is an attempt to prevent lawsuits from clogging the courts.

19. Allied dental professionals are not automatically covered by the dentist's malpractice insurance. Malpractice insurance is available from the dental auxiliary's professional association.

## CRITICAL THINKING GROUP ACTIVITY RESPONSE

Based on the virtue of truth, cheating is considered wrong. Using ethical conduct to prevent cheating is a voluntary personal choice and is not always a legal mandate. For example, cheating on an examination is not against the law but rather violates school policy. Although it is not illegal to cheat on a test, a school can set ethical standards or policies for acceptable behavior. Many schools require students to pledge to these policies, which are sometimes called an honor code. Anyone who observes cheating is bound by the honor code to report it because ethical conduct requires it.

Ethical behaviors to prevent cheating on an examination are to cover your paper and to keep your eyes on your own examination. A person suspected of cheating on an examination would not be following the honor code and could be denied continuance in a program of study.

## CHAPTER 6

1. Oral healthcare providers have the option of determining whom they will accept as a patient into the practice, must provide care to all accepted patients, and must refer unaccepted patients to an appropriate healthcare provider. Their decisions may be based on financial fact finding or the degree of treatment needed.
2. Client is an alternative word for patient.
3. Posting the Patient Bill of Rights informs patients of the dental office's legal duties.
4. The three forms of consent differ in how they are given. By coming into a dental practice office for treatment, implied consent is given for the physical contact necessary for an oral examination, diagnosis, and consultation. Informed consent arises after the practitioner provides information regarding the healthcare procedure and associated risk to allow for intelligent decision making. Expressed consent is permission given orally or in writing to allow a procedure to be performed.
5. The oral healthcare provider must be licensed and meet all legal requirements to engage in the practice of dentistry. The dentist must use reasonable care and skill in diagnosis and treatment by using standard drugs, materials, and techniques. For those procedures considered experimental or outside the standard of care such as

laser dentistry, the provider must obtain written informed consent. Patient treatment must be completed within a reasonable length of time. The provider must not abandon patients and is obligated to care for all the needs of the patient. Care for the patient must be arranged in case of an emergency when the dentist is unavailable. The dental team member must do only those services consented to by the patient. The provider must refer unusual cases to a specialist. The dental team member must provide adequate patient instructions. The provider must charge a reasonable fee for services rendered. The dental team member must achieve a reasonable result. The dental team member must maintain the client's right to privacy and confidentiality.

6. The patient's duties are to provide accurate information about his or her health history and status, pay a reasonable fee for services rendered within a reasonable time, keep appointments, cooperate in care, and follow instructions.
7. The Americans with Disabilities Act prohibits discrimination against disabled people by stating that physical barriers in existing facilities must be removed or alternative methods of providing services must be offered in most practice settings.
8. The first prosecuted case of child abuse in the United States was pursued under the laws for the prevention of cruelty to animals.
9. Signs of physical child abuse include unexplained lacerations, bruises, and welts (in various stages of healing); unexplained burns such as cigarette or patterned burns; unexplained fractured bones; fear of parents or of going home from school at the end of the day; wariness of adult contacts or inquiries; and inconsistency in the report of how an injury occurred when asked open-ended questions.
10. Signs of emotional child abuse include speech disorders; failure to thrive; lags in physical development; habit disorders (rocking, sucking, biting); neurotic behaviors (hysteria, obsession, phobias); extreme behaviors (passive or aggressive); and suicide attempts.
11. Signs of sexual child abuse include bruising of the palate; unexplained sores around the lips; and oral signs of venereal disease.
12. Signs of child neglect include hunger; poor hygiene; constant fatigue; filthy clothing or clothing inappropriate for the weather; untreated

physical conditions such as caries, abscesses, or oral pain; lack of supervision for long periods of time; alcohol or drug abuse; and abandonment.

13. Spousal abuse is the misuse of power and control by one spouse over the other. During the tension-building phase, stress and pressure increase and end in an explosion of violence. The honeymoon phase occurs after the violence and may be characterized by gift giving. The violence usually escalates over time.

14. Elder abuse is the exploitation of or any act or omission that causes injury to people age 60 years or older.

15. Abuse of the disabled may be detected through such signs as inadequate dental care or oral hygiene, bruxism, or a fear of dental equipment, rubber dams, impressions, or the smell of latex.

## CASE STUDY QUESTION RESPONSES

1. B. The first statement is false and the second statement is true.
2. C. Home fluoride rinse

## CHAPTER 7

1. A sole proprietorship is a business in which one person is the business owner, called a proprietor. A partnership is a business in which two or more people own the business and are called partners. A corporation is a business in which the owners are employees of the business.

2. Corporations have benefits such as different tax laws; can provide retirement accounts; and protect the shareholders, board of directors, and officers from debts and legal liability, thus reducing the risks associated with business ownership.

3. Business plans describe a business, measure performance over time, set forth goals, and project growth potential for prospective grantors, lenders, or investors.

4. All dental practices have patient reception, treatment, and consultation areas. The business owner may decorate the dental office in a theme based on location of the practice or as a reflection of his or her personality.

5. Because judgments are made within minutes of an encounter, dental practices look at the environment to make it appealing to the patient's senses. Appearance of the office, air quality, noise,

and temperature are monitored to a comfortable environment for the patient.

6. Business tasks performed in the dental office include public relations, patient management, records management, maintenance of accounts receivable and accounts payable, and the operation of office equipment.

7. The business dental assistant should have a basic knowledge of dentistry, interpersonal communication skills, good personal appearance, integrity, dependability, and a positive attitude.

8. Business dental assistants produce written materials, treat patients as individuals, prepare and maintain records, maintain accounts receivable and accounts payable, and operate the dental office software program.

9. All patients are greeted by name immediately, treated respectfully, and told whether there will be a waiting time.

10. It is good public relations to great the patient with respect and polite personal attention. In addition, established reception procedures may deter crime.

11. The office manager directs employees, schedules staff, plans meetings, and performs office functions.

12. Staff conferences are used to discuss daily operations, communicate, maintain efficiency, and conduct in-service activities.

13. Ergonomic designs and equipment provide physical comfort for patients and dental personnel in the dental operatory.

14. The conference room is used to conduct a patient conference or consultation and to educate the patient.

15. The private office area is used to conduct confidential business such as patient treatment planning.

## CHAPTER 8

1. Telecommunications encompasses the systems and services that involve the transmission of words, sounds, or images in the form of electronic signals via landline or mobile telephones, facsimile, computer, webcams, radio, television, microwave, or satellite, using telephone companies, Internet service provider companies, and insurance clearinghouses.

2. It has been estimated that over 95% of the dental office's business is received from telephone

calls, meaning first telephone impressions are very important.

3. The telephone is answered before the end of the second ring.

4. Open questions require an explanation and closed questions require short responses.

5. Restating information verifies that the correct information was received.

6. Patients in an emergency situation will report having discomfort, swelling, and/or bleeding. Emergency patients are seen the day of the call for palliative treatment.

7. Documentation of telephone usage helps determine why the patient is calling, assesses whether a dental emergency is or was occurring, creates a legal record, and determines telephone usage.

8. Facsimile machines transmit digital or photocopy images for sending a prescription to a pharmacy, placing a purchase order, and sending/receiving insurance company information and product sales information.

9. Personal computers use integrated dental software programs to perform business practice procedures such as word processing, accounting procedures, producing graphics, appointment scheduling, treatment planning and diagnosis, insurance claims processing, and record assessment findings. They also provide Internet access.

10. Accounts receivable; accounts payable; insurance claims processing; pretreatment estimates; appointment scheduling; recare/preventative management; patient financial accounts; patient billing and financial management; practice production analysis reports; letter writing; prescription writing.

11. Patient records consist of financial account data and patient information such as personal history. Account information is further divided by insurance coverage information.

12. Treatment rendered is entered on the routing slip or superbill. These forms serve as a billing and treatment record. As a billing record, information on current balance, fees for services rendered, insurance codes, and posted payments are listed. As a treatment record, recare status, procedures performed, next appointment procedures, and procedure descriptions are listed. The routing slip/superbill can be used as a walk-out statement for the patient or attached to an insurance claim for payment processing.

13. Daily: transaction listing, personnel production summary (one per provider), listing of charges and payments (day sheet), insurance claims filed, summary of procedures performed, listing of new patients added, listing of new/modified recalls, bank deposit slip, transferred to installments.

Monthly: purged recalls report, purged insurance claims, purged installments, account activity detail report, cash receivables aged trial balance (by provider), insurance claims status report (by provider), installment a/r aged trail balance (by provider), monthly provider summary, monthly practice summary, practice management reports—combined and individual.

Yearly: account history detail report, accounts receivable reports, superbill/MTD statement/YTD statement, account history (2 years), monthly statement (mailer or standard), accounts receivable aged trial balance, accounts receivable past due listing.

14. Correspondence such as letters can be merged with information from patient and treatment records for improved public relations. Computerized practice management systems are also used to input patient data such as dental charting, periodontal examination, appointment scheduling, and preoperative and postoperative treatment instructional aids and handouts. This can improve staff and patient interaction and rapport development for public relations. Inventory control management can also monitor inventory stock, use, expenses, and purchasing online.

## CHAPTER 9

1. To become an advanced dental hygiene practitioner, the dental hygienist would continue in and complete an advanced course of study of diagnostic, preventative, restorative, and therapeutic services.

2. Minimal intervention philosophy follows the medical model to treat disease therapeutically. In dentistry, it separates treatment into surgical and nonsurgical interventions for the treatment of microbial-based infections such as caries and periodontal diseases.

3. The nonsurgical approach to oral healthcare delivery using therapeutic agents and regimens for caries and periodontal disease is the dental hygiene scope of practice. Caries therapeutics and regimens are billable dental hygiene proce-

dures performed by dental hygienists. Periodontal disease therapies and regimens to stop the infection process include the nonsurgical periodontal treatments at the heart of soft tissue management programs administered by dental hygienists. When these interventions are not successful, referral to the appropriate oral healthcare provider (general dentist or periodontist) becomes necessary for surgical care.

4. (A) Assessment: data collection procedures using office forms or the computer. (B) Diagnosis: dental insurance diagnostic and procedural insurance coding. (C) Treatment planning: appointment scheduling system documented on a variety of paper forms or computer programs; case presentation using a multimedia approach, such as an intraoral camera to photograph the appearance of the oral conditions; cosmetic imaging; and CD-ROM educational programs that include photos, graphics, animation, and sound to appeal to all levels of learning. (D) Implementation of dental hygiene services: financial arrangements based on plans available from the practice are maintained in an office system. Communication systems: staying current on treatment modalities, technology, governmental regulations; continuing care; customer service; and public relations. Accounting and insurance systems and, in the case of independent practice, all practice management systems are used. (E) Evaluation of care: continuing care, patient education, examinations, consultations, and office survey are systems to evaluate care.

5. Independent practice is the dental hygienist who owns a dental hygiene practice. An alternative practice dental hygienist is an employee of a dentist, an employee of another registered dental hygienist in alternative practice, an independent contractor, a sole proprietor of an alternative dental hygiene practice, an employee of a primary care clinic or specialty clinic, or an employee of a clinic owned or operated by a public hospital or healthcare system. In collaborative practice, the dental hygienist practices under general supervision with one or more consulting dentists.

6. They allow dental hygienists to provide care to underserved populations.

7. The dental hygiene diagnosis can be based on human needs deficits, client oral hygiene needs, statements regarding necessary care, or the identification of conditions that are treated by the dental hygienist.

8. Dental spas offer a blend of medicine with dentistry plus a number of services such as hair, skin, hand, and foot care; hair removal; massage; makeup; and/or fashion advice.

9. The association between a visit to the dental office and pain makes some clients avoid seeking dental care because of their fear. Human needs and deficits, Maslow's hierarchy of needs, and other methods explain the basics of what humans need and want. The dental office spa takes into account that care and comfort are primary needs. Amenities to meet these needs take into consideration all the senses—touch, smell, sight, sound, and taste. By focused attention on care and comfort, spas help put the patient at ease and strive to make him or her comfortable.

10. Notes about private conversations should be written in the patient's chart to document referrals to other healthcare providers, domestic violence programs, suicide hotlines, or local departments of social services. Simple notes regarding discussions serve as a reminder of the conversation.

## CHAPTER 10

1. Accounts receivable, accounts payable, petty cash control, and barter exchange.

2. The accounts receivable office system is the management of production fees that are owed to the dental practice, payment or credits received, and the summation of unpaid money due to the dental office. The accounts payable system is the recording of check and cash disbursements from the dental practice or independent practice bank account.

3. Monitoring bookkeeping systems helps prevent errors, fraud, or embezzlement.

4. Walk-out statements are financial accounting paper forms to communicate to the patient services performed and money exchanged. Routing slips are financial accounting paper forms to communicate to the business office the charges incurred by the patient.

5. Transactions are any account activity, including fees charged, payments received, exchanges of goods/services, or account adjustments.

6. A daily transaction summary report is used to review for errors in posting.

7. Proof of posting is a daily summary procedure to add the day's receivables to the previous day's balance to determine the total accounts receivable balance.
8. A disbursement journal is a special ledger book designed to reflect the business transactions in a dental practice related to operational costs.
9. Money received should be accounted for and deposited into the practice's account at the bank daily to reduce the opportunity for missing funds.
10. Monthly disbursement summary sheets are paper forms used to record itemized totals of expenses.
11. Ledger control sheets are used for banking, payroll, and other expenses.
12. The petty cash fund is used for incidental purchases and usually contains $50 to $100. Cash control journals are used to itemize cash-in and cash-out transactions.
13. Cash transactions should be handled by one individual to lessen the likelihood of cash shortages.
14. Several people should have the ability to perform transactions in the accounting systems, including banking.
15. The embezzlement of office funds costs the industry millions of dollars a year and can be eliminated with control systems and monitoring that makes it difficult to steal money. It is recommended that all personnel be bonded, with bonding coverage reviewed yearly. New employees should have their references and financial stability evaluated before bonding.

## CHAPTER 11

1. (A) Cross coding: the filing of medical insurance claims for dental procedures. (B) Co-payment: a percentage of the treatment cost that is required to be paid by the patient. (C) Usual, customary, and reasonable (UCR): traditional fee for service plans to pay a set amount for a procedure code number as determined by the insurance carrier. (D) Schedule of benefits: a fee schedule for a specified amount to be paid for a procedure code number as determined by the carrier; the patient is financially responsible for the difference between the carrier payment and dentists' fee. (E) Subrogation: the communication process between two insurance carriers when there is dual coverage. (F) ADA attending dentist's statement dental insurance form: the standardized dental insurance claim form used to submit dental insur-

ance claims for payment or preauthorization for services to be performed. (G) CMS-1500 medical insurance form: the standardized form used to submit medical insurance claims. (H) Fee for service: the dental practice that requires the patient to pay for treatment in advance based on a fee schedule. (I) Preauthorization: a detailed listing of procedure codes to be performed sent to the carrier for review before beginning any treatment to determine the patient's eligibility, covered services, payment amounts, co-payments, deductibles, and plan maximums. (J) Bundling: the grouping of related procedure codes based on multiple appointments. (K) Narrative report: a letter that provides information on diagnosis and treatment sent to the insurance carrier. (L) Explanation of benefits: an itemized statement of details regarding benefit payment information, reasons for a rejected claim, and how payment was made according to the plans' benefit guidelines. (M) Insurance fraud: the intentional attempt to falsify insurance claims.

## CHAPTER 12

1. Practice production helps control and monitor why the dental practice spends money, where the money is spent, and how much is spent.
2. The hygiene department drives the practice by providing distinctive services. Without a strong hygiene department, the office will experience slow growth.
3. Primary dental hygiene procedures have high production value and should represent at least half of the daily hygiene production amount. Secondary dental hygiene procedures have lower production value and represent all other comprehensive dental hygiene services. Tertiary dental hygiene procedures are performed at no cost, yet are necessary for patient care.
4. Production blocking is the setting aside of time each day for primary procedures.
5. One industry benchmark for production in the dental hygiene department is that it account for one third of the practice's total production.
6. Dental hygiene production is based on the growth markers of forecasting, total quality management, service design and process, inventory, scheduling, and production analysis reports.
7. Total quality management in the service sector system is a commitment to excellence in service

delivery to meet the dental consumer's expectations and keep the consumer satisfied.

8. Service design is the selection and delivery of labor-intensive care that is individualized and unique to the patient to improve health. The focus of the dental hygienist is to provide the patient with good customer service.

9. Legal delegation of duties to a dental assistant enhances production totals by increasing the number of patients scheduled and thus production.

10. Spending less money on supplies improves the bottom line of operational costs.

11. Personal care products, drugs, medicaments, and therapies that may be available only from the dental office are promoted and sold to the patient. It is good customer service to individualize patient care based on the patient's needs and wants and to enhance his or her health and well-being.

12. Practice net margin is the proportion of gross billings remaining after all costs have been paid.

## ANSWERS FOR "DETERMINING PRODUCTION" ASSIGNMENT

1. Production totals for a single-booked schedule.

**Woody Trail**

| | |
|---|---|
| 4 bitewing x-rays | $61 |
| Adult prophylaxis | 84 |
| Periodic examination by DDS/DMD | (40) |
| Adult fluoride | 35 |
| Dispense breath malodor kit | 25 |
| Dispense sonic toothbrush | 125 |
| Patient education | no charge |
| Total | $330 |

**Luke Warm**

| | |
|---|---|
| Upper and lower right periodontal scaling and root planing | $400 |
| Local anesthesia | no charge |
| Dispense chlorhexidine | 15 |
| 8 site-specific antibiotic injections | 280 |
| Total | $695 |

**Lucy Little**

| | |
|---|---|
| Full-mouth x-rays | $120 |
| Periodontal maintenance | 120 |
| Dispense take-home fluoride | 10 |
| Adult fluoride | 35 |
| Patient education | no charge |
| Total | $285 |

**Bill Board**

| | |
|---|---|
| Full-mouth x-rays | $120 |
| Periodontal maintenance | 120 |
| Dispense take-home fluoride | 10 |
| Adult fluoride | 35 |
| Patient education | no charge |
| Total | $285 |

**Bill Fold**

| | |
|---|---|
| Office visit for observation | $35 |
| Periodontal débridement per tooth (unspecified periodontal treatment by report) | 20 |
| Site-specific antibiotic injection | 35 |
| Total | $90 |

| | |
|---|---|
| **Half-Day Total** | **$1,685** |

2. Production totals for a double-booked schedule.

**Woody Trail**

| | |
|---|---|
| 4 bitewing x-rays | $61 |
| Adult prophylaxis | 84 |
| Periodic examination by DDS/DMD | (40) |
| Adult fluoride | 35 |
| Dispense breath malodor kit | 25 |
| Dispense sonic toothbrush | 125 |
| Patient education | no charge |
| Total | $330 |

**Luke Warm**

| | |
|---|---|
| Upper and lower right periodontal scaling and root planing | $400 |
| Local anesthesia | no charge |
| Dispense chlorhexidine | 15 |
| 8 site-specific antibiotic injections | 280 |
| Total | $695 |

**Lucy Little**

| | |
|---|---|
| Full-mouth x-rays | $120 |
| Periodontal maintenance | 120 |
| Dispense take-home fluoride | 10 |
| Adult fluoride | 35 |
| Patient education | no charge |
| Total | $285 |

**Bill Board**

| | |
|---|---|
| Full-mouth x-rays | $120 |
| Periodontal maintenance | 120 |
| Dispense take-home fluoride | 10 |
| Adult fluoride | 35 |
| Patient education | no charge |
| Total | $285 |

## BOX A.1 *Annual Production Totals for the Double-Booked Day*

| | |
|---|---|
| Hour | $2,131 per half day ÷ 4.5 hours per operatory = $473.56 |
| Day | $473.56 per hour × 8 hours per day = $3,788.44 |
| Week | $3,788.44 per day × 4 days per week = $15,153.76 |
| Month | $15,153.76 per week × 4 weeks per month = $60,615.04 |
| Quarter | $60,615.04 per month × 3 months per quarter = $181,845.12 |
| Year | $60,615.04 per month × 12 months per year = $727,380.48 |

**Bill Fold**

| | |
|---|---|
| Office visit for observation | $35 |
| Periodontal débridement per tooth (unspecified periodontal treatment by report) | 20 |
| Site-specific antibiotic injection | 35 |
| **Total** | **$90** |

**Jade B. Green**

| | |
|---|---|
| Child prophylaxis | $60 |
| 2 bitewing x-rays | 61 |
| Child fluoride | 35 |
| Periodic examination by DDS/DMD* | (40) |
| **Total** | **$156** |

**Holly Berry**

| | |
|---|---|
| Periodontal maintenance | $120 |
| Dispense take-home fluoride | 10 |
| Periodic examination by DDS/DMD* | (40) |
| **Total** | **$130** |

**Robin Bird**

| | |
|---|---|
| Full-mouth débridement | $145 |
| Dispense chlorhexidine | 15 |
| **Total** | **$160** |

| | |
|---|---|
| **Half-Day Total** | **$2,131** |

The difference between the single-booked hygiene day and the double-booked hygiene day is $2,131 – $1,685 = $446.

3. The single-booked day total production after the cancellation of Luke Warm is $990 (compared to $1,685). The double-booked day total production after the cancellation of both Luke Warm and Robin Bird is $1,276 (compared to $2,131). The effect of a cancellation is lost opportunity for

* Periodic examination fees are credited to the dentist, not the dental hygienist.

the provider, the patient who canceled, and patients waiting to come into the office.

4. The production totals for the double-booked day with no cancellations by category are provided in *Box A.1*. These totals are estimates that reflect a well-established private practice working 32 hours/week, 4 weeks/month, with no vacations, cancellations, and no-shows in a fee-for-service office that includes a dental assistant. The totals do not reflect participation in insurance programs, pro bono services, and seasonal and economic downturns.

5. This independent practice would require five or six employees.

6. The production totals for the double-booked day with two cancellations per day by category are provided in *Box A.2*. Comparisons are to the results provided in *Box A.1*.

## CHAPTER 13

1. The oral healthcare provider is not a creditor when customers pay for purchased goods or services at delivery.

2. There are many complex aspects of credit law that may be better determined by banks, lending institutions, and credit companies than by the dental office staff.

3. Incidental credit is a type of credit extended for 90 days. The debt is not subject to any finance charge or interest during that time. Many dental office payment plans are based on the amount to be paid within 90 days.

4. Even though a patient has dental insurance, it is essential to make financial arrangements. Dental insurance is a third-party lender with reimbursement to the dentist or to the patient. If the plan is one under which the reimbursement is sent to the dentist, the dentist files the insurance

> **BOX A.2** *Annual Production Totals for the Double-Booked Day with Two Cancellations Per Day*
>
> Hour
> $1,276 per half day ÷ 4.5 hours per operatory = $283.56
> (compared to $473.56)
>
> Day
> $283.56 per hour × 8 hours per day = $2,268.48
> (compared to $3,788.44)
>
> Week
> $2,268.48 per day × 4 days per week = $9,073.92
> (compared to $15,153.76)
>
> Month
> $9,073.92 per week × 4 weeks per month = $36,295.68
> (compared to $0,615.04)
>
> Quarter
> $36,295.68 per month × 3 months per quarter = $108,887.04
> (compared to $181,845.12)
>
> Year
> $36,295.68 per month × 12 months = $435,548.16
> (compared to $727,380.48).

claim with the carrier and the patient pays his or her anticipated percentage.

5. Cash, check, or credit card payment at each appointment; cash or check payment of entire amount before treatment begins receives a courtesy fee reduction of 5%; loan from a bank, credit card, or finance company; multiple payment plan to be completed within 90 days; pro bono oral healthcare services; senior citizen discount of 10%; statement billing.

6. Payment options take into consideration office policy, socioeconomic status of the patient, and operational costs of the office.

7. The federal Truth in Lending Act states that healthcare providers become creditors when procedures are performed at a cost that exceeds $100 and the fee is not paid within 90 days. The federal Equal Credit Opportunity Act bars discrimination in all areas of credit to make credit available fairly and impartially. The federal Fair Debt Collection Practices Act states that collection calls to a person demanding payment cannot be made at the workplace, but telephone contact with the workplace can be made to determine if a person is employed there and to set up a convenient time to call at home to discuss the account.

8. Federal law provides protection for people across jurisdictions and states; state laws may vary.

9. Patients who move from dental practice to dental practice; state they have dental insurance but after verification procedures are found to not be covered; overreact when asked to pay; complain or find fault with the care received; change jobs in a short period of time; move often; have family problems such as separation or divorce; have a large number of children; or have dental needs caused by accidental injury, as well as those whose insurance is expiring who ask for care to be done in a short period of time.

10. The fee-for-service practice demands payment at the appointment time in the form of cash, check, credit card, or payment from another lending source.

11. Account aging reports are generated to identify patients who have not paid for services, and analyze how much is owed and for what length of time.

12. The most successful method of preventing collection problems is to inform the patient via the treatment plan for each procedure planned of the estimated cost and of the amount they must pay at the end of each appointment.

13. Collection activity begins with informed consent forms that include pricing, and progresses to monthly statements, assorted sticker messages placed on statements, a series of collection letters, telephone calls, a collection agency, and small claims court.

14. Collection agencies use the copy of the patient's driver's license, Social Security number, credit report, registration information, and financial records to make contact with the financially

responsible parties. They charge a fee for their services (usually half of what they collect).

15. If the patient appears in court, he or she will have to pay the court clerk after the hearing. If the patient does not show up in court, a lien can be placed at his or her place of employment to garnish the wages until the debt is repaid. If the patient is not employed, the court can seize property to be sold at public auction until the debt is paid.

## CHAPTER 14

1. Records management is the organization, maintenance, and protection of client information, either electronically or on paper. Data collection, documentation, storage, retrieval, and maintenance is complex and must be organized for quality assurance and risk management, which requires advanced education and training.

2. Active files are current records of patients who have been seen within a 3-year period. Inactive files are the records of patients who have stopped treatment or have not been seen for 3 years.

3. (A) Alphabetical: recommended for up to 10,000 patient files. (B) Numerical: recommended for over 10,000 patient files. (C) Terminal digit: recommended for over 50,000 files.

4. Patient records are stored on computer and require back-up procedures to save data. Digital records are stored on the computer. Document imaging and bar coding use computer technology.

5. Bar coding allows control of tracked items such as patient files, x-rays, imaging, or other diagnostic test results. Computer software generates bar code labels, printing equipment produces labels, and handheld scanners read bar-coded items to track the movement of patient information.

6. Electronic imaging allows for a cost-effective way to handle documents and share information with employees and business associates. Electronically generated files eliminate the need for paper, photographic and/or x-ray film, and storage equipment; they also serve as a disaster recovery strategy by allowing the backup storage of documents off site.

7. The changes mandated by HIPAA came about after complaints were made to the U.S. Congress regarding the sale by healthcare providers of patient personal information to companies for use in direct marketing of supplies and services to the patient.

8. The dental office is required to keep health information private, to notify patients regarding privacy practices, and to inform patients of their legal rights.

9. Patients have a legal right to look at or request a copy of their records and make any additions to their file. Requests must be placed in writing using an appropriate HIPAA form. In the instance of a copy request, a reasonable fee may be charged for duplication of the patient records.

10. The business associate may perform legal, actuarial, accounting, consulting, data aggregation, management, administration, accreditation, or financial services using protected health information. A written agreement with each separate business associate allows for the use and disclosure of private health information to complete the associate's fiduciary duties while protecting the patient's private health information.

11. The correct indexing order is Patty O'Cover, Keri Onward, Kay O'Pectate, Bill Overdeaux, Roger Overendoute, and Al Oye.

12. The correct indexing order is J. R. Johnson, J. T. Johnson Jr., John Johnson, John Robert Johnson III, John Thomas Johnson II, Johnny Johnson Sr., and John St. John.

## CHAPTER 15

1. Appointment scheduling is best performed by one person because errors occur when many people make appointment reservations.

2. Production blocking for primary procedures allows open time necessary to schedule these high-production-value appointments.

3. Difficult cases are best scheduled during the peak effectiveness time of the provider. For example, the morning person will perform better early in the day, whereas the afternoon or evening person will perform better later in the day.

4. The top priority dental hygiene patient is the patient of record who is in an active course of periodontal therapy.

5. Giving the patient a written reminder and telling him or her of the importance of the reserved time slot reinforce the message that the patient is expected to show up for the appointment. Confirmation of appointments 24–72 hours in

advance by a staff person or an automated service is a courtesy performed for the patient and reduces last-minute cancellations and no-shows.

6. Legitimate reasons or causes patients report in regard to missed appointments include illness, death, unforeseen business obligations, and slow traffic.

7. Nonlegitimate reasons for broken appointments include lack of money, fear, absentmindedness, or lack of value attached to healthcare issues.

8. A cancellation list contains the names of people who need an appointment or who can come on short notice before their scheduled appointment.

9. Daily treatment schedules list the patient name, appointment time, services to be rendered, and a phone number to call in the event of delayed arrival. They are placed in every operatory, lab, lounge, front desk, and even the darkroom. Easy access to the schedule helps keep the staff members informed of the patients who are expected to arrive.

10. When the oral healthcare provider encounters a patient with needs beyond his or her expertise, it is necessary to use the services of another healthcare provider or specialist.

## CHAPTER 16

1. (A) Advance appointment recare system: the advance appointment recare system is the scheduling of the next appointment at the end of the current appointment. (B) Continuing care: this office system helps maintain patient oral health and appearance, prevent pain and disease, protect previous treatment, and reduce the need for extensive/expensive dental treatment. (C) Mailed notice recare system: the mailed notice recare system is the mailing of a preprinted decorative postcard to inform the patient it is time to call to schedule a hygiene appointment. (D) Recall: this office system helps maintain patient oral health and appearance, prevent pain and disease, protect previous treatment, and reduce the need for extensive/expensive dental treatment. (E) Recare systems: recare systems are a component of the appointment scheduling system meant to inform the patient of record that it is time to schedule a dental hygiene visit. (F) Telephone call recare system: the telephone recare system makes contact with the patients via the telephone to schedule recare appointments.

2. Recare procedures maintain patient oral health and appearance, prevent pain and disease, protect previous treatment, and reduce the need for extensive/expensive dental treatment.

3. The advance appointment recare system is the scheduling of the next appointment at the end of the current appointment. The mailed notice recare system is the mailing of a preprinted decorative postcard to inform the patient it is time to call to schedule a hygiene appointment. The telephone recare system makes contact with the patients via the telephone to schedule recare appointments.

4. The advance appointment recare system is recognized as the most effective method because it is a time saver and patients have scheduled their own appointments and made the commitment to return.

5. The mailed notice recare system is least effective owing to the cost of postage for large mailings and the lack of patient response, making it necessary to place follow-up telephone calls.

6. A recare tracking system monitors patient contact to determine whether appropriate attempts to schedule have been made to avoid any possibility of abandonment.

7. The computer identifies patients needing appointments on a computer-generated list; prints labels, envelopes, or postcards; and produces mail merge letters.

8. (A) August. (B) October. (C) May. (D) December. (E) September.

## CHAPTER 17

1. Gross pay is total wages earned during a pay period before deductions, whereas net pay is total wages earned during a pay period after deductions. Wages are the total earnings at an hourly pay rate during a pay period. Salary is the total earnings at a fixed rate during a pay period regardless of the number of hours worked.

2. The two components of payroll are earnings and deductions.

3. On the first day of employment and every time there is a change, employees complete the Employee's Withholding Allowance Certificate known as the IRS Form W-4 for exemptions.

4. Each pay period federal income taxes, Social Security taxes, and Medicare taxes are withheld.

5. Additional deductions that may be taken from an employee's gross pay include health insurance payments, disability insurance, repayment of an office loan, parking fees, and state and local taxes.

6. Each year, the employer pays the federal income tax withheld, Social Security tax, Medicare tax, state tax, unemployment tax, worker's compensation tax, and local taxes.

7. Federal government forms mailed to the dental office include the W-2 Wage and Tax Statement, W-3 Transmittal of Income and Tax Statements, W-4 Employee's Withholding Allowance Certificate, Federal Depository Receipts, Form 941, Quarterly Federal Tax Return Report, Federal Unemployment Tax Form (FUTA) and Circular E: The Employer Tax Guide tables.

8. State government forms mailed to the dental office include the Quarterly Tax Return Report, State Unemployment Tax Form, and the Employer State Tax Guide Tables and worker's compensation forms.

9. A check from the federal depository account is written to the IRS to pay the quarterly taxes.

10. Withdrawal of taxes to the federal government from the dental practice's federal depository account is documented by the federal depository receipt form.

11. Every year the Employee's Withholding Allowance Certificate Form W-4 and the W-2 Wage and Tax Statement are filed for employees.

12. When a practice is being audited, a federal agent of the IRS may arrive at the office with a federal subpoena to enter into the office, or a notice is sent via the postal service. Usually the dentist will ask that legal counsel, an accountant, and a bookkeeper be present for any proceedings.

## CRITICAL THINKING GROUP ACTIVITY ANSWER

- If you are working for an hourly wage: $100,000 per year ÷ 52 weeks = $1,923 per week ÷ 40 hours per week = $48 per hour.

- If you are working on commission at one third of production with 2 weeks of vacation: $100,000 per year ÷ 50 weeks = $2,000 per week ÷ 5 days per week = $400 in earnings per day × 3 = $1,200 a day for production. Average periodontal scaling and root planing per quadrant is $200; thus, you must treat three patients with two quadrants of periodontal scaling every day for 50 weeks to meet a yearly production goal of $300,000 and a salary of $100,000.

- If you are working on commission at one quarter of production with 2 weeks of vacation: $100,000 per year ÷ 50 weeks = $2,000 per week ÷ 5 days per week = $400 in earnings per day × 4 = $1,600 a day for production. Average periodontal scaling and root planing per quadrant is $200; thus, you must treat four patients with two quadrants of periodontal scaling every day for 50 weeks to meet a yearly production goal of $400,000 and a salary of $100,000.

- If you are working on commission at 35% of production with 2 weeks of vacation: $100,000 per year ÷ 50 weeks = $2,000 per week ÷ 5 days per week = $400 in earnings per day × 3.5 = $1,400 a day for production. Average periodontal scaling and root planing per quadrant is $200; thus you must treat 3 patients with two quadrants of periodontal scaling plus other services equaling $200 every day for 50 weeks to meet a production goal of $350,000 and a salary of $100,000. That's a lot of scaling!

## CHAPTER 18

1. Inventory control systems are used to monitor purchasing, to maintain supply and equipment levels, and to enable a steady flow of production.

2. Expendable supplies generally cost less than $50; nonexpendable supplies cost more than $50.

3. Capital items generally cost more than $1,000 and include the operatory equipment and office furniture.

4. Professional supplies are expendable and nonexpendable items used in the operatory and laboratory.

5. Purchasing office supplies in advance spreads the cost throughout the year and makes better use of the supply budget. By selecting the best purchase rate and quantity, the staff is able to consider the total cost of the order as well as the capital available for cost effectiveness.

6. Dental offices make purchases via mail order, telephone calls, fax, or online ordering.

7. To adequately maintain inventory, the maximum and minimum level of inventory needs are determined based on rate of use, shelf life, cost, delivery time, and storage space available. Establishing reorder time and purchasing quantity for

maximum and minimum inventory help avoid any overstocking or lack of a supply item.

8. To maintain inventory, the following information is needed: item name, preferred brand, item description, date purchased, purchase source, catalog number (if applicable), amount purchased, unit cost, reorder time.

9. Dental supply houses are usually set up with the following divisions: business office supplies, drugs and medications, equipment sales, gold, installation/service/repair, merchandise and miscellaneous supplies, sales representatives, tooth.

10. Depending on the supply item, supplies are purchased from a business supply company (office items); dental manufacturer (dental materials and equipment); dental supply house (dental materials and equipment); grocery, discount, or department store (coffee, cleaning supplies); medical supply company (masks, gloves, gauze); occupational safety supply company (safety items, OSHA products); pharmacy (prescription drugs and first aid supplies); professional association (patient education materials); toy manufacturing company (gifts for pediatric patients); or uniform manufacturer (clothing).

11. Packages and shipments are opened and inspected in a confined area of the dental office. Once the package is opened, a packing list and/or shipping invoice is dated and checked against the merchandise received.

12. Invoices are verified for missing items, substitutions, and any items that were not shipped.

13. Any items that are returned to the company are documented on a credit slip/voucher sent from the supplier.

14. Expiration dates are checked to determine an item's shelf life to prevent expiration and the inability to use the item.

15. Incoming merchandise is placed behind currently stocked supplies.

16. Special storage conditions include lead-lined boxes for radiographic film, cool/dark/dry areas for impression materials, refrigeration for medicaments, and a room temperature storage location for developer and fixer chemicals.

17. Storage of chemical, combustible, and flammable items are unique for each product to allow for workplace safety and fire prevention.

18. Right-to-know laws provide standards for identifying and communicating information about hazards in the workplace to employees.

19. The Material Safety Data Sheet (MSDS) is a form that describes product contents and potential health hazards from exposure to enable the safe handling and the use of chemical products by employees.

20. Employee rights with respect to an MSDS are accessibility to the MSDS, nondiscrimination for exercising his or her rights, and notification and direction for locating a new or revised MSDS that arrives in a shipment.

## CHAPTER 19

1. Client communication is the transfer of an idea from one person to another person. Patient conversations are centered on dental wants and needs; less than 25% are social in nature.

2. Children respond best when talked to in the same tone of voice used for adults. Communication is different with children because they live in the present and do not visualize the future. They understand the literal word and facts but do not fully understanding all concepts.

3. Adolescents respond best when talked to in the same tone used for adults. Avoid being judgmental of their attitude or appearance and develop trust and open communication.

4. Allow older people to finish speaking; use listening techniques; and modify communication techniques if there are cognitive deficiencies, sensory disturbances, physical impairments, or age-related discrimination.

5. Sensory impairment conditions include learning disabilities and visual and hearing impairments.

6. Communication-challenged individuals are those with a language barrier, learning disability, or hearing impairment. Adaptation is usually required in communicating with them, such as using appropriate terminology; talking through an interpreter; looking directly at them; relying on printed materials; and minimizing background noise. The professional may use cognitive, psychomotor, and affective teaching techniques; speak slowing to facilitate lip reading; and use gestures and visual aids.

7. The case study, in which dental hygiene students prepare and present a clinic patient profile to an audience of peers, helps develop critical thinking and communication skills.

8. Research papers, table clinics, and poster sessions are assigned to dental hygiene students to

develop writing skills and higher cognitive critical thinking skills and provide public speaking practice and experience.

## CHAPTER 20

1. Patients consider dental professionals as experts; therefore, remaining credible and gaining trust are fundamental to developing good public relations.
2. Patients do not trust those who lack values, clinical competence, honesty, and inspiration.
3. The patient will not believe or trust the healthcare provider who does not engender trust and credibility.
4. Freedom from pain and anxiety are critical because they are associated with trust and credibility. Patients dislike and distrust dentists, and the fear of pain is frequently stated as the number one reason why people postpone and avoid dental visits.
5. Marketing in dentistry is the development and implementation of plans to disseminate healthcare information to promote the purchase of oral healthcare services and products. It is getting the patient to trust, agree to necessary treatment, enjoy the process, and refer friends and family.
6. Internal marketing is promoting the office to potential prospects inside the practice, whereas external marketing is promoting the office to potential prospects outside the practice.
7. A true–false survey allows for a yes or no answer, a Likert-scale survey allows rating on a scale of 1 to 5, from positive to negative, and an open-question survey allows for written explanations.
8. Practice management owners hire experts to analyze the practice management systems and personnel to improve office systems and communication.
9. As a target audience, it has been determined that women spend the market share of money on OTC products and drugs.

## CHAPTER 21

1. Dental practices engage in public relations writing to disseminate specific information; often such print material is used to promote the practice as well to the public at large.
2. Broadcast media disseminate information over radio and television/cable, as well as the Internet.
3. Broadcast media may be used as a source of advertising directed to a preselected target audience to promote the dental practice.
4. Print media in the form of newspaper, magazine, journal, newsletters, or yellow pages use written materials to disseminate information to reach a broad market, whereas brochures and flyers are directed toward specific individuals.
5. Print advertising in the form of a welcome letter, brochures/pamphlets, flyers, newsletters, or direct mail marketing pieces are included in welcome packets.
6. Most dental practices are privately owned businesses and a yearly report may be used to document ROI, analyze the terms of partnership, as a statement of accomplishments, or as a report sent to grant-funding authorities.
7. A feature article is the main story of a group based on a theme. A profile is a main story about a person, product, service, and/or organization. Editorials are essays written to disseminate information based on a personal opinion.
8. A newsletter can be distributed externally and internally to disseminate information to clients and the public about the dental practice, allied dental personnel, nonpractice information, and office policy.
9. Publications and materials created, produced, or printed in the office include business cards, letterhead, brochures/pamphlets, flyers, and direct marketing mail.
10. News releases are sent to print and broadcast outlets to publicize noteworthy information such as an honorary award earned by a provider, when the team sponsored by the dental practice wins a championship title, when the dental practice is recognized as a provider of care to a special-interest group, or when the practice offers a new high-tech procedure.
11. PSAs are broadcast written public relations activities used to disseminate information on a single topic; they provide a service to the public and also represent a form of advertising because the sponsoring practice is mentioned at the end of the announcement.
12. Billboards, indoor or outdoor lighted signs, lettering, neon signs, portable signs, vinyl banners, and vinyl graphics and decals are all types of outdoor signage; some are more permanent than others.

## CHAPTER 22

1. Written documentation on forms and letters of all financial transactions, clinical instructions and recommendations, referrals, and public relations activities are considered legal documents serving as proof that the standard of care has been implemented and followed.
2. The services rendered form is where progress notes for each contact with the patient are recorded in ink, transcribed, or typed into the patient's record.
3. The basic supplies necessary for business mailings include a quality bond paper containing the practice logo and catch phrase with matching envelopes.
4. A final photocopy is placed in the patient file for reference. An electronic copy can be saved as well but should not replace the photocopy.
5. The dental office may generate birthday letters/cards, marketing letters and aids, narrative reports, new patient welcome letters, patient education materials, postoperative letters regarding results and photographs, recall letters, referral letters, and thank-you letters and cards.
6. Business letters are properly folded into thirds and placed into an envelope with a preprinted or typed return address; the envelope should be legibly addressed to the intended recipient.

## CHAPTER 23

1. Policy and procedure manuals, found in businesses, professional organizations, and government, outline business operational information for employees.
2. Vision statements are short written declarations of an ideal and a unique image of the future. Mission statements are declarations of what the practice wants to accomplish, whom it serves, and what makes it unique based on its strengths and weaknesses. Philosophy statements are expanded mission statements that reflect core values.
3. Procedure protocols contain information about and steps to follow in a certain set of circumstances.
4. The performance review is a discussion of skill development, attitude/work habits, communication skills, and professional development. Skill development is the eagerness to learn and progress. Attitude and work habits are about accepting criticism, having a good appearance and grooming, helping coworkers, being enthusiastic, making efficient use of time, and following directions. Communication skills include being an active team member, participating in staff meetings, having good verbal skills, and being credible and trustworthy. Professional development relates to attending continuing education courses and keeping up to date.
5. The personnel section of the office manual provides information on compensation. A compensation package may include some or all of the following: the assigned workload, salary/wage compensation per year, bonus pay, commission pay, FICA withholding, accidental death/life/dental/medical insurance, commuting reimbursement, education expense reimbursement, malpractice insurance, paid time off (vacation, national holidays, bereavement, election day, jury duty, maternity/medical leave, personal leave, sick days), parking reimbursement, pension/profit-sharing contributions, payment of professional association dues, short- and/or long-term disability, uniform allowance, and workers' compensation.
6. A job description identifies those tasks necessary to perform to and exceed the employer's needs. When a written job description is available, communication regarding job performance is based on factual information.
7. Contracts are used to obtain the services of independent contractors, who are self-employed individuals providing specified services under the terms of a legal agreement to do so.

## CHAPTER 24

1. Academic skills are those skills necessary to prepare for prospective training and education and to acquire, keep, and progress in a job. Employers seek applied communication, mathematics, science, and computer skills, and the ability to use technology.
2. Personal management skills are those skills necessary to develop responsibility and dependability. Employers seek skills such as maintaining positive self-esteem, maturity, job commitment, using enthusiasm to do the best on the job, taking pride in working, making decisions, acting honestly, exercising self-control, and having good work habits.

3. A significant way to instill positive self-esteem in others is to use praise and encouragement.

4. Improving negative thoughts can be done by making a list of events or relationships that produce a negative feeling to recognize what influences negative feelings. Listing and finding alternatives, changing negative self-talk, accepting things that cannot be changed, and helping others are additional techniques to improve negative thoughts.

5. A self-assessment is an individual's questioning about needs and values used to develop a life strategic plan and ascertain the situations and relationships needed to flourish in the working environment.

6. People set goals for three reasons: personal attainment, job-related attainment, and learning or performance.

7. Processing skills are those skills necessary to use knowledge and learn new concepts. Employers seek teamwork, problem solving, decision making, recalling, comprehending, applying, analyzing, synthesizing, and evaluating knowledge skills.

8. An employee's positive attitude makes for a pleasant co-worker as do taking care of one's personal appearance, acting in a safe and healthy way, respecting the rights of others, and taking responsibility for one's behavior.

## CHAPTER 25

1. Workers change jobs every 5–8 years and change careers 3 times in their lifetime.

2. Career planning is an ongoing process of change that occurs throughout an individual's lifetime as personal interests and environment change owing to new experiences, furthering one's education, and making new personal contacts. Planning for change makes the transition easier.

3. Job search strategies include targeted communications/direct marketing, networking, indirect marketing, and job research.

4. Networking is asking all of the people you know for their advice and support on how to find employment.

5. The best people to start networking with are those found in your immediate circle.

6. Occupational research is the investigation of job descriptions, employment statistics, education and credentialing requirements, and employment outlook. This helps find employment by making contacts in an area of interest.

7. Business research is an investigation of the healthcare industry in general to enable you to respond to questions and demonstrate a broad knowledge base. This allows for discovering employment options.

8. Organizational research is an investigation of a particular place of employment. This leads to better performance during the interview.

9. Contacting multiple sources of employment improves the chance for interviewing and employment offers.

10. The most common reason why people change jobs is poor communication with the employer or fellow workers. Other common reasons are a desire for a life change and personal happiness.

## CHAPTER 26

1. Functional résumés emphasize skills, achievements, and accomplishments versus dates of employment. Chronological résumés furnish dates of all employment experiences and education in a time sequence. Combination résumés use both styles to emphasize qualifications and grab the reader's attention.

2. A descending chronological list of former employers, with emphasis on the skills that transfer from one environment to another, is a sound strategy to use when you have held more than three jobs.

3. Personal information at the end of the résumé includes activities or interests.

4. Reference lists should include three to six individuals, along with their personal information and their relationship to the job seeker.

5. A résumé is a one-page history of personal information, education, experience, accomplishments, and other qualifications. A curriculum vita is a multipage biographical historical summary emphasizing professional background, qualifications, and accomplishments.

6. Curriculum vitae are used when applying for positions in education, medicine, research, and related fields.

7. A portfolio is a collection of academic and credentialing documents, achievement awards, and records of accomplishments used during the

interview process to depict a profile of personal growth.

8. The letter of application may be sent with a résumé or vita when responding to job postings, vacancy announcements, and advertisements. It emphasizes special abilities or connections not mentioned in the résumé/vita.

9. Sign the letter in ink with your proper name above the signature line.

10. When a question does not apply, write N/A, which means "not applicable," on the line or draw a straight line in the space to acknowledge that the line was read and it does not apply to the circumstances; this shows the employer that the question was read and understood.

11. If a mistake is made, draw one line through it and write the correction next to it.

12. Read the form completely before answering any questions to reduce the chance of making errors.

13. Yes.

## CHAPTER 27

1. The interviewee may be required by the potential employer to take skills tests or complete application forms. He or she should also prepare to present a professional image, practice answering and asking questions, know how to use telecommunications equipment, and find out about the practice. He or she should anticipate interview tactics and be able to respond to difficult and illegal questions, tell personal stories, and interview the employer.

2. Communicating competency at a job interview begins with a professional appearance because judgments regarding a person's character are made within the first minute of contact.

3. Employment skills tests may include typing; basic mathematics; and English proficiency in reading, spelling, and grammar.

4. Contact with the dental office may be by telephone to schedule an interview. Prospective employers use the telephone to save time, determine the interest level of applicants, and schedule interviews. Prospective employees use the telephone to save time, find information about job openings, network, save on transportation costs, and market skills.

5. Good posture communicates to the interviewer interest and attention. Facing the interviewer and smiling indicates a cheerful and friendly disposition. Frequent eye contact and a nod of the head communicate understanding and confidence. Nervous habits detract from interview performance.

6. Interview tactics are arriving 15 minutes before the scheduled time, waiting patiently, offering a firm handshake, not sitting until the interviewer sits, sitting in the chair closest to the interviewer, not accepting gum or a cigarette when offered, and engaging in small talk.

7. There are three courses of action to take when asked an illegal question: (1) Ignore that it is an illegal question and answer it. (2) Respond, "How does that information relate to this position?" or "I do not think that information is relevant to this job." (3) Contact the Equal Employment Commission to report the potential employer.

8. Asking questions during the interview helps determine whether or not you want to work there and shows interest.

9. Interview data worksheets keep track of the job search and help evaluate interview performance.

## CHAPTER 28

1. A clear understanding of the job description helps match interests and ability.

2. Full-time employment is defined as 40 hours of continuous work per week. Overtime pay at a rate of $1\frac{1}{2}$ times the regular rate is required by law for any time worked over 40 hours in a workweek for nonexempt employees. The U.S. Fair Labor Standards Act sets the minimum wage at $5.15 per hour.

3. Difficult moral dilemmas can occur when dental professionals are asked to perform illegal duties and functions by their employer. Discussing employer expectations in advance may prevent uncomfortable situations.

4. At all times, the allied dental professional is required to adhere to all federal and state occupational safety and health laws.

5. The most common benefit is paid vacation time. Other benefits are continuing education, free dental care, healthcare insurance coverage, holiday pay, life insurance, malpractice insurance coverage, paid parking, paid personal days, pension plan participation, payment of professional association dues, profit sharing, severance pay,

short- or long-term disability insurance, sick leave and pay, and a uniform allowance.

6. Writing a confirmation letter legally completes the employment negotiations.

7. Writing a declination letter closes the negotiation process and allows you to reapply to the dental practice in the future.

8. Yes, because it includes the job description and defines the expectations of the employer.

9. An employee must be at least 16 years old to work in most nonfarm jobs; youngsters 14 and 15 years old may work outside school hours no more than 3 hours on a school day and 18 hours in a school week.

10. Many employers require drug testing as a condition of employment to determine illegal drug use owing to its effect on absenteeism and healthcare costs.

## CHAPTER 29

1. Formal oral communication is the oral exchange of instructions, information, or ideas. Formal written communication is the written or transmitted exchange of messages that follows a chain of command. Informal communication is the spread of information via talking and writing.

2. Individuals differ in terms of their internal clocks. Take the time of day into consideration when communicating with coworkers, realizing that some will be more attentive in the morning and others, in the afternoon.

3. A low attention level may affect proper message transfer.

4. Two common issues that affect work relationships are co-dependence and counterdependence.

5. With positive interdependence, people are connected within a group, and the group cannot succeed without the help of each member.

6. In the first few minutes of any interaction, each individual assesses the other following a sequenced process, including the manner in which a person is touched. Touch is used to reassure someone, is therapeutic, and shows more concern than the spoken word.

7. The ability to recognize when autocratic communication occurs helps in the understanding that male employers may communicate using power over female employees instead of authority and influence.

8. The most common assertions are straightforward statements used to raise an issue with someone for the first time, using direct sentences to convey a need or stand up for one's rights.

9. Listening to the thoughts and opinions of coworkers helps in understanding and responding to them.

10. Communication distance should occur outside an individual's personal space, usually an arm's length distance, to make him or her comfortable.

## CHAPTER 30

1. The dental team will consist of people with a mix of the 16 different personality types, and individuals are not necessarily the same each day. Thus, communicating with coworkers and developing working relationships with each personality type can be challenging.

2. Creativity and innovation improve productivity, work quality, and employee job satisfaction. Creativity also helps when planning for the future and developing mission statements.

3. Staff meetings keep the group focused on the practice's goals. Effective communication takes practice, and the staff meeting provides a forum for everyone's input and helps staff prepare for change.

4. Strategies include controlling, compromising, avoiding, or accepting stress.

5. Conflict is a negative aspect of work that affects everyone in the dental office by upsetting the equilibrium of the group.

6. The federal Equal Employment Opportunity Commission (EEOC) guidelines, based on Title VII of the Civil Rights Act of 1964, define two types of sexual harassment: quid pro quo and environmental.

7. The performance review is a private meeting between the employee and the employer to discuss job accomplishment, shortcomings, and goals.

8. Any worker or employer may sever employment at any time for any reason without warning.

9. No.

10. Managing failure includes analyzing what went wrong, regrouping emotionally, reflecting on what occurred, reevaluating goals, and determining a course of action.

# Index

Page numbers in *italics* denote figures; those followed by "t" denote tables; and those followed by "b" denote boxes